AF413033

FUTURE OF INTELLIGENT AND EXTELLIGENT HEALTH ENVIRONMENT

Studies in Health Technology and Informatics

Volume 118

Volume 2 in the subseries:
Future of Health Technology Series
Editor: Renata G. Bushko

Vol. 1   R.G. Bushko (Ed.), Future of Health Technology

Recently published in SHTI

Vol. 117. C.D. Nugent, P.J. McCullagh, E.T. McAdams and A. Lymberis (Eds.), Personalised Health Management Systems – The Integration of Innovative Sensing, Textile, Information and Communication Technologies

Vol. 116. R. Engelbrecht, A. Geissbuhler, C. Lovis and G. Mihalas (Eds.), Connecting Medical Informatics and Bio-Informatics – Proceedings of MIE2005

Vol. 115. N. Saranummi, D. Piggott, D.G. Katehakis, M. Tsiknakis and K. Bernstein (Eds.), Regional Health Economies and ICT Services

Vol. 114. L. Bos, S. Laxminarayan and A. Marsh (Eds.), Medical and Care Compunetics 2

Vol. 113. J.S. Suri, C. Yuan, D.L. Wilson and S. Laxminarayan (Eds.), Plaque Imaging: Pixel to Molecular Level

Vol. 112. T. Solomonides, R. McClatchey, V. Breton, Y. Legré and S. Nørager (Eds.), From Grid to Healthgrid

Vol. 111. J.D. Westwood, R.S. Haluck, H.M. Hoffman, G.T. Mogel, R. Phillips, R.A. Robb and K.G. Vosburgh (Eds.), Medicine Meets Virtual Reality 13

Vol. 110. F.H. Roger France, E. De Clercq, G. De Moor and J. van der Lei (Eds.), Health Continuum and Data Exchange in Belgium and in the Netherlands – Proceedings of Medical Informatics Congress (MIC 2004) & 5th Belgian e-Health Conference

Vol. 109. E.J.S. Hovenga and J. Mantas (Eds.), Global Health Informatics Education

Vol. 108. A. Lymberis and D. de Rossi (Eds.), Wearable eHealth Systems for Personalised Health Management – State of the Art and Future Challenges

Vol. 107. M. Fieschi, E. Coiera and Y.-C.J. Li (Eds.), MEDINFO 2004 – Proceedings of the 11th World Congress on Medical Informatics

Vol. 106. G. Demiris (Ed.), e-Health: Current Status and Future Trends

Vol. 105. M. Duplaga, K. Zieliński and D. Ingram (Eds.), Transformation of Healthcare with Information Technologies

Vol. 104. R. Latifi (Ed.), Establishing Telemedicine in Developing Countries: From Inception to Implementation

Vol. 103. L. Bos, S. Laxminarayan and A. Marsh (Eds.), Medical and Care Compunetics 1

ISSN 0926-9630

Future of Intelligent and Extelligent Health Environment

Edited by

Renata G. Bushko

Future of Health Technology Institute, Hopkinton, MA, USA

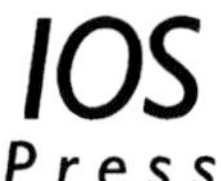

Amsterdam • Berlin • Oxford • Tokyo • Washington, DC

ISBN 1-58603-571-1
Library of Congress Control Number: 2005909821

Publisher
IOS Press
Nieuwe Hemweg 6B
1013 BG Amsterdam
Netherlands
fax: +31 20 687 0019
e-mail: order@iospress.nl

Distributor in the UK and Ireland
IOS Press/Lavis Marketing
73 Lime Walk
Headington
Oxford OX3 7AD
England
fax: +44 1865 750079

Distributor in the USA and Canada
IOS Press, Inc.
4502 Rachael Manor Drive
Fairfax, VA 22032
USA
fax: +1 703 323 3668
e-mail: iosbooks@iospress.com

Future of Intelligent and Extelligent Health Environment
R.G. Bushko (Ed.)
IOS Press, 2005

Preface

"The Future of Intelligent and Extelligent Health Environment" book brings you closer to the world where technology on our body, in our body and all around us enhances our health and wellbeing from conception to death. This environment is emerging now with intelligent caring machines, cyborgs, wireless embedded continuous computing, healthwear, sensors, healthons, nanomedicine, adaptive process control, mathematical modeling, and common sense systems.

Human body and the world in which it functions is a continuously changing complex adaptive system. We are able to collect more and more data about it (wearable body monitors will be soon in each household just like toothbrushes) but the real challenge is to infer local dynamics from that data. Intelligent Caring Biomechatronic Creatures and Healthmaticians (mathematicians serving human health) have a better chance of inferring the dynamics that needs to be understood than human physicians.

Humans can only process comfortably three dimensions while computers can see infinite number of dimensions. Will we enjoy doing medical science if computers become better at it than us? We will need to trust the distributed network of healthons, Intelligent Caring Creatures, and NURSES (New Unified Resource System Engineers) – designers who inbuilt medical intelligence in our external environment – creating Health Extelligence.

We need new vocabulary to push forward in a new way – healthons are tools combining prevention with diagnosis and treatment based on continuous monitoring and analyzing of our vital signs and biochemistry. The "Healthon Era" is just beginning. Authors of the chapters of this book all are on the cutting edge of thinking in their respective fields. They all sense the Healthon Era and push forward to create a better life for us all.

At Future of Health Technology Summit™ 2003 Space Elevator example was used to show how seemingly impossible conceptual designs could become real. Celestial hospitals and errorless healthcare are possible. We may need to use bionic arms and extended cognition to do that but if we spend as much time designing our preferred future as we do researching the past we can get there in no time.

Developments like robo-docs, robo-cats, and space elevators are not just exotic; they are a reaffirmation that with creative thinking we can go a long way to the discoveries that will allow us to fix our healthcare system and set it on a high road for the future.

The dream of an intelligent caring creature is closer to reality considering that Timothy Bickmore's relational agent can help you with your fitness training, Yulun Wang's robotic doctor can help you even from a remote location (remote presence); Astro Teller's BodyBug™ can collect your lifestyle data and tell you what to eat and how much to sleep. We are closer and closer to the world with healthons on your body, in your body and all around you; where not a doctor but your primary care healthmatician warns you about an approaching headache; and where NURSE programs your intelligent caring creatures so they can talk to your cells and stop disease in its tracks.

Renata G. Bushko
Editor, Future of Health Technology book series
Founder, Future of Health Technology Institute
Hopkinton, MA, USA

Acknowledgements

You will be able to get closer to the intelligent and extelligent heath environment thanks to the creative spirit of all superb chapter authors. Thank you all for your dedication to building a better future. Please refer to the list of names below.

I would also like to thank those who will take the time to read this book and engage in creating the vision of the future. As the editor, I invite you to send your ideas and comments to the Future of Health Technology Institute at Bushko@fhti.org and join FHTI's annul summit to define health technology agenda for the 21st century.

Editor
Renata G. Bushko, M.S.
Bushko@fhti.org
Director, Future of Health Technology Institute
www.fhti.org

"Future of Intelligent and Extelligent Health Environment" Authors List:

David Andre, Ph.D.
Timothy Bickmore, Ph.D.
Matthew M. Burton, M.D.
Victor A. Capoccia Ph.D.
Aubrey de Grey, Ph.D.
Tim Ganous
Alison S. Gottlieb, Ph.D.
David H. Gustafson, Ph.D.
Teresita B. Hernández, Ph.D.
Bradford W. Hesse, Ph.D.
Stephen S. Intille, Ph.D.
Thomas R. Kosten, M.D.
Animesh Kumar
Kent Larson
Alexander Libin, Ph.D.
Elena Libin, Ph.D.
Lynne Maher, RGN, BSc Hons, MBA
Cindy Mason, Ph.D.

Benjamin L. Miller, Ph.D.
George B. Moseley III, MBA, JD
Aaron Oppenheimer
Tara E. Palesh
Salil H. Patel
Alex Pentland, Ph.D.
Rosalind W. Picard, Ph.D.
Paul E. Plsek
Nina M. Silverstein, Ph.D.
Richard N. Spivack, Ph.D.
Jeffrey V. Sutherland, Ph.D.
Astro Teller, Ph.D.
Willem-Jan van den Heuvel, Ph.D.
Elizabeth Van Ranst, M.S.S.S.
Kevin Warwick, Ph.D.
Stephan V. Wiet, Ph.D.
Jean A. Wooldridge, M.P.H.

About
the Future of Health Technology Institute
"Common Sense in Health"

The Future of Health Technology Institute, 4 Lamplighter Lane, Hopkinton, MA, 01748, US, www.fhti.org is the health technology think-tank dedicated to defining the health technology agenda for the 21st century. Renata Bushko (Bushko@fhti.org) founded Future of Health Technology Institute in 1996 and has since chaired ten annual Future of Health Technology Summits™. These summits engage creative minds from the technology and healthcare fields in envisioning the future of technology for global healthcare. Under her leadership, the Future of Health Technology Institute has become as one of the most forward thinking health technology research and training organizations.

Specific goals of the Future of Health Technology Institute are:

1. Develop a vision of future health care supported by current and future health technologies.
2. Define distinct promising health technology research areas.
3. Demonstrate that technology driven cost increases in healthcare can be stopped and possibly reversed by a new allocation of research and development resources.
4. Define productive areas for research and development that will have potential impact on healthcare.
5. Identify new technologies that are practical and necessary in health and wellness maintenance.
6. Identify research and development needed to meet future health challenges.
7. Identify current products best for preparing 21st century healthcare.

Future of Health Technology Summits™ are about:

1. Stopping disease before it even begins
2. Stopping suffering before tears occur
3. Stopping symptoms before they hurt
4. Stopping medical errors before they kill

We can do that by:

1. Beginning to seriously think about the long-term future
2. Beginning to manage randomness of the technology creation and adoption process
3. Beginning to address health crisis situation as a national and international emergency

Future of Health technology Institute's "3I™" – Inspiration-Incubation-Insight™ method simulating the discovery process is used to stimulate creative thinking at annual FHTI's summits.

Elevator to the Future

Renata G. Bushko
December 5, 2003

Racing to the future;
Counting days and nights;
Nanoseconds divided more than thousand times.

For better;
For brighter;
For braver and smarter.

Guess,
Act,
And guess again.
Do not be afraid.

Laser light will cut inside,
Sharp and agile,
Growing from outside,
Blooming from within,
Changing how we spin.

Spin and stop,
Stop and spin,
Find the way to win.
Find the way to help
The confused human race.

Then fly above the anyon,
Dance with epigenetic intron now,
Let our being merge with the unknown kind.

Human Soul
Sculptured by the Suffering

Renata G. Bushko
November 17, 2004

Deep inside the crystal forms;
Higher up – it shines like gold;

Never ending stream of souls;
Going over giant walls;
Sliding down the sky of fears;
Begging for the end of tears.

Never ending stream of love;
Going higher than the clouds above;
Climbing up the pearls of thought;
Begging for the friendly soul – forgot.

Never ending stream of wants;
Going deeper than the pain;
Climbing never-ending maze of passion;
Begging for the fruit of random gaze.

Beauty born out of shinning walls;
Going to the mystery light where we all want to be at once;
Climbing up to distant stars;
Looking back just one more time;
Saying:
"Here I am – pure love sculptured by the suffering,
looking for another human being".
Found.
Completed.
Done.
Infinity of the human heart.

Contents

Preface v
Renata G. Bushko

Acknowledgements vi
Renata G. Bushko

About the Future of Health Technology Institute "*Common Sense in Health*" vii

Elevator to the Future viii
Renata G. Bushko

Human Soul Sculptured by the Suffering ix
Renata G. Bushko

Goals and Unsolved Problems

Healthons: Errorless Healthcare with Bionic Hugs and No Need for Quality Control 3
Renata G. Bushko

Consumers Era – Sociotechnological Environment

The Prospects for Medical Technology in the Next Decade 15
George B. Moseley III

Innovation in Telehealth and a Role for the Government 32
Richard N. Spivack

Present and Future Challenges in Medical Data Management: Economics,
Ethics, and the Law 43
Salil H. Patel

Healthons Era – Technology on Our Body, in Our Body and All Around Us

Healthwear: Medical Technology Becomes Wearable 55
Alex Pentland

Interfacing Biology and Computing for Health: The Future of Home Diagnostics 66
Benjamin L. Miller

Designing and Evaluating Home-Based, Just-in-Time Supportive Technology 79
Stephen S. Intille and Kent Larson

Health. Care. Anywhere. Today 89
David Andre and Astro Teller

How Do We Get the Medical Intelligence Out?   111
Aaron Oppenheimer

Cyborgs Era – Implants, Merging Humans with Machines and Caring Machines

Future of Computer Implant Technology and Intelligent Human-Machine Systems   125
Kevin Warwick

Future of Caring Machines   132
Timothy Bickmore and Rosalind W. Picard

Cyber-Anthropology: A New Study on Human and Technological Co-Evolution   146
Alexander Libin and Elena Libin

Hi-Tech Cure and Care Era – Examples: Future of Cancer and Addiction Control

Harnessing the Power of an Intelligent Health Environment in Cancer Control   159
Bradford W. Hesse

Future of Anti-Addiction Vaccines   177
Thomas R. Kosten

Automating Addiction Treatment: Enhancing the Human Experience and
Creating a Fix for the Future   186
*David H. Gustafson, Tara E. Palesh, Rosalind W. Picard, Paul E. Plsek,
Lynne Maher and Victor A. Capoccia*

Long Life Era – Extending Human Life-Span and Future of Caring for Elders

A Strategy for Postponing Aging Indefinitely   209
Aubrey de Grey

Future of Caring for an Aging Population: Trends, Technology, and Caregiving   220
Stephan G. Wiet

Promoting Safe and Comfortable Driving for Elders   231
Elizabeth van Ranst, Nina M. Silverstein and Alison S. Gottlieb

Global Digital Healthcare Era – Enhancing Healthcare with Soft Technologies

Global Medicine Technology   247
Cindy Mason

Shaping a Healthy Future: Megabyte, Not Mega Bite!   257
Teresita B. Hernández

Digital Literacy in a Landscape of Data: A Plea for a Broader Definition for
Citizens and Patients   263
Jean A. Wooldridge

Adaptive and Errorless Era – Adaptive Healthcare Process Management

Situated, Strategic, and AI-Enhanced Technology Introduction to Healthcare   273
  Renata G. Bushko

Towards an Intelligent Hospital Environment: OR of the Future   278
  Jeffrey V. Sutherland, Willem-Jan van den Heuvel, Tim Ganous,
  Matthew M. Burton and Animesh Kumar

Framework for Measuring Adaptive Knowledge-Rich Systems Performance   313
  Renata G. Bushko

The Authors

Biographies of the Authors   327

Author Index   335

Goals and Unsolved Problems

Future of Intelligent and Extelligent Health Environment
R.G. Bushko (Ed.)
IOS Press, 2005

Healthons: Errorless Healthcare with Bionic Hugs and No Need for Quality Control

Renata G. BUSHKO, M.S.
Director, Future of Health Technology Institute, Hopkinton, MA, USA

Abstract. Errorless, invisible, continuous and infrastructure-free healthcare should become our goal. In order to achieve that goal, we need to rapidly move from current episodic and emergency-driven "healthcare delivery system" to an intelligent and extelligent health environment. That requires introduction of distributed affective Intelligent Caring Creatures (ICCs) consisting of healthons. Healthons are tools combining prevention with diagnosis and treatment based on continuous monitoring and analyzing of vital signs and biochemistry. Unlike humans, who posses only two or three dimensions of thinking, healthons can assure errorless health because of their adaptability, flexibility, and multidimensional reasoning capability. ICCs can do "the right thing" based on (1) state-of-art medical knowledge, (2) data about emotional, physiological, and genetic state of a consumer and (3) moral values of a consumer. The transition to the intelligent health environment based on ICCs requires the solutions to many currently unsolved healthcare problems. This paper lists the unsolved problems (by analogy to mathematical unsolved problems list) and explains why errorless healthcare with bionic hugs and no need for quality control is possible.

1. Errorless, Invisible, Continuous and Infrastructure-Free Healthcare

A concept of errorless healthcare is based on the broad definition of an error:

Definition 1: Individual Error

Error occurs when we could have had a positive impact on person's life assuming current state of medical science, knowledge and resources but we fail to do so.

Definition 2: Inter-generational Error

Error occurs if we could have had positive impact on populations' health but we failed to achieve that because of inappropriate allocation of resources.

E.g. If we invested in nonomedicine the day that Dr. Eric Drexler described it, we could be saving lives with much more advanced nanorobots today. If we, as a society, decide to delay research on postponing aging or common sense knowledge representation, we may create an inter-generational error that costs us millions of lives.

It is not enough to set a goal to reduce the number of medical errors, which is what happens with many improvements programs. These medical errors must be eliminated. We strive for errorless space missions. The same should happen in health care. The life of an astronaut is equally important as the life of any other person.

The invisible feature of new healthcare means that it is handled in an unobtrusive way that does not disturb the normal lifestyle of the consumer.

Infrastructure-free and continuous healthcare means that it goes on anywhere and all the time. Healthcare becomes life-care.

2. Intelligent Caring Creatures and Healthons

Affective Intelligent Caring Creatures (ICCs) are needed to achieve errorless, invisible, continuous and infrastructure-free healthcare, something that is impossible within the current organization of the healthcare system. ICCs consist of "healthons" that consumers carry in their bodies, on their bodies (intelligent health environment) and that are embedded in their homes, offices, cars, plains, furniture and robo-pet assistants (extelligent heath environment). Healthons are tools combining prevention with diagnosis and treatment based on continuous monitoring and analyzing of our vital signs and biochemistry of the body. Healthons in 2050 will be like vitamins or tooth brushes in 2005 – broadly available and used by everyone. There will be one difference, however, because they will be able to talk to each other and, if desired by the consumer, they will be able to explain what is happening with consumer's health at any moment. It is very important that the designers of ICCs include the "explain on human level" feature in the products they produce. Otherwise, we will be left out by the omnipotent machines.

2.1. Examples of Healthons

Memory glasses are a good example of a healthon: a consumer wears them and his/her recognition of people increases 50% without any conscious effort by the consumer. Another example is a nanooptical sensor placed in the brain that can monitor glutamate and that allows for feedback on the progress in the learning in children (glutamate is a neurotransmitter secreted by nerve cells that influences sensory perception, learning and memory).

A Robopet jumping on its elderly owners lap to remind him/her about his/her medication or exercise schedule, an artificial nose extension sensing allergents before they cause negative reaction, or Professor Shioyama's electronic eye translating the visual input into instructions of how to cross the street for the blind, or a second skin (e.g. BodyMedia's bodybugg™ or continuous thermometer) suggesting diet change are also good examples. Artificial red cells that can help us stay underwater for two hours without an oxygen tank or the relational agent that explains the work of other healthons in a virtual medical visit via Nomad-like glasses and realistic OLED display are yet additional examples.

The best example of a healthon that combines diagnosis, therapy and treatment is "surgical injection" developed by Philips Medical Systems: an injectable chemical agent (Apomate) identifies the portion of the heart experiencing the heart attack, and the same agent delivers VasoEndothelial Growth Factor to the region of the heart attack to cause new blood vessels to grow thus repairing the heart non-invasively.

Cellular healthons are possible because of fast progress in nanotechnology. One of the examples is nanomolecular tagging technology – molecular bar-coding system – invented by Krasen Dimitri that allows tagging, identifying, and counting individual molecules.

2.2. Adaptiveness – the Key to Errorless Healthcare

The key attribute that guarantees an errorless health maintenance process is adaptability, which could be achieved by common sense knowledge representation with analogical reasoning engine. Adaptive biomechatronic and nono-biomechatronic ICCs, non-brittle and non-human, will have a better chance of avoiding errors than humans. Investment in the creation of non-brittle ICCs with common sense will generate extensive benefits in health-care where the compartmentalization and the enormous size of new medical research is prohibiting a single un-aided human mind from being effective.

3. Big Need for Software

In the ICCs era, there will be no need for healthcare quality control, but instead a great need for software quality control. Everything from nonomolecular devices in our bodies to rela-tional agents explaining to us nanorobot's actions will contain software programs. Intelli-gent Caring Centers (equivalent to current hospitals but without patients because of infra-structure-free healthcare organization) will reprogram and upgrade Intelligent Caring Crea-tures. Intelligent Caring Centers will be run by healthmaticians (mathematicians that serve human health) and NURSES (New Unified Resource Systems Engineers) who also take care of healthon allocation according to the medical needs and the ethical convictions of the population. Significant investment in software development methodologies is needed to conquer the software bottleneck and to make sure that we can take advantage of all newly available hardware. Healthmaticians and NURSES must remember to include the "explain on human level" feature in all ICCs – even those who can program themselves based on the experience they have had. These learning ICCs can self correct, and some of them can set their own goals. Because of that, healthmaticians developed an "Emotion in Motion" en-gine that can indirectly influence ICCs to set humanitarian goals.

4. Deriving Dynamics from Medical Data – the Key to Errorless Healthcare

We cannot currently derive the dynamics of the system from data about our body and genes. There is a better chance that machines can do that before we – mere humans – can. This is what medical science is trying to do "manually," using previous experience, isolated data points, and a lot of guessing. It is like trying to find an ant in a 5000 square-foot house.

What if we have all possible data about the way our body functions gathered by wear-able or implantable devices? Does it change much? Yes – but only if we can reason on the data and derive dynamics of the phenomena that manifested itself by that data.

Intelligent Caring Creatures and healthmaticians have a better chance of inferring the dynamics that need to be understood than human physicians. Humans can only process comfortably in three dimensions while computers can see an infinite number of dimensions. We will need to trust the distributed network of Intelligent Caring Creatures and NURSES who built the medical intelligence into our external environment. The time that it takes to accept the fact that machines decide about the healthcare process will determine the time that it takes to achieve errorless healthcare.

5. Talking to Our Cells – Nanocommunication

What if we had a digital model of a human including the functioning of each and every cell? What if a wearable computing paradigm applied to each and every cell? Cells would be making a decision to "wear" the nanomonitor or not; to undergo nanosurgery or not; to die or not. Cells would be reporting to organs and to their owners (us) about the probability of a mutation that may cause a problem (e.g. cancer) later on. Or should we forget about reporting all together – why waste the time doing that – let's give our cells the power to fix themselves and to communicate only with other cells that perform related functions. This would mean invisible healthcare – similar to the invisible disease creation process. Real-time electrical detection of single viruses is already possible – we are moving in the right direction. We are also moving rapidly from the era of robotic surgery to nanosurgery. A high-speed ultrasensitive bar-coding system for identifying individual molecules by NanoString Technologies gets us closer to knowing ourselves on a cellular level and talking to our cells.

6. Bionic Hugs – Unlimited Supply of Care – Remote Presence

Errorless, infrastructure-free healthcare could be possible with an army of bionic helpers – a type of specialized Intelligent Caring Creatures who replace current nursing and are made available in any amount to all who need physical or emotional help. From a simple hand-shake to a sophisticated dialog, bionic intelligent caring creatures will be able to help.

Bionic pets will play an important role too. The human need for affection and friendship will be fulfilled even for those who cannot care for a real pet. Robo-pets will also serve medical roles – gathering data about the consumer and reminding about healthy behaviors and disease management routine in chronic conditions. With robotic-pets encouraging an active lifestyle, childhood obesity will be a long forgotten history.

7. Extelligent Adaptable Environment

Most of us will still have a chance to live in an extelligent environment that will change depending on the emotional and physical state of the consumer. With the use of OLED wall-sized programmable displays wirelessly communicating with body sensors, it will soon be possible to design healing environments that are so much underutilized. For example, a patient who loves outdoors but has to stay immobile for some time could program his room as a tent with windows showing pine forest and wind moving the branches and an occasional blue bird's call. The walls could also be self-programmable based on diaries from the past describing most positive energizing experiences.

Objects that we use in every day life will talk to each other, to the walls, cabinets, our second skin and nanorobots inside our bodies. They will be working together to create the most favorable living environment for each of us.

8. Remote Presence and Trust in Invisible Healthcare

Physical and virtual remote presence will extend to unthinkable proportions. What if a new type of a human/machine doctor – "doctoron" could care for 100 patients with the similar disease at the same time? Of course, that would be needed only if consumer chooses to know each and every step of the care process. Most consumers will choose to lead a normal, uninterrupted life style instead of checking on the doctoron's decisions. It will be more and more so within our capability to extend our life spans indefinitely. There will be no need to double-check our human/machine doctorons or even use them. Most people will delegate control to their cells directly.

Just like computers are used in mathematical proofs (computer performs tasks that are not possible to be verified by humans), they will be also used this way in healthcare – without us understanding each and every step of the reasoning and computation behind a decision. But we need to be in control – we need to understand qualitatively what is happening and our biggest current responsibility as human beings is to make sure that it will happen – that new brave human/machine systems will be able and will be willing to share their findings with us human beings.

9. Getting There – Example of Turning Existing Infrastructure into HealthStructure

Before we all wear body monitors in the form of second skin, we would all be healthier if we could get a quick medical checkup while pumping gasoline at the gas station. Our blood pressure at least should be measured every time we stop at the gas station and we should also be checked for sleepiness and alcohol level (breathalyzers) to determine if we should continue driving. Falling asleep at the wheel causes a large percentage of accidents. We could imagine facilities for those who need to take a nap or rest (Sleeping chambers) right at the gas stations.

10. Unsolved Health Problems

By analogy to mathematics where there is always a list of unsolved problems to guide the young generation of mathematicians, Future of Health Technology Institute conducted an "unsolved health problems" survey in 2003–5. The results are listed in the table below. All survey participants were also asked to state what will we gain if we solve that problem and what will we lose if we do not solve it. Solving these problems will get us closer to errorless, invisible healthcare with bionic hugs and no need for quality control.

Table 1. Unsolved Health Problems – Based on HFTI's Unsolved Problems Survey 2003–5.

Unsolved Problem	What will we gain if we solve this problem?	What will we lose if we do not solve this problem?
Lack of clean water in much of developing world.	Reduced (especially child) mortality rates.	Lives
Lack of drugs resulting from human genome.	Cures for previously untreatable, fatal illnesses.	Funding for genetic research
Really effective interfaces with human users.	Efficiency	Usability
Significant (in magnitude) replacement of human professionals by machines.	Enormous increase in efficacy/productivity and better "results"/outcomes.	Status quo
Translation from the Laboratory to the Bedside: many innovations seem to never to get past the "proof of concept demo" phase.	We may see more of these projects make a difference in clinical treatment.	We will waste a lot of our intellectual capital on projects that don't make it to the bedside.

Table 1. (Continued.)

Unsolved Problem	What will we gain if we solve this problem?	What will we lose if we do not solve this problem?
Lack of tools to build causal models that integrate all pieces of medical and process information; information systems that can help us to integrate all information into causal models, test the models against available information, and help us do thought experiments to devise new hypothesis to test.	If we are able to overcome the problems of how to build, interpret and validate what will often be massively underspecified models of physiological systems, then we will be able to accelerate the process of discovery.	We will continue to build an increasingly fragmented knowledge base and many important discoveries will not get translated into useful understanding.
Independent nanorobots with smart software controls.	Stop disease before it develops.	Lives.
Anticipating human and system failures so that processes can be devised to prevent these failures.	We will be better able to optimize the care we can give with the clinical advances we have in hand.	Medical errors will continue to limit our ability to give the best care possible with the current clinical knowledge.
Structured capture of clinical data (history, physical examination, progress notes, procedure reports, discharge summaries.	Increased formal encoding of phenotype information to enable research, clinical care, decision support, etc.	We will continue the present process of having this information unavailable. Some could be captured through natural language processing techniques, but structured data capture also encourages more discipline and thoroughness in recording, and provides more opportunity for timely decision support.
Personal longitudinal integrated health record.	This will foster improved continuity of care, access to relevant information to care providers, better decision making, decreased errors (e.g., overlooking an allergy or ordering of a medication conflicting with another), and the ability to track a patient's care over time, issue reminders, recommendations for improved health, etc.	We will continue the present process of fragmented, incomplete, inefficient management of episodes of care without ever having a complete picture of the health status of a patient.
Comprehensive structured population health data bases.	This will provide the ability to do analyses of screening tests, genome-phenotype correlation, outcomes analyses, technology assessments, and clinical prediction/prognosis.	Continued current state of limited comparability and size of datasets.
Application of cutting edge technologies for Primary Prevention i.e. implanted calorie counter/blood sugar monitor with beeper or such for weight loss, nicotine or drug aversion implants etc to give ongoing feedback and stimulus for behavior change. The simple low cost pedometer is a good example, but perhaps taken to a higher level or personalized monitoring.	Decrease in incidence of chronic illness and money spend for chronic illness, care and improved quality of life.	Individual quality of life and economic stability in health care costs as current population ages with chronic illnesses due to behavior factors.

Table 1. (Continued.)

Unsolved Problem	What will we gain if we solve this problem?	What will we lose if we do not solve this problem?
Cost benefit ratio analysis of health technologies.	Truly beneficial and cost effective health technology applications.	Increasing personal and 3rd party costs for marginal efficacy – "technology for technology sake".
Inadequate distribution of current technologies, based on geography, income etc.	Equity in world health.	Continued Inequitable distribution which may eventually be the death of us all i.e. SARS AIDS etc. spreading world wide without available monitoring and prevention measure
Lack of coordination. This problem crosses all applications of technology, whether business, aerospace, or medical. In medicine, the cost of mistakes is already too high.	A specific example of positive coordination among medical systems includes the sharing of patient information among pharmaceutical and patient records so that errors in prescriptions, both in hospital and out of hospital are reduced, if not eliminated. But also that same mechanism of sharing, can provide a uniform source of information across many platforms, many software systems, so that validation and cross checking among the different systems may be simplified and when errors are detected, more easily tracked.	If we do not attack the problem of coordination, we risk additional sources of error, loss of our ability to track errors, and loss of time, not to mention increases in medical error and possible law suits.
Lack of recognition that not all medical problems can be solved with "more technology"... sometimes, "LO TECH", is a more cost effective and patient friendly. E.g., providing access to meditation classes can reduce the cost of medication for chronic medical conditions such as high blood pressure and pain management.	Reduce patient load, empower patients, create first steps in the cultural shift to one where patients begin to take an ACTIVE rather than PASSIVE role in their own health.	Continuing on the path we are on is no longer an option. Health insurance costs are not going down. Not only are Americans uninsured they are also underinsured.
Effective use of media such as TV and the internet to raise awareness and engage the average consumer into healthcare. Make being healthy "trendy"; make it "attractive". This requires administrators to make this a line item in the budgets, a non-technical issue, but implementation is technical.	It will take time to help consumers reach for self care in their medicine cabinets rather than pills, but eventually we can hope to see an improvement in the overall health of human race reducing the costs of chronic conditions and the incidence of health problems.	We will continue to see the deterioration of health status. The cost of insurance, and the cost of Hi-tech healthcare need to be offset by low tech, such as dietary habits, practice of meditation, and so on.
Regenerative Medicine: ability to apply stem cells to address regenerative medicine.	Find cures for millions that suffer and sometimes die prematurely from degenerative illnesses.	Billions of dollars spent on unpromising therapy as well as incalculable human misery.
Background noise in biological agent detection system.	Ability to rapidly detect pathogens to isolate populations from further exposure.	Millions of lives lost to infectious disease epidemics that may be able to be curbed with early detection.

Table 1. (Continued.)

Unsolved Problem	What will we gain if we solve this problem?	What will we lose if we do not solve this problem?
Growing new Telomeres from stem cells.	Potentially slow down the aging process.	Immortality
100% Electronic infrastructure for medical records.	Greater portability of data, greater collation of data for research, longitudinal tracking of health information, and potential reduction in medical errors.	Privacy lapses, consumer apprehension.
Wide-spread mobile computing in medical care.	Instant access to reference and clinical information, greater evidence-based healthcare.	Fragmentation of technological application in well-funded vs. poorly-funded settings; physician resistance and lack of acceptance of new computing technology.
Personal understanding of preventative health lifestyles.	Lower heath costs and better quality of life.	Unbounded cost of health care.
Adequate pricing of health care	Reduction of serious ethical problems in health care pricing.	Lost market pressure for improved health care costs with monies being extracted for drugs and procedures no care and health.
Inpatient medical error as the third leading cause of death. Medication error is the largest subcomponent and by itself is the fourth leading cause of death. 60% of medication error is caused by physician ordering and 30% is caused by nurse administration.	Eliminate of a substantial portion of 220,000 unnecessary inpatient deaths per year and millions of persons maimed or incapacitated in some way. Elimination of a portion of about 1M unnecessary outpatient deaths. Elimination of about half of patient visits and hospitalization by proper disease management.	220,000 unnecessary inpatients deaths and millions of outpatient deaths and disabilities. About $500 Billion in unnecessary healthcare costs.
Outpatient medical error (even higher than inpatient error, perhaps by an order of magnitude)	Human Lives	See above
Disease management errors – the iceberg of which medical error is the visible tip. E.g., many unnecessary amputations on diabetics performed every year in the U.S., caused by improper follow-up.	Human Lives	See above
Bringing the bio-med hypothesis builders and the tech developers closer (educational challenge).	Fast progress and better penetration of innovations into practice.	Slow progress
A reliable protein/proteomics database for NORMAL human serum. (Surprisingly, from the many decades doctors have looked for signs of disease in the blood, the normal constituents – proteins-in blood are very poorly known, both qualitatively and quantitatively. Before we can exploit nanotech & high throughput methods, we really must get a handle on what the range of normal proteins is in peripheral blood.)	Human Lives – Reduction in unnecessary anxiety about "symptoms" that are part of normal variation not a sign of disease.	Lack of individualized biochemistry understanding and treatment.

Table 1. (Continued.)

Unsolved Problem	What will we gain if we solve this problem?	What will we lose if we do not solve this problem?
Expediting tech transfer from lab to clinic (administrative, governmental challenge).	Reduction in suffering.	Wasted human effort.
Finding the genetic basis of the telomerase-independent telomere extension seen in about 10% of human cancers.	We'll be able to control telomerase-independent cancers (including half of all sarcomas, for example) by gene therapy in the same way that we will be able to control telomerase-dependent cancers by gene therapy against the telomerase genes.	We will fail to give people longer healthy life spans and reverse aging in order to reverse aging comprehensively enough to keep people alive and healthy for a few decades more than now, which will be enough to let us improve the therapies further and keep us alive indefinitely.
Making the 13 protein-coding mitochondrial genes work when placed in the nucleus.	We'll be able to ignore the accumulation of mitochondrial mutations during aging, because they will be harmless – the proteins that are made from the mitochondrial DNA will be made from nuclear copies of the genes so the mitochondria will still work.	We will fail to give people longer healthy life spans. See above
Finding microbial enzymes to break down the cholesterol analogues that cause atherosclerosis and maybe Alzheimer's disease.	We'll be able to treat all major diseases that are caused by the accumulation of garbage inside cells. That includes atherosclerosis, macular degeneration and probably most types of neurodegeneration.	We will fail to give people longer healthy life spans. See above.
Lack of machines with common sense that could take care of us	Well cared for population. Increased health status of the population.	Worldwide healthcare crisis due to lack of care givers. Unnecessary suffering.
Lack of comprehensive working easy to use framework for performance evaluation of adaptive complex systems.	Faster progress towards errorless healthcare.	Slow progress towards errorless healthcare.
Maintaining long-term engagement between users and health dialog systems (caring machines), especially crucial for chronic disease management systems in which we need people to use the system regularly for the rest of their lives.	Increased speed of acceptance of caring machines.	No good communication between people and caring machines.
Encoding of behavioral medicine concepts and theories into shareable computational ontologies, to support information sharing and re-use.	Exponential growth of the use and utilization of the caring machines.	Limited use of caring machines.

11. Conclusions

Utilizing Intelligent Caring Creatures (ICCs) to achieve errorless healthcare requires departure from thinking that the only entity that can justify a medical action is an un-aided human being. Once we are ready to delegate management of our health to ICCs we need to make sure that they are able and willing to explain their multidimensional reasoning. Compiling a list of "unsolved problems" helps moving towards errorless healthcare. It would be useful to have awards system for solving currently unsolved healthcare problems to make healthcare errorless, invisible, infrastructure-free and continuous sooner – to enter a healthon era. The Worldwide Marathon for Health: Healthon Initiative initiated by FHTI will start that process.

Acknowledgements

The author gratefully acknowledges participants of Future of Health Technology Summits 1996–2005 – especially those who responded to FHTI Unsolved Problems Survey.

References

Future of Health Technology Summit – Proceedings 1996–2005, www.fhti.org Future of Health Technology, IOS Press, 2002, Ed. Renata G. Bushko.

Consumers Era – Sociotechnological Environment

Future of Intelligent and Extelligent Health Environment
R.G. Bushko (Ed.)
IOS Press, 2005

The Prospects for Medical Technology in the Next Decade

George B. MOSELEY III, MBA, JD
*Faculty, Institute of Cybermedicine, Harvard Medical School
Lecturer in Health Law and Management
Harvard School of Public Health, Cambridge, MA, US*

"Some grocery stores have better technology than our hospitals and clinics."

Tommy Thompson, Secretary of Health and Human Services

What drives up premiums?

"There's absolutely no debate. It's medical technology, whether it's machines or new drugs. The reason it is so hard to control costs is because medical technology is almost a religion in America. All of us want the latest and the best, and we want it now, and we want it in our own community."

Drew Altman, President, Henry J. Kaiser Family Foundation
(Boston Globe, 7.18.04.)

Abstract. Powerful forces encourage the growth of medical technology (health benefits, private equity capital, public funding, pervasive academic research, consumer demand, specialist training, reimbursement mechanisms, and industry competition). Countervailing forces that inhibit growth are the costs of the technology, difficulty in evaluating clinical and cost effectiveness, unequal patient access, and misuse, overuse, and underuse. While technology funding sources continue to expand, so do the methodologies for technology assessment.

They are part of a broad movement to better manage the diffusion of medical technology. Specific proposals include more centralized planning, more discriminating federal funding, drug price controls, curtailing insurance reimbursements, more selective adoption of new technologies, and more rigorous attention to cost effectiveness. Savvy develops of and investors in new medical technology will anticipate these changes and take them into account in their planning.

1. Introduction

The U.S. has a love-hate relationship with health care technology.

One of the distinguishing features of Western medicine and US health care in particular has been its reliance on medical technology, in the form of new drugs, procedures, medical devices, and diagnostic equipment. The demand for innovations that might enhance or prolong life seems insatiable, and vendors pour a steady stream of new products and services into the health care marketplace to meet that demand.

Many patients look to new medical technology as the answer to their health care problems; it also is a primary driver of health care cost increases. Some people believe that there is always room for new innovation in medical care: others feel that more effort should be devoted to making the current technology accessible to more patients.

In the dynamic, ever-changing world of US health care, the environment for this technology will transform dramatically over the next several years. For developers, vendors, and users, it would be wise to consider the new prospects for health care technology.

2. Types of Health Care Technology

It is important to be clear about what constitutes "health care technology". The now defunct Congressional Office of Technology Assessment defined the term as "drugs, devices, medical and surgical procedures used in medical care, and the organizational and supportive systems within which such care is provided".[1]

A laundry list of some new technologies recently deployed in the health care field might look something like this.

Type	Example
Diagnostic	Fetal monitor
	Automated clinical laboratories
	Magnetic resonance imaging
Survival (life threatening)	Cardiopulmonary resuscitation (CPR)
	Liver transplant
	Autologous bone marrow transplant
Illness management	Renal dialysis
	Pacemaker
	PCTA (angioplasty)
Cure	Hip joint replacement
	Organ transplant
	Lithotripter
Prevention	Implantable automatic cardioverter-defibrillator
	Pediatric orthopaedic repair
	Vaccines for immunization
System management	Computerized physician order entry (CPOE)
	Telemedicine
	Electronic medical records
Facilities and clinical settings	Intensive care unit (ICU)
	Outpatient surgery centers
	Modern home health care
Organizational delivery structure	Managed care
	Integrated delivery systems
	Preferred provider organizations

However, this list is a little too large and diverse to grapple with effectively. The properties of these various technologies, as well as their roles in the health care system, raise different questions and present different challenges. For purposes of discussion, it helps to divide them into two broad categories.

---

[1] U.S. Congress. OTA. 1982. *Strategies for Medical Technology Assessment. Publication.* no. OTA-H-181. Washington, DC: U.S. Government Printing Office.

One is Medical Technology (MT), concerned with clinical treatment of disease; the other is Information Technology (IT), concerned with management of health care delivery logistics, and analysis and administration of health care financial/clinical operations. Information technology includes the applications in the areas of system management, facilities and clinical settings, and organizational delivery structure; MT encompasses the other items.

Looked at in this way, the two apparently contradictory quotes on technology at the beginning of this article make more sense. In complaining about excessive costs, Drew Altman was talking about Medical Technology, implying that there is too much of it. Tommy Thompson was referring to Information Technology and arguing that it should be more widely adopted. This is an important and useful distinction.

This discussion concentrates on the medical side of health care technology. It begins with an overview of the forces within the health care industry that are encouraging and restraining the spread of technology. It then looks at the infrastructure and principles through which medical technology is evaluated for possible implementation. Special attention is given to the primary source of criticism of that technology: its cost impact, including how it can both increase or decrease it. Finally, there are some predictions about future trends in health care technology diffusion within the U.S., coupled with suggestions for developers of new technology.

3. Forces Encouraging the Growth and Spread of Health Care Technology

There are several powerful factors working in favor of broader diffusion of health care technology.

3.1. Health Benefits

These are sometimes substantial, other times only incremental. They range from vaccines against the polio and hepatitis B virus to new surgical treatments like organ transplantation and the implantation of pacemakers. Other benefits are replacements for certain hormonal and vitamin deficiencies, catheterization, bypass surgery, and angioplasty for the surgical treatment if heart attacks, and selective serotonin reuptake inhibitors (SSRIs) for the treatment of depression. Increasingly, these benefits are being promoted through direct-to-consumer advertising.

3.2. Equity Capital

Equity capital continues to be available for at least later stage applied research ventures.[2] For most of the 1990s, medical and health care companies were among the leading recipients of venture capital (VC), receiving almost 21% of all VC funds in 1992. This share dropped to 5% (1999) during the dot.com boom years. When the Internet bubble burst, funding interest shifted back to medical and health care-related companies (11% of total VC investments in 2002) and biotechnology companies (6% in 2002). Although the preference for later stage expansion and acquisition financing continues, substantial shares of available seed money have gone to medical and health care-related (20%) and biotechnology companies (15%).

---

[2] National Science Foundation, *Science and Engineering Indicators – 2004*, pp. 6–27 to 6–31.

3.3. Government and Foundation Funding

Government and foundation funding for basic and applied research in medical technology is substantial and increasing. The total National Institutes of Health (NIH) research expenditures, the bulk of which are in life sciences (medical, biological, and agricultural), increased steadily every year from 1970 ($1.1 billion) to 1999 ($13.9 billion).[3] The increases since then have been dramatic: $17.2 billion in 2000, $19.7 billion in 2001,[4] $22.7 billion in 2002, and $26.2 billion in 2003.[5]

3.4. Academic Research

Academic research institutions are empowered to license and commercialize any technology developed with public funds. The Bayh-Dole Act of 1980 (Public Law 96–517) allows universities to elect to retain title to, and obtain a patent on, an invention resulting from federally funded research. A university then may license the invention to a third-party private business for the purposes of development and commercialization. The process is referred as "technology transfer". This Act was a significant factor in the increase in membership of the Association of University Technology Managers (AUTM) from 113 in 1979 to 2,178 in 1999,[6] the increase in the number of citations of scientific articles in patent applications in the life science fields of biomedical research and clinical medicine (an indicator of the link between research and practical application) from 17,009 in 1995 to 49,619 in 2002,[7] the increase in the share of academic patents with biomedical relevance[8] granted from 22% in the early eighties to 39% in 2001,[9] the increase in number of new patents filed from 2,497 in 1991 to 7,741 in 2002, and the increase in new license agreements executed during the same period from 1,280 to 4,673.[10]

3.5. Consumer Demand and Public Expectations

Public opinion surveys of the citizens of the U.S. and several European countries show that Americans have much higher expectations of what medical technology can do to cure illness.[11] Two-thirds of Americans are "very interested" in new medical discoveries, compared to an average of 44% of adults in 12 European countries. 22% of Americans say that

---

[3] U.S. Department of Health and Human Services. 2002. *Health, United States, 2002*. Publication No. (PHS) 02-1232. Hyattsville, MD: USDHHS.

[4] American Academy for the Advancement of Science, Reports VII through XXVI, based on OMB and agency R&D budget data. *Table I-16. Historical Tables: Federal R&D by Agency, FY 1990–2002 (REVISED July '01) (budget authority in millions of dollars)*. Available at http://www.aaas.org/spp/rd/xxvi/tbi16r.pdf (accessed on 3.4.05.).

[5] American Association for the Advancement of Science, Science and Technology in Congress, March 2003. *Congressional Action on R&R in the FY2003 Budget (Budget Authority in millions of dollars; March 7, 2003)* Available at http://www.aaas.org/spp/cstc/pne/pubs/stc/stc03-03.pdf (accessed on 3.4.05.).

[6] Council on Governmental Relations, October 1999, *The Bayh-Dole Act: A Guide to the Law and Implementing Regulations*. Available at http://www.ucop.edu/ott/bayh.html (accessed 2.18.2005.).

[7] National Science Foundation, *Science and Engineering Indicators – 2004*, Appendix Table 5-52.

[8] Patent classes 424 and 514 – drug, bioaffecting, and bodytreating compositions, and class 435 – chemistry, molecular biology, and microbiology.

[9] U.S. Patent and Trademark Office (USPTO), *Technology Assessment and Forecast Report: U.S. Colleges and Universities, Utility Patent Grants, 1969–2001* (Washington, DC, 2001).

[10] AUTM Frequently Asked Questions, available at http://www.autm.net/aboutTT/about_TT_faqs.cfm (accessed 2.18.2005.).

[11] Kim, M., Blendon, R.J., and Benson, J.M. 2001. "How Interested Are Americans In New Medical Technologies? A Multicountry Comparison". *Health Affairs* 20 (5): 194–201.

they are "very well informed" about new medical discoveries, versus 12% of Europeans. In the US, 34% of the people believe that "modern medicine can cure almost any illness for people who have access to the most advanced technology and treatment", while only 11% of German citizens feel that way. 35% of Americans believe that "being able to get the most advanced tests, drugs, and medical procedures and equipment is absolutely essential"; only 21% of Germans share that view. Nearly half (47%) of Americans "disagree that it is impossible for any government or public or private health insurance to pay for all new medical treatments and technologies", compared to 36% of Europeans.

3.6. Specialist Physician Training and Practice

It is frequently argued that there are too many specialist physicians in the U.S. health care system. The ratio is approximately one-third generalists to two-thirds specialists, the reverse of what it is in other industrialized countries.[12] Specialists normally receive their residency training in acute care hospitals that typically deploy the latest medical technology. Upon graduation, the specialists manifest a "technological imperative" – a desire to have access to state-of-the-art medical innovations regardless of the cost.

3.7. Reimbursement Mechanisms

Financing of health care through private insurers insulates both patients and providers from personal accountability for utilization of high-cost, high-tech services and, in some cases, encourages it. To the extent that it still exists, fee-for-service payment of physicians and full cost reimbursement of hospitals aggravates the phenomenon.

3.8. Competition Among Hospitals

Hospitals and other provider institutions project perceptions of higher quality to patients and payors by acquiring and promoting the latest technology. In the competition to recruit specialists who will refer patients, medical care centers often promise to obtain new technology and offer high tech procedures.

3.9. Direct Marketing or Promotion of the New Technology to Purchasers and Patients

The manufacturers of medical technologies are spending increasing sums of money on marketing and promotion to build demand for their products. The traditional practitioners of this strategy have been the drug companies, initially, for many years, through detail men contacting physicians and, more recently through direct-to-consumer (DTC) advertising. In 2001, the U.S. pharmaceutical industry spent the following amounts on various forms of promotion:[13]

---

[12] Shi, L., and Singh, D.A. *Delivering Health Care in America, A Systems Approach, Third Edition*, Ch. 4, Health Services Professionals, p. 130, Jones and Bartlett Publishers (Sudbury, MA, 2004).
[13] Press Room, Total U.S. Promotional Spending by Type, 2001. IMS Health, Integrated Promotional Services™, and CMR, 2002. Available at http://www.imshealth.com/ims/portal/front/articleC/0,2777,6599_9285_1004963,00.html (accessed 3.4.05.).

Journal Advertising	$425 million
Hospital Promotion	$702 million
DTC	$2,679 million
Physician Office Promotion	$4,789 million
Total Promotion	$8,595 million

In addition, the retail value of free samples given out was $10,464 million. The spending on DTC alone was expected to reach about $5 billion in 2004.[14]

4. Forces Inhibiting/Restricting the Growth and Spread of Health Care Technology

Although the growth and spread of medical technology seems irresistible, some forces are emerging that may inhibit that growth.

4.1. Cost to Implement the Technology

This is far and away the most significant factor causing policymakers to question the blind acceptance of every new medical technology. The costs related to the implementation are:

- Capital costs of acquiring the technology and its related equipment.
- Training or hiring of physicians and technicians in the new skills required to operate the technology.
- Facilities may require renovation or expansion to accommodate new technology.
- Greater utilization of the technology when covered by insurance, as a result of the phenomena of moral hazard and provider-induced demand.

Many industries have been affected by the introduction over the last two decades of new technologies. In nearly all cases, the result was a reduction in production costs and labor force requirements. The opposite has been true in health care, where both labor and capital costs have risen.[15]

Generically, the increases in spending on technology are due to three factors: price increases for existing technology, utilization increases for existing technology, or higher prices of new technology that replaces old technology.

It is estimated that medical technology innovations account for as much as one-third of the total increase in real medical costs. Numerous studies over the past decade have produced widely-varying results on the contribution of medical technology to health care cost inflation. The most recent analysis found that the technology contribution, over a 38-year period, ranged from 4% to 64%.[16] There is a strong consensus among researchers that technology diffusion is one of the strongest drivers of long-term growth in health care costs.

It is important to note that some medical technologies have produced measurable cost savings. Some examples are:

---

[14] DTC Perspectives Magazine. January 13, 2005. Are We Really Spending So Much? Available at http://www.dtcperspectives.com/content.asp?id=230 (accessed on 3.4.05.).

[15] Iglehart, J.K. 1982. The Cost and Regulation of Medical Technology: Future Policy Directions. In *Technology and the Future of Health Care*, ed. J.B. McKinlay, 69–103. Cambridge, MA: MIT Press.

[16] Mohr, P.E., C. Mueller, P. Neumann, S. Franco, M. Milet, L. Silver, and G. Wilensky. 2001. *The Impact of Medical Technology on Future Health Care Costs*. Report to the Health Insurance Association of America and the Blue Cross and Blue Shield Association, March 13. Bethesda, MD: Project Hope.

- Replace earlier, more costly treatments (implantable infusion pumps and lasers)
- Avoid lifelong medication and prolonged disability (coronary artery bypass graft)
- Reduced hospitalization (antiretroviral therapies for AIDS patients)
- Reduced average length of hospital stay (treatments in home and outpatient settings)
- Reduced admissions for inpatient psychiatric care (antidepressant and antipsychotic drugs)

4.2. Difficulty in Evaluating Cost Benefit and Balancing with Clinical Effectiveness

There are two methodologies for evaluating the cost impact of medical technologies – cost-effectiveness and cost-benefit analyses. These are explained more fully below. Actually conducting such analyses is a challenge.

It is only within the last few years that the methodologies have been taken seriously and practiced rigorously by payors, providers, vendors, and researchers. The monetarization of very subjective qualities, like a more accurate diagnosis or quicker recovery from surgery, almost defies common sense – and yet it must be done. With multiple institutions engaged in the assessment of medical technology, it is not easy to reach consensus on the standards or indices to be used. One commonly used measure is the quality-adjusted life year (QALY), defined as the value of one year of high quality life. It might be used in assessing increases in life expectancy. It currently is assigned a somewhat arbitrary worth of $100,000.

4.3. Diversion of Knowledge Resources

It can be argued that the intense concentration on the development of new medical technologies has distorted the allocation of scientific knowledge resources. The dramatic growth in the number of new ventures in biotechnology has created employment opportunities that have drawn talented researchers away from other important fields of scientific exploration. The large volume of federal funds devoted to medical research has left less money available for research in the areas of engineering, environmental science, and the physical sciences. In turn, universities have emphasized the creation of new research programs and facilities in the life sciences; their graduate students are choosing careers in the same fields, at the expense of other worthy research paths.

4.4. Unequal Distribution of New Technologies Among the Patient Populations

There are significant geographic and financial barriers to equitable access to medical technology. The very high cost of some technologies – either for the treatment itself, as in the case of drugs, or for the equipment to deliver the treatment, as in the case of diagnostic imaging – makes them unaffordable, and therefore unavailable, to patients who lack insurance that might pay for them or whose insurance does not cover them. Some high tech medical equipment (imaging again is a good example) is so expensive that only medical centers with a high volume of demand for its use can justify its purchase. These are inevitably located in more densely populated urban areas. Residents of more sparsely populated rural areas may have to travel considerable distances to gain access to such equipment.

4.5. Misuse, Overuse, and Underuse of Medical Technology

Documentation of inappropriate use of medical technology leads many to question the rapid pace of its diffusion.[17] *Misuse* occurs when the technology provider commits an error and the system in which he practices is not adequate to prevent either the error or the resulting injury.

One arguable cause of *overuse* of technology is a fee-for-service payment mechanism that rewards the delivery of greater volumes of service units. In addition, some physicians are enthusiastic believers in the value of the services they are most familiar with and seek to apply them at every opportunity. This may include delivering a new technology to a patient for whom it is not clinically indicated in the belief that its application in a case for which it was not tested is a natural extension of the cases for which it was tested and found appropriate. Clinical studies may eventually be conducted to justify the physician's belief – or to contradict it. The physician's patients may also insist that some overt action be taken when rest and watchful waiting are the best prescription.

There are several possible explanations for *underuse*. Financial barriers, like lack of insurance, lack of coverage for the particular technology, or high deductibles or co-payments, may make the technology unavailable. The treating physician may have been unable (for lack of time or other resources) to acquire and digest the necessary clinical information about the technology to know to use it in a particular case. A few patients, rather than embracing every new medical technology, fear innovative treatments and choose to avoid them.

The primary tool for reconciling the conflicting forces acting on the diffusion of health care technology is Technology Assessment. This is a process for examining and reporting on the most relevant properties of technology, both in absolute terms and in comparison among competing technologies.

First, some background on who conducts research on medical technology and who funds it. This is followed by a review of the current state of medical technology assessment.

5. Sources of Medical Technology Research

Research on new medical technologies is conducted by:

- Academic health centers (colleges and universities)
- Private research institutes (Howard Hughes Medical Institute, Whitehead Institute for Biomedical Research)
- Government laboratories (NIH, Agency for Healthcare Research and Quality)
- Public Health departments
- Pharmaceutical, biotechnology, medical device, and durable medical equipment companies
- Contract research organizations (CROs) – typically for drug companies
- Practice-based researchers and networks
- Public and private hospitals
- HMO-based researchers and networks
- Community health centers

The first three sources tend to conduct basic and applied research, while the remainder are engaged primarily in developmental research.

---

[17] Becher, E.C. and Chassin, M.R. 2001. "Improving the Quality of Health Care: Who Will Lead?". *Health Affairs* 20 (5): 164–179.

6. Sources of Medical Technology Research Funding

There are three major sources of funding for medical technology research.

6.1. Federal Government

Spent $16.2 billion (0.17% of GDP and 0.95% of total federal outlays) on life science and medical research in 1999. The bulk (86%) of this spending passed through the NIH; the rest was handled by the U.S. Department of Agriculture and the National Science Foundation (NSF). The NIH funding in FY2003 was about $27 million. In 2000, 53% of the NIH grants went toward basic research, 34% to applied research, and the remainder for development. Only 18% of all NIH funds support its own intramural research. Academic institutions receive nearly 60%, hospitals and medical foundations get 17%, and 5% goes to industry.[18] The Agency for Healthcare Research and Quality (AHRQ) budget request for FY 2004 was $279 million.[19] It is spent primarily on research into the financing organization, quality, and utilization aspects of health care delivery.

6.2. Academic Institutions

In addition to the funds that universities receive from the NIH (approximately 59% of all their research funding), they also obtain research money from state/local governments (8%), industry (7%), internal sources (19%), and other external sources (7%).[20] The aggregate total was $26.3 billion in 1998. Of this amount, 45.6% went toward research in the biological and medical sciences. The total also was divided among basic research (68.7%), applied research (24.1%), and development (7.2%).

6.3. Private Industry

Corporate spending on R&D in health and medicine-related industries reached $28.1 billion in 2001,[21] divided as follows:

Pharmaceuticals and medicines	$10.1 billion
Medical equipment and supplies	$5.9 billion
Health care services	$1.1 billion
Scientific R&D services	$10.9 billion

The category "scientific R&D services" comprises companies that specialize in conducting R&D for other organizations, such as many biotechnology companies and often on a contract basis. The internal spending in this category was augmented by $3.4 billion in federal funding.

The scientific R&D services industry accounted for slightly more than half of the reported total of $7.4 billion of biotechnology research in 2001. Biotechnology R&D in turn made up 3.7% of all U.S. industrial R&D in 2001.[22]

---

[18] Zinner, D.E. "Medical R&D At The Turn Of The Millenium". *Health Affairs* 20 (5): 202–209.

[19] Testimony on the President's Fiscal Year 2004 Budget Request for AHRQ before the House Subcommittee on Labor-HHS-Education Appropriations, by Carolyn M. Clancy, M.D., Director, AHRQ, available at http://www.ahrq.gov/about/cj2004/cjtest04.htm (accessed on 2.22.05.).

[20] National Science Foundation, Division of Science Resources Studies, Science and Engineering Indicators – 2000, *National Patterns of R&D Resources* (Arlington, VA; biennial series).

[21] National Science Foundation, *Science and Engineering Indicators – 2004*, Appendix Table 4-2.

[22] National Science Foundation, *Science and Engineering Indicators – 2004*, Appendix Table 4-4.

The pharmaceutical industry allocates about 13% of its annual revenues to R&D. The medical device industry devotes roughly 7%.[23]

For these entities researching, financing, or marketing new health care technology, it is important to understand how such technology enters the health care system. This requires looking at the key decision makers who determine whether it will be adopted, covered, reimbursed, and provided. This includes the procedures and criteria for making those decisions. The process is called "technology assessment".

7. Medical Technology Assessment Agencies

Most who work in the health care industry are familiar with following entities. One thing to notice about this list is that it is a "list" of several agencies. Most of them are assessing the same innovations, often simultaneously, and not using the same criteria. In other industrialized nations, the assessment, diffusion and utilization of new medical technology is managed centrally to control the effect on costs.

- Food and Drug Administration (drugs and medical devices)
- American Medical Association – Diagnostic and Therapeutic Technology Assessment (DATTA) Program
- Blue Cross and Blue Shield Association – Technology Evaluation and Coverage Program
- Managed care organizations – technical assessment committees
- Pharmaceutical companies – "pharmaco-economics" departments
- Private technology assessment and rating firms

Examples of the private assessment firms are ECRI (www.ecri.org) and Hayes (www.hayesinc.com) are two leading examples. MCO's contract with them for independent evaluations of new technologies or new applications of existing technologies. For strategic planning purposes, they increasingly are seeking forecasts of technologies that will emerge in the future. These assessment companies oblige.

8. Medical Technology Assessment Criteria

The criteria employed in medical technology assessment fall into four basic categories.

- Efficacy
- Safety
- Cost-Effectiveness
- Cost-Benefit

In practical terms, "efficacy" is the health benefit derived from a technology and is usually synonymous with "effectiveness". This is not an easy variable to quantify. Traditionally, health outcomes were measured in terms of mortality and morbidity rates. Psychosocial and functional factors are now taken into consideration, but they are harder to translate into numbers. A great deal of work is going into efforts to define and measure what it is that we try to achieve when administering medical care.

---

[23] Neumann, P.J. and E.A. Sandberg. 1998. Trends in Health Care R&D and Technology Innovation. *Health Affairs* 17 no. 6: 111–119.

The "safety" criterion aims to prevent any unnecessary harm from the technology. Some negative side effects are acceptable, but they must be substantially outweighed by the benefits.

Both efficacy and safety are assessed through clinical trials – carefully designed research studies in which human subjects participate under controlled observation. They typically extend over three or four phases involving increasingly larger groups of subjects and taking.

Traditionally, technology assessment ended with these two criteria. In fact, the FDA's approvals are still based solely on efficacy and safety. The ratings of the AMA's DATTA program are indicative of the output of such efforts.

- *Established*: Accepted as appropriate by the practicing medical community for the given indication in the specified patient population.
- *Promising*: Given current knowledge, the effectiveness of this technology appears to be appropriate for the given indication in the specified patient population.
- *Investigational*: Evidence insufficient to determine appropriateness: warrants further study. Use of this technology for the given indication in the specified patient population should be confined largely to research protocols.
- *Doubtful*: Given current knowledge, this technology is inappropriate. As the given results of long-term follow-up accumulate, this interim rating will change.
- *Unacceptable*: Regarded by the practicing medical community as inappropriate for the given indication in the specified population.

The assessment firm, Hayes, grades new technologies from A to D. The grades have the following definitions and are given in the following percentages of cases.[24]

A "Absolutely rock solid." Safety is clearly backed up by long-term studies. Efficacy and appropriate patient recipients are specified. (10%)

B "Very promising." Results must be available from randomized controlled trials with good safety and efficacy results. "It works for sure on some, but not so sure on others." (25%)

C "Promising but not there yet. Sometimes it will hang there and be proven effective with more studies, and other times it goes down and goes away." Until further study is carried out, insurance coverage is unlikely. (All other technologies get C's or D's.)

D The evidence shows that it doesn't work, or isn't safe, or there is "just not enough published evidence to make any other rating."

One of the largest purchasers of health care services, and medical technology, is the federal Centers for Medicare and Medicaid Services (CMS). This agency receives advice on which new technologies to cover from the Medicare Coverage Advisory Committee, which is composed of six multi-stakeholder panels concerned with diagnostic imaging; drugs, biologics, and therapeutics; durable medical equipment; laboratory and diagnostic services; medical and surgical procedures; and medical devices and prosthetics. The committee evaluates the effectiveness of each new technology by comparing it to existing technologies and placing it in one of eight categories.[25]

1. Breakthrough technology: The improvement in health outcomes is so large that the intervention becomes the standard of care.

---

[24] Carroll, J. February 2004. "Brave New World, Old-Fashioned Fear". Managed Care Magazine. At http://www.managedcaremag.com/archives/0402/0402.newtech.html (accessed on 2.28.05.).

[25] Executive Committee Working Group, Medicare Coverage Advisory Committee. *Recommendations for Evaluating Effectiveness*. First version: February 21, 2000. Revised and approved by the Executive Committee, September 25, 2002. Available at http://www.cms.hhs.gov/mcac/recommendations.asp (accessed on 2.28.05.).

2. Substantially more effective: The new intervention improves health outcomes by a substantial margin as compared with established services or medical items.
3. More effective: The new intervention improves health outcomes by a significant, albeit small, margin as compared with established services or medical items.
4. As effective but with advantages: The intervention has the same effect on health outcomes as established services or medical items but has some advantages (convenience, rapidity of effect, fewer side effects, other advantages) that some patients will prefer.
5. As effective and with no advantages: The intervention has the same effect on health outcomes as established alternatives but with no advantages.
6. Less effective but with advantages: Although the intervention is less effective than established alternatives (but more effective than doing nothing), it has some advantages (such as convenience, tolerability).
7. Less effective and with no advantages: The intervention is less effective than established alternatives (but more effective than doing nothing) and has no significant advantages.
8. Not effective: The intervention has no effect or has deleterious effects on health outcomes when compared with "doing nothing" (e.g., treatment with placebo or patient management without the use of a diagnostic test).

Some health plans are interested in the future effects of a new technology. ECRI's Health Technology Forecast meets the demand with "1 to 5" ratings on the potential impact in the areas of utilization, cost, diffusion, health care delivery, and patient care.[26]

Technology manufacturers and vendors feel the weight of these assessment ratings. Low grades or rankings can permanently damage the marketability of a new product. It might be a good idea to keep these possible assessment outcomes in mind as a technology is being researched and developed.

Most of these assessment schemes do not place much emphasis on the cost implications of new technologies. Until recently, there has been resistance from manufacturers to having their products evaluated on this basis and a reluctance on the part of health plans explicitly to ration on the basis of cost. That is changing. As a result of the growing concern over the soaring costs of health care in general, and technology costs in particular, greater attention is being given to cost-effectiveness and cost-benefit analyses.

"Cost-effectiveness" (CE) analysis evaluates the additional or marginal benefits derived from the additional or marginal costs to be incurred, especially when they are *not expressed in monetary terms*. These are the types of variables that are considered.

Non-Monetary Costs (resource inputs)
- Staff time
- Number of service units
- Space requirements
- Degree of specialization required

Non-Monetary Benefits (health outcomes)
- Efficacy of treatment
- Prognosis or expected outcomes
- Disease cases averted
- Life years saved
- Life expectancy increase
- Hospitalization and sick days avoided

---

[26] Ibid.

- Early return to work
- Quality of life
- Patient satisfaction

In contrast with CE analysis, "cost-benefit" analysis is used when both the costs and benefits can be measured in monetary terms. The common denominator of money permits more rigorous quantitative analysis than CE analysis. If projected benefits exceed costs, the additional spending on medical care is deemed worth the expense.

Although these two analytical methodologies may seem sophisticated, the science of measuring the influence of medical advances on health care spending is not well developed. Surprisingly little is known about the cost-effectiveness of even well-established health care technologies. Furthermore, our understanding of the contribution of all new technologies to the steady increase in health care spending is imprecise, at best.

Although the willingness of provider and payor organizations to acknowledge the costs of the new medical technologies that they offer, and to balance those costs against clinical benefits, is a step in the right direction, these measures still are not the equivalent of the investment analysis techniques employed by well-run businesses in other industries. Over the next decade, health industry organizations can be expected to apply the following procedures to either their technology assessment or their general resource allocation process.

- Calculate the return on investment (ROI) in the proposed new technology. This need involve no more than using the monetary plusses and minuses from a cost-benefit analysis, making time adjustments, and dividing the latter into the former to come up with a rate of return on the funds spent on the new technology.
- Compare the ROI's for several different technologies being considered for implementation at one point in time. Put into practice those technologies with the highest ROI's.
- Compare even the highest-ROI technologies with the cost of the capital that will be used to buy them. Acquire only those technologies with ROI's that exceed the cost of capital.

These calculations will not necessarily ignore the societal and public health benefits of a new technology. These will either be translated into monetary terms (as is already being done in cost-benefit analysis) or used as a non-monetary factor in the decision-making balance.

9. Proposals to Manage the Diffusion of Medical Technology

Because of the negative aspects of medical technology noted above, particularly its cost, there have been numerous proposals to restrain or manage the widespread adoption of new medical technology. Not all of them will be put into practice, but they are indicative of an accelerating movement. Individuals and organizations with a stake in med tech R&D would do well to stay informed about the success of these proposals.

- **Institute more centralized planning to determine how much technology will be made available and where.** This is the approach taken by most other industrialized countries, including Canada. The goal would be to reduce the multiplicity of entities, public and private, with often conflicting standards, currently playing some role in technology management. The result need not be a single omnipotent agency. The planning might be carried out at the federal or state level, by public or private organizations, with clearly defined authorities and mandates. They likely would combine some degree of control with the existing assessment function.

- **Limit and more discriminatingly allocate federal funding for medical R&D.** This would require quelling the sometimes politically-motivated, bipartisan Congressional support for increasing the NIH budget, which in turn would depend on some abatement in the public eagerness for medical technology. Perhaps this will happen when the Congress attempts to reconcile the conflicting roles of the federal government as financer, regulator, and purchaser of medical research and its products.

- **Expand the FDA's drug and device approval mandate to include cost-effectiveness criteria.** This initiative would prevent cost-ineffective products from ever reaching the market. The challenge would be to reach agreement on the cost-effectiveness or cost-benefit analysis methodology to be employed and the level of effectiveness or benefit that would have to be met to qualify for approval. This is complicated by the fact that some technologies become more or less cost-effective once they are put into practice.

- **Impose controls on pharmaceutical prices, and incidentally make less money available for research and development of new drugs.** These sorts of controls would have to be imposed by the federal government. The move would be controversial and vigorously resisted by the drug companies. The controls would have the immediate effect of reducing the costs of drugs to both patients and health plans. As a secondary effect, there would probably be a decline in the drug companies' revenues. They would have less internally generated capital to invest in R&D and presumably would devote available funds to the development of the most cost-effective drugs.

- **Change the patterns of medical training, with a greater emphasis on primary care practice.** This would begin with a reduction in the number of specialty residency slots for medical graduates, and an increase in the number of primary care opportunities. It has been argued for many years that the U.S. has too high a proportion of specialists who are paid more and consume more resources. Their specialization prepares them to rely extensively on technology-based products, services, and equipment.

- **Curtail insurance payments for cost-ineffective medical treatments.** Health plans have traditionally been criticized by their members for denying coverage for new, sometimes experimental, even untested technologies, usually drugs. What is proposed is that the plans begin to gather reliable data on the cost-effectiveness of all available technologies – tested or untested – and use them to make hard decisions on their adoption. This would include ending coverage for technologies that, with the passage of time and the introduction of newer technologies, are no longer cost-effective.

- **Translate proven utilization procedures for new technologies into practice guidelines as quickly as possible.** As physicians become more comfortable and experienced with practice guidelines, they can be used as tools for steering the doctors to the appropriate use of medical technologies. This will work best if the necessary guideline is prepared and disseminated just as soon as the technology becomes available. A well-crafted guideline will specify the technology's application for those patients and conditions for which it has been tested. Other creative, but untested uses would not be authorized.

- **Take cost-effectiveness calculations into account when promulgating practice guidelines.** This takes the previous proposal a step further and asks that cost-effectiveness or benefit be a factor in shaping all guidelines. This does require always choosing the lowest cost course of treatment, but rather balancing carefully the cost with all other considerations.

- **Provide reimbursement for technologies only when they are used according to protocols.**[27] Once proper utilization of a technology has been codified in a practice guideline or protocol, the health plan can provide incentives to providers to use it accordingly. The most powerful is to withhold coverage or reimbursement unless usage complies with the guideline.

- **Preliminary coverage of new technology in exchange for vendor funding support for assessments.** Under this proposal, health plans and other payors would cover new technologies that had passed initial tests for efficacy and safety in return for the willingness of the technology's manufacturer to pay for more sophisticated assessment that also addresses cost-effectiveness. This would be done with the understanding that the coverage might be ended if the final assessment was unsatisfactory.

- **Take cost-effectiveness calculations into account when choosing which new technologies to offer and reimburse under a health benefits plan.** All good health plans confirm the safety and efficacy of new technologies before offering them to their members. Until now, there have been few reliable cost-effectiveness data if plans wished to consult them. As these analyses are more frequently prepared for innovative new products, the plans are more likely to include them in their coverage decisions.

- **Technology purchasers demand cost-effectiveness studies from technology vendors.** Whether health plans or providers, the purchasers of new technologies can insist on seeing a cost-effectiveness or cost-benefit analysis before they will even consider acquiring or adopting them. Such studies could become a mandatory component of the marketing package for medical technology.

- **Technology purchasers broadcast their desire for technologies that reduce overall costs.** Implicit in the request by purchasers for cost-effectiveness studies would be their preference for cost-saving technologies. This preference could be made explicit and emphatic.

- **Health care plans engage in aggressive education of both patients and providers, particularly physicians, on the appropriate use of medical technology.** Even with the timely conduct of technology assessments that incorporate cost-effectiveness or cost-benefit analyses and the translation of the results into practice guidelines, work needs to be done to change the attitudes of both the consumers (i.e., patients) and providers (i.e., physicians) of medical technology. This best will be accomplished through a combination of education and incentives. It will take some time.

- **Use several of these measures to limit the development of certain technologies while they are still in the pipeline.** This would involve using early-stage cost-benefit studies to set priorities for the development and distribution of technologies. The sooner in the new technology R&D process that restraints can be applied that might result in a project's termination, the better for all involved. The research funder, whether a public or private entity, does not waste money, and the researchers do not waste time and effort, on a technology with little prospect of implementation.

- **More thoughtfully distribute large, costly technologies around the country according to population and epidemiologic characteristics.** More centralized planning techniques would take into account population densities and distribution, as well as the specific disease treatment needs, in deciding the right number and geographic location of new technologies to deploy.

---

[27] Moloney, T.W., and D.E. Rogers. 1979. "Medical Technology – A Different View of the Contentious Debate over Costs". *New England Journal of Medicine* 301 (26): 1413–19.

- **More aggressively identify and eliminate the use of technologies that have lost, or never had, clinical value.** Additional cost savings would be realized by the withdrawal from usage of older technologies made obsolete by post-introduction tests showing their cost or clinical inadequacies or by newer replacement technologies.

- **Generally refine the science of technology assessment and expand its use.** This would be accomplished in several ways: develop and reach consensus on standards for measuring key technology characteristics, initiate collaboration among assessment institutions in carrying out the analyses, generate and disseminate good, timely data on emerging technologies, and broaden training and expertise in conducting technology assessments.[28]

10. Near-Term Trends in Medical Technology Diffusion

A good number of those proposals are likely to be implemented over the next decade, though it is hard to predict which ones. There are a few trends that seem virtual certainties.

- "Appropriate" technology applications encapsulated in medical practice guidelines. More and more of the practice of medicine is being taken over by practice guidelines. They make good sense, when properly researched and prepared, and physicians are becoming more comfortable with them. If anything, it will be easier to write and disseminate a practice guideline for a new technology whose efficacy has just been studied.

- Payors for health care services will start paying serious attention to cost-effectiveness or benefit criteria in deciding which new medical technologies to cover. As these methodologies become more accurate and reliable, assessment of the cost implications will become commonplace in all decisions to add, continue, or drop medical technologies.

- Patients being made more fiscally responsible for the health care, including medical technology, that they demand and consume. The hot new trend in combating overall health care cost inflation is consumer-driven health care. As it becomes more widespread, it will result in patients being much more cost-conscious than they have been in the past. They will scrutinize more closely recommendations that they receive expensive new high technology medical treatments.

- Technology assessment to be performed by fewer less self-interested entities, using national standards. There is likely to be a strong push to create a smaller number of more professional and objective assessment organizations employing more sophisticated methodologies that produce more commonly accepted results. Prospective technology buyers will turn to these organizations for guidance in their purchase decisions.

- Growing general emphasis on "value" (balance of cost and effectiveness) by health care payors (public agencies, health plans, and employers). Although the dialogue on health care still focuses largely on cost concerns, the flood of data in the last few years about quality deficiencies is leading steadily to a more balanced discussion about the kinds of health care services that deliver the greatest overall value. This thinking will certainly be applied to new medical technologies.

---

[28] Luce, B.R., and R.E. Brown. 1995. "The Use of Technology Assessment by Hospitals, HMOs, and Third Party Payers in the U.S." *International Journal of Technology Assessment in Health Care* 11 (1): 79–92.

11. Recommendations for Researchers, Developers, Vendors, and Purchasers of New Medical Technology

In light of the likely and possible changes in the ways that new medical technology is evaluated for approval, coverage, and implementation, there are several steps that savvy technology developers and manufacturers should take.

- When embarking on a new course of research likely to culminate in a marketable medical product, be sure that you are familiar with the legal and administrative hurdles that must be passed, ranging from FDA approval and technology assessment by an industry association or private assessment firm, to the coverage decision by health plans.
- When contemplating several new courses of biomedical research, research the specific expressed needs of health plans, providers, and patient advocacy groups. Perhaps interview or survey them directly. Enhance the likelihood that there will be a market waiting for the new technology when it emerges. As a general rule, lean toward technologies that save costs when implemented.
- Become familiar with cost-effectiveness analysis methodologies and follow their development as they become more sophisticated. When the final configuration and characteristics of the technology being researched become clear, perform on it the kind of analyses that assessment agencies and ultimate purchasers are likely to use. Compare the analysis results with the standards used by those agencies and purchasers. Be prepared to halt development of the technology if it appears that it will not meet the requirements – efficacy, safety, cost-effectiveness – of potential buyers.
- It has been possible, to some degree, to drive the demand for a new medical technology through marketing or promotional efforts. This will become a less viable strategy as purchasers and insurers more rigorously and objectively evaluate their technology purchase decisions.
- There is a good chance that the flows of money for development of different areas of medical technology will shift. Track those changes and try to synchronize R&D efforts accordingly. There is no point in pursuing research that may lose funding.
- Learn about the decision-making procedures and criteria of key medical technology constituents – whether funders, investors, assessors, or buyers. Aim to meet their needs.

The environment for medical technology in the U.S. is evolving rapidly, and becoming somewhat less hospitable. The researchers, developers, and manufacturers that succeed over the next several years will be those that anticipate the coming changes and prepare for them.

Future of Intelligent and Extelligent Health Environment
R.G. Bushko (Ed.)
IOS Press, 2005

Innovation in Telehealth and a Role for the Government[1,2]

Richard N. SPIVACK, Ph.D.[3]
Economist, Economic Assessment Office of the Advanced Technology Program,
National Institute of Standards and Technology, US Department of Commerce

Abstract. The convergence of information technology and telecommunications, including Internet technologies, is emerging as a key tool to drive increased efficiency and effectiveness in health systems worldwide. With part of its roots in medical research for military and space applications, telemedicine is expected to make it possible to link medical expertise with patients in the most distant locations-providing clinicians with valuable new tools for remote monitoring, diagnosis, and intervention.[4]

1. Introduction

A 1997 Kaiser Permanente study of telehealth concluded that "technology in healthcare can be an asset for patients and providers and has the potential to save costs; therefore, this technology must be a part of continuous planning for quality improvement."[5]

Innovation in healthcare technologies can contribute to increased access to and improved quality of care, reduced costs, and better national security. With healthcare expenditures of over $1.5 trillion accounting for 13 percent of U.S. GDP in 2002,[6] even incremental improvements in delivery can have a significant economic impact. Although telehealth technologies currently account for a small segment of all healthcare technologies (an estimated $380 million out of $71 billion nationwide and $169 billion globally), innovation in this area could spur significant improvements in sector productivity and quality of life.[7]

---

[1] I am indebted to the following people for editorial support, Lorel Wisniewski, Stephanie Shipp and Connie Chang.

[2] This chapter is based on the following report prepared for the U.S. Department of Commerce. "Innovation, Demand and Investment in Telehealth," by David Brantley, Karen Laney-Cummings, and Richard Spivack. The full report is available at: http://www.technology.gov/reports/TechPolicy/Telehealth/2004Contents.

[3] Richard Spivack is an economist in the Advanced Technology Program's (ATP) Economic Assessment Office, which focuses on evaluating the long term results of ATP funding. Richard's research focuses on examining ATP's Health Care Information Technologies which has resulted in his publication of several articles on the topic of telehealth.

[4] "Technology Forecast" from *Medical Device Link*, at http://www.devicelink.com/mddi/archive/00/01/012.html.

[5] Barbara Johnston, *RN, MSNM&L;* Linda Wheeler, *RN, MSNM&L;* Jill Deuser, *RN, MBA;* Karen H. Sousa, *RN, PhD* "Outcomes of the Kaiser Permanente Tele-Home Health Research Project" from the *Archives of Family Medicine,* January 2000. View the 1997 study at: http://archfami.ama-assn.org/issues/v9n1/ffull/foc8072.html#a4.

[6] "U.S. Statistics in Brief," *Statistical Abstract of the United States 2003*, U.S. Commerce Department.

[7] Table A-2, "Health Insurance Coverage Status and Type of Coverage by Selected Characteristics: 2000," U.S. Censure Bureau, can be viewed at: http://www.census.gov/prod/2001pubs/p60-215.pdf.

Today, after more than 30 years since the introduction of telehealth, that potential still has not been fully realized. This Chapter assesses telehealth technology and research and identifies barriers to innovation that have impeded its potential and identifies a role for the government.

2. Telehealth Technologies

Telehealth focuses on the transfer of basic patient information over networks and the diagnosis, treatment, monitoring, and education of patients using systems that allow access to expert advice and patient information. A technical definition of telehealth technology includes devices and software that enable healthcare providers and educators to diagnose, consult with, monitor, treat and educate patients and consumers remotely. In order for the devices and software to be effective, however, it is necessary to integrate technology with healthcare applications and clinical procedures. The integration of devices and applications with clinical processes must then be integrated with provider workflow or protocols that would add value to a network of providers and patients. This innovation continuum may be characterized as a five stage process:

Need identified	=>	Applications developed	=>	Devices developed	=>	Integration with clinical protocols	=>	Programs developed

Effective functioning requires proper infrastructure including the physical facilities, setup, and equipment used to capture, transmit, store, process, and display voice, data, and images. Examples of infrastructure devices and systems required to support telehealth include:[8]

- "Capture" devices such as digital and video cameras, radiographs (e.g. x-ray images), and physiologic monitors (e.g. EKGs, oxygen saturation monitors);
- Basic telecommunications and networking of computer systems;
- Communications software, including electronic mail and browsers for the World Wide Web, and forms of telecommunications, including videoconferencing, remote data monitoring and file transfer, applicable to medical care in remote or rural areas; and
- Electronic data storage facilities (e.g. disk arrays to store patient records and/or digital images).

Current telehealth technologies can be grouped into nine broad categories which include remote monitoring, diagnostics, video conferencing, digital imaging, information technologies (IT), networking/interfaces, robotics/remote controls, store-and-forward, simulation and training. Table 1 presents examples of devices and software and applications representative of organizations that are active in each of these areas.

The telehealth technologies in Table 1 may be classified according to the point in time when the encounter is transacted: *store-and-forward* (asynchronous) and *interactive* (synchronous). *Store-and-forward* technology is a lower-cost method of transmitting images by computer; currently this technology is most frequently used for transmitting radiological and dermatological pictures, and is employed by hospitals and clinics across the country. Store-and-forward technology allows the provider to perform a procedure, store the material, notes, etc. for a later use, or forward this material to another location for further activ-

---

[8] Guler, Nihal Fatma and Elif Derya Ubeyli. "Theory and Applications of Telemedicine." *Journal of Medical Systems*, vol. 26, No. 3, June 2002. p. 202.

Table 1. Current Telehealth Technologies.

Technology	Examples of Devices and Software	Examples of Applications	Innovators
Remote Monitoring	Sensors Instruments Ultrasound	Bio-defense Telehomecare	Laboratories Sensor manufacturers Telemedicine centers Military/Veterans Adminstration
Diagnostics	Otoscope Stethoscope EKG	Consultations Telehomecare	Medical device manufacturers
Video-conferencing	Cameras (Videocams, Webcams) Computer-based desktops Portable communications and data systems	Consultations Teledermatology Telementalhealth	Videoconferencing manufacturers
Digital imaging	Instruments Media (e.g. film, magnetic tape) Scanners/Viewers Digital cameras Videocams with scopes	Telepathology Teleradiology Teledentistry Teledermatology TeleENT, TeleGI	Laboratories Instrument manufacturers Media manufacturers
IT	Data storage systems Servers Software/Informatics/ Middleware	Electronic medical record Data mining Syndromic surveillance Web portals Decision-support systems Administration	IT manufacturers Systems integrators Software developers Database developers Webmasters
Networking/ Interfaces	Hubs, routers, servers "Black boxes" System software	Interoperability Internet/intranet Hub and spoke networks Mobile data transmission	IT/telecom manufacturers System integrators
Robotics/Remote Controls	Instruments Controls Viewers	Telesurgery Telepathology Homeland security	Instrument manufacturers Control manufacturers Defense Advanced Research Projects Agency (DARPA)
Store-and-Forward	Data/image/video/audio card capture/scanners Computer/camera/microphone & image management software	Electronic medical record Report generator	Card capture manufacturers Scanner manufacturers Software developers
Simulation and Training	Multi-media graphics Software Audio-visual	eLearning Curriculum Conferencing	Multimedia firms Software developers

ity. *Interactive* telehealth implies face-to-face interaction with a patient, health professional, or both, and requires some combination of audio, full-motion video, and still images. Although these categories are sometimes used in conjunction with one another, store-and-forward technologies are more widely used due to lower start-up and sustainability costs, and increased flexibility and productivity in scheduling encounters and managing workload.

Leaders in the field of telemedicine/telehealth suggest that the current state of technology is moving from its second generation into its third.[9] The "*first generation*" can be traced as far back as the 1950s. "One of the earliest uses was at the University of Nebraska where psychiatric consultations were conducted on two-way closed-circuit TV using microwave technologies."[10] The *second generation* might be dated from 1989, when then Secretary Bowen of the Department of Health and Human Services (HHS) directed the Health

---

[9] A generation is defined as a period of time in which stakeholder interests and technological development are at a similar stage. A generation changes when breakthroughs occur in technologies and innovation moves quickly to a different level.

[10] For more history of telehealth, see Telecommunications for Nurses, *2nd Edition*, Armstrong and Frueh (editors), "An Overview of Telemedicine: Through the Looking Glass," (D.S. Puskin), Springer Publishing, 2003.

Resources Services Administration (HRSA) and the Centers for Medicare and Medicaid Services (CMS)[11] to fund a telemedicine project called "the MedNet Project" (now Health-Net) at Texas Tech University. Until then, telehealth was limited to a few medical specialties such as radiology and focused on either store-and-forward or video conferencing applications. That first generation was characterized by specialized devices that did not interface easily with other devices and have not integrated well with clinical protocols. This lack of "interoperability" and technical know-how frequently led to user dissatisfaction and may have created a negative image of telehealth products and services within the traditional medical community.[12]

With the *second generation* of telehealth technologies, users demanded greater ability to integrate with legacy systems and peripheral devices, and manufacturers responded with multi-application systems. Successful first generation telehealth applications, such as monitoring, radiology and video consults, were joined by other specialty applications such as dermatology and pathology. Most first and second generation technologies were based in some way on remote monitoring, video conferencing, or digital imaging technologies.

At the beginning of the 21st century technological advances in videoconferencing and digital imaging are now well into a *third generation* of telehealth. Several factors account for the faster pace of innovation in these technologies and their attendant applications: the underlying technologies are multi-use, the broadcast infrastructure is stable, cost effectiveness is more evident, and their market is much broader than simply healthcare.[13]

3. Innovators and the Federal Role

Telehealth research since 1975 has included a mix of public and private sector R&D, clinical studies, and demonstration projects. Federal departments and agencies, state and local governments, universities, private foundations, manufacturers, insurers, and other sources provide varying amounts and forms of research funding. Technology and research efforts span a wide range of organizations and medical specialties, from military medical commands to rural clinics, from major medical centers to the needs of sparsely populated regions and territories. This diversity (and fragmentation) complicates quantitative analysis of R&D expenditures, as well as the collection of information about current and required R&D and technology transfer.

Public sector research and innovation are centered on applications (including software) and programs, but not devices. Federal civilian and state R&D is most often associated with "demonstration grants." Attempts have been made to quantify public investment in telehealth in the past, but have been largely unsuccessful because agencies are not required to either collect or report on their telehealth investments. Although data are not easily identifiable, it is estimated that, in FY2001, federal agencies spent at least $332 million for military and civilian telehealth research and programs. That amount grew in FY2003 as recent legislation included funding for telehealth infrastructure, programs, and projects, and, because of telehealth's potential role in homeland security, as homeland security research, program development, and procurement were funded.

Table 2 summarizes federal funding for telehealth initiatives by federal agency for FY 2000–2001. Over eighteen agencies or bureaus were involved in telehealth initiatives during

---

[11] Formerly the Health Care Financing Administration.

[12] Mark Newburger, CEO of Apollo Telemedicine and a panelist at the U.S. Department of Commerce Technology Administration's Roundtable discussion "Innovation, Demand and Investment in Telehealth," June 19, 2002 in Washington D.C.

[13] Many technologies have found their way into healthcare from a variety of business backgrounds, e.g., inventory tracking technologies are also useful in tracking patient records as well as a patient's lab results.

Table 2. Federal Telehealth Research Funding (FY2000–01).

Department	Agency or Bureau	Nature of Research or Program	Nature of Technologies	FY2000 Funding $million	FY2001 Funding $million
Agriculture	Rural Utilities Service	Program grants	Distance learning and telemedicine	25	25
Commerce	National Telecommunications and Information Administration (NTIA)	Demo Projects	Network Infrastructure	15.5	15.5
	NIST Advanced Technology Program (ATP)	High-risk, enabling technology development and commercialization	All technologies	3	3
Defense	Defense Research Projects Administration (DARPA)	Applied	All technologies	<1	<1
	Telemedicine and Advanced Technology Research Center (TATRC)	Applied	Remote access, warfighter	100	100
	Army Medical Department (AMEDD)	Applied	Web-based triage	3.1	3.6
	Navy	Applied	Shipboard applications	*	20
	Air Force	Applied	Several	*	11.5
Energy	Sandia	Applied	Robotics	*	*
	Sandia	Applied	Diagnostic devices	*	*
	Oak Ridge	Applied	Sensors	*	*
	Oak Ridge	Pure	Sensors	*	*
U.S. Department of Health and Human Services	Agency for Health Research and Quality (AHRQ)	Evaluation	***	*	*
	Health Resources and Services Adminstration (HRSA)-Office for the Advancement of Telehealth (OAT)	Demo Projects[14]	***	34.5	34.7
	HRSA-Office of Rural Health Policy (ORHP)	Demonstration projects	AHEC, Community Health Centers, Rural development	*	13
	Center for Medicare & Medicaid Services (CMS)	Demo Project	***	6	6[15]
	U.S. Food & Drug Administration (FDA)	Demo Projects	***	*	*
	National Institutes of Health (NIH) National Library of Medicine (NLM) National Institute for Biomedical Imagining & Bioengineering (NIBIB)**	Applied Demo projects	Next generation Internet	45	45
Justice	Bureau of Prisons	Clinical	Consultations Cost-benefit	*	*
National Aeronautics and Space Administration (NASA)	Various	Pure Applied	Remote monitoring	10	10
Veterans Administration (VA)	Various	Applications Clinical	Ongoing programs Efficacy Studies	45	45
Federal Communications Commission (FCC)	Universal Service Administrative Company (USAC)	Subsidies	ERate	*	18
* Funding amounts not available ** Began telehealth initiatives in FY2003 *** No particular names have been chosen			TOTAL	287	332

[14] These figures are the latest amounts available and include Congressional earmarks.

[15] Amounts for the Center for Medicare & Medicaid Services represent one year of a five-year, $30 million demonstration grant managed by Columbia Presbyterian.

this period. The Defense Department and HHS receive the greatest share of the funding as the U.S. Army possesses the world's largest telehealth research program, and the U.S. Public Health Service is the largest in the world and comprises a significant part of the HHS budget.

The Department of Veterans Affairs (VA) operates the nation's largest civilian telehealth program, conducting more than three hundred thousand teleconsultations annually. Like the Department of Defense, the VA is considered a "closed system" that includes patients, providers and payers, and is not significantly affected by the need to annually compete for grant funding. Therefore, it offers the size and stability necessary to provide one of the best available "testbeds" for research, development, standards, clinical efficacy and cost-benefit studies, and needs assessment. The VA is also considered unique among telehealth programs because of its leadership in taking on the role of "early adopter" of healthcare technologies, and in its being adequately funded to procure and integrate telehealth with clinical medicine on a very broad scale.

Most states and some local governments fund telehealth research, programs and procurement, generally with the goal of supporting program infrastructure, project development, or feasibility studies. A number of states have developed statewide public and private strategies for increasing access to quality healthcare through telehealth technologies. In several cases, states have organized "taskforces" responsible for assessing needs and factors affecting telehealth adoption and deployment.

4. Identifying Technologies

It was not until the National Research Council and Institute of Medicine issued "Crossing the Quality Chasm: A New Health System for the 21st Century"[16] that the concept of a national health information infrastructure began to acquire traction. The Council's report was followed by "Information for Health: A Strategy for Building a National Health Information Infrastructure (NHII)" by the National Committee on Vital and Health Statistics.[17] In June 2003, HHS convened a conference that brought together representatives from all stakeholders to develop a consensus for a national action agenda, which was then published and widely disseminated, and offered as a guide to the further development of NHII.[18]

Consideration of such an infrastructure would include the converging technologies of telehealth, healthcare informatics, and eHealth as well as other healthcare devices and applications. The nation's interstate highway system, banking (ATM and credit card) network, and Internet are good examples of current national infrastructures, and may, in fact, provide models for national health infrastructure development.

With a few exceptions, little effort or coordination has yet been directed toward the "front end" identification of research, clinical healthcare or homeland security requirements for telehealth. This is not unexpected, however, since the focus of healthcare is healing and not technology. The healthcare industry is largely disaggregated, and providers focus on their own services and patients rather than on national needs or priorities. Issues such as reimbursement and the availability of clinical studies would facilitate provider's decisions

---

[16] "Crossing the Quality Chasm: A New Health System for the 21st Century," Committee on Quality Health Care in America, 2001, Washington D.C., National Academy Press.

[17] "Information for Health: A Strategy for Building a National Health Information Infrastructure (NHII)" by the National Committee on Vital and Health Statistics. U.S. Department of Health and Human Services. Washington, D.C. November 2001.

[18] For more information on "Developing a National Action Agenda for NHII" see: http://www.nhii-03.s-3.net/welcome.htm.

regarding technology needs. In addition, increased attention to homeland security has underscored a need supported by President Bush that the technology be multi-use.[19]

The events of September 11, 2001 reinforce the concept that telehealth technology must meet the primary requirements of being both multi-use and interoperable. To accomplish these requirements most effectively and efficiently, homeland security and clinical healthcare needs must be integrated at every possible level, locally, regionally and nationally. As a first step a needs assessment process will not only identify current "gaps," but will also identify technology and information needs not currently being addressed and which require additional effort and/or investment in research, development, testing, and evaluation.

Some activities that would contribute to telehealth needs assessment are currently under way. The National Library of Medicine, for example, evaluates commercial telehealth, informatics and eHealth products. The Office for the Advancement of Telehealth (OAT) of HHS requires its grantees to meet periodically to discuss lessons learned, and uses the proposal process as a method of assessing technology needs. It has also developed guidance for strategic planning, technical guidelines for purchasing equipment for specific telehealth applications, and is currently developing a series of technical assistance documents for its grantees to guide them in assessing needs.

Early efforts to develop a national health technology and information infrastructure include the Information Infrastructure for Healthcare (1994–1997) of the U.S. Department of Commerce National Institute of Standards and Technology Advanced Technology Program (ATP). The Information Infrastructure for Healthcare was an ATP focused program that provided funding for infrastructural technology development to enable enterprise-wide integration of information among all sectors of the healthcare industry. Of 221 proposals submitted under three competitions to this program, 32 multi-year awards were made to 79 participants, totaling $295 million in R&D funding ($146 million from ATP, and $149 million from industry). Funded projects included informatics tools to automate, validate, and distribute clinical best practice guidelines for an array of medical situations for practitioner use; tools to enable community-wide, computerized information sharing of multi-media information across local area and wide-area networks; and an interoperable, open-system architecture to connect independent, and often legacy, healthcare information systems.[20]

A number of technologies from the focused program have found their way into the market place. Several Harvard affiliated hospitals have adopted *Baby Care Link*, a technology that enables parents to view patient information about their children from remote locations, and *Care Web*, a collection of web sites offering healthcare advice and direction to people of all ages. In another project the Connecticut Hospital Association (CHA) was initially approached by a healthcare research joint venture for their services in providing needed data. The data were provided and the CHA went on to develop a for-profit division, Chime, to pursue further development of necessary information technologies for the telehealth industry. Chime-Net, a subsidiary of Chime, has established a strategic alliance with Passport Health Communications Inc. of Nashville, Tenn., to provide electronic-based insurance eligibility, benefit coverage, claim status, and address verification transactions to Connecticut healthcare providers through their private data network.[21]

ATP has continued to fund projects in telehealth since the conclusion of the focused program in healthcare information infrastructure. Seven additional projects from open com-

---

[19] Phil Bond, Under Secretary for Technology United States Department of Commerce, address to the American Telemedicine Association conference, Orlando, FL., April 2003.

[20] For more information, see Bettijoyce Lide and Richard N. Spivack, "Advanced Technology Program Information Infrastructure for Healthcare Focused Program: A Brief History," (NISTIR 6477), February 2000.

[21] For more information on the many telehealth services offered by the Connecticut Hospital Association please refer to <http://www.chime.org/>.

petitions totaling $27 million in which industry has contributed $14 million, continues ATP's involvement in this area. Examples of recent ATP awards in telehealth include:

- the combination of surgical robotic systems with telemedicine to allow a mentoring surgeon to physically interact with an in-training surgeon from a remote location and guide the in-training surgeon through complex minimally invasive surgical procedures;
- development of a software architecture for physicians and researchers that automatically extracts patient data from electronic medical records and generates a list of patient problems, and displays information in ways that support diagnostic and therapeutic decision making;
- development of a wallet-sized, wireless server for America's mobile workforce that will provide medical personnel with secure, instant access to all e-mail and automatically updated data files, everywhere.[22]

5. Homeland Security and the Role of Telehealth

A major activity of the Department of Homeland Security's Office of Science and Technology is coordinating research, development, science and technology activities among multiple agencies, and identifying homeland security research, science, and technology requirements. Interagency teams tasked with evaluating federal needs for homeland security infrastructure have been convened in several critical areas, but not, as yet, for healthcare. It is important that any consolidation of healthcare technology requirements for homeland security be integrated considering other private and public stakeholders, including such research organizations as the Army's Telemedicine and Advanced Technology Research Center (TATRC). Cooperation among users in requirements definition as well as research and development could well result in multi-use breakthrough innovations for homeland security, public health and clinical healthcare technologies.

Telehealth technologies offer the opportunity to not only augment the "first response level" but also empower successive levels of authority in crafting an overall response network. Such a network would require: 1) updated, open-platform systems; 2) high-speed networks; 3) workstations; 4) industry-standard applications; 5) standardized nomenclatures and taxonomies; 6) data security tools and protocols; and 7) computer-based patient records.[23] While each of these requirements is being addressed in some fashion by researchers and federal organizations, there has been little coordination with each other or within the telehealth community.

Homeland security technology needs include sensors and surveillance devices, related information systems for syndromic surveillance, and alert capabilities. One of the leading examples is the Real-time Outbreak and Disease Surveillance (RODS) system developed by the University of Pittsburgh's Center for Biomedical Informatics and funded by the National Library of Medicine, the Agency for Healthcare Research and Quality (AHRQ), the Centers for Disease Control and Prevention (CDC), and the Defense Advanced Research Project Agency (DARPA). RODS is essentially a proven telehealth technology that could be used as the basic platform supporting national Chemical, Biological, Radiological and Nuclear Resource Links (CBRN/E) development programs.

---

[22] For a more complete description of these technologies as well as others funded in the ATP go to <www.atp.nist.gov>.

[23] Simpson, Roy L. "Our First Line of Defense Against Bioterrorism." *Nursing Management* 2002 May 33(5): 10–13. p. 12.

Of the total 736 projects awarded to high risk, enabling projects from 1990 through May 2004, the National Institute of Standards and Technology's Advanced Technology Program (ATP) has provided $290 million in cost-shared funding to 106 projects for research and development of important technologies with direct application to Homeland Security. ATP projects in the area of Homeland Security include:

- an automated security surveillance system that combines closed circuit video cameras, radio-frequency identification technology, and computer modeling and analysis of human behaviors, with the aim of achieving rapid, reliable detection of suspicious events warranting the attention of security personnel;
- a large-area digital X-ray inspection system with heretofore-unavailable accuracy for near error-free screening of cargo and sealed container freight at airports, seaports, and other points of entry;
- a system to guarantee telephone call delivery and dial tone in order to maintain telecommunications continuity during and following terror attack, natural disaster, equipment failure, or human error.[24]

Beyond surveillance and detection, other areas of focus for innovation and adoption related to development of a technology infrastructure for homeland security include telecommunications, information, and training networks which link providers and institutions. Deploying these technologies and programs, and providing training to the nation's public health providers to meet their new homeland security responsibilities, present both financial challenges and opportunities to increase access to quality healthcare for medically underserved areas. Linking sensors to central receivers or monitors and linking those facilities, in turn, to centralized databases requires telecommunications infrastructure that does not exist in much of the nation's rural and remote areas. Although wireless communications may provide a partial answer (Oak Ridge Laboratory's "Sensor Net" uses wireless telephony, although over a relatively limited area), most sensor research and development has yet to address interfaces or integration with public health systems.

6. Standards Requirements

The integration of technology with medicine may be the single greatest current research need for the telehealth community.[25]

Increasing the interoperability of devices and the integration of telehealth with clinical medicine and other healthcare technologies is a near term focus of telehealth innovation. Standards are a means by which interoperability is achieved. Interoperability is the ability of two or more systems to interact with one another and exchange information in order to achieve predictable results. Innovations in this area include the integration of networks with programs, of devices with applications, of applications with clinical protocols, and of technologies with business processes. For telehealth to improve productivity, increase quality and reduce costs, the following three levels of interoperability are needed:[26]

- Interactions among stations or applications developed by independent vendors;
- Connectivity among medical devices and other "peripherals" developed by independent vendors; and

---

[24] For a more complete description of these technologies as well as others funded in the ATP go to <www.atp.nist.gov>.

[25] Jon Linkous, Executive Director, American Telemedicine Association, September 2002.

[26] Col. Ron Porapatich's address at the American Telemedicine Association conference, Los Angeles, CA., December 2002.

- "Plug and play" components developed by multiple vendors for independent vendors.

The use of open standards and wide publication will facilitate interoperability, eventually enabling most applications to link back to electronic clinical patient record databases.

Problems associated with interoperability are due in large part to the fragmented nature of telehealth, many participants each having different requirements or solutions and each applying different technical standards. The healthcare industry is not unique in having multiple standards that are developed by various organizations. Other organizations face similar situations and challenges with respect to electronic business specifications. Healthcare is unique, however, in the diversity of standards such as: infrastructure standards, clinical information standards, and business information standards, as well as standards within each medical discipline, only some of which are comparable. Healthcare is also unique in that, due to the number and diversity of providers and technology suppliers, interoperability is significantly more challenging.

Some vendors' telehealth systems are similar enough that physicians need not be fully retrained when they move to a new delivery system or combine services with another provider. But the lack of compatibility among many homegrown systems has limited just how far many telehealth services can extend. On a national level, compatibility is essential to constructing a larger infrastructure of healthcare service. The National Institute of Standards and Technology (NIST) works with industry, research, and government organizations to make emerging information technologies, including telehealth technologies, more usable, more secure, more scalable, and more interoperable. NIST has identified healthcare as a "strategic focus area" and is working with private organizations to assist in the development of standards. Through NIST developed tests, test methods, measurements and related material, both the implementers and the users of telehealth technologies can objectively measure, compare and improve their systems.

Faster connection and transmission speeds have increased the capabilities of telehealth applications overall, but without standards (or the ability to integrate patient information among various internal or external systems) many telehealth services cannot be performed within or across delivery systems. Standards form the building blocks of effective health information systems and are essential for efficient and effective public health and healthcare delivery systems.

Adoption of standards that make it easier for telehealth systems to interoperate with other hospital information systems and easier to integrate technology with routine care should encourage physicians to adopt telehealth applications. Without standards that make telehealth technologies easier to use or that enable interoperability among disparate systems, physicians are unlikely to embrace advancements in telehealth applications.[27]

7. The Future for Telehealth

As the need for providers to transmit data increases, the need for higher speed and higher capacity telecommunications such as broadband becomes as important as securing additional resources for further research and development. Speed and capacity are but two areas of need for an industry that is still in its infancy. In the case of broadband technologies, advantages for the Internet and voice-over-internet applications include the "always on" feature required for store and forward applications. Higher capacity bandwidth is also important for accuracy and clarity in digital imaging applications such as teleradiology, teledermatology and pathology.

---

[27] Kelly, Becky. "Telemedicine Begins to Make Progress." *Health Data Management*, Jan. 2002, p. 76.

Inadequate private sector resources have led to a number of "public-private partnerships" for research, development, testing and promotion of products. As discussed earlier, the Army's Telemedicine and Advanced Technology Research Center conducts much of its research with private sector "partners" and the Advanced Technology Program makes awards to companies to develop telehealth technologies deemed too high-risk for private sector investment. These arrangements increase the probability that the technologies will be commercialized. In the case of the Advanced Technology Program, the emphasis is on both the acceleration of technology and the commercialization of enabling technologies leading to national economic benefits.

Government already plays a role in developing and delivering telehealth services as well as offering assistance in standards development. In some cases the role is that of investor in R&D where the private sector may consider the investment technically "too risky". In other cases telehealth is used as an adjunct to regular health services. Support in standards development, guaranteeing that standards are complete, unambiguous and testable, is crucial to an industry that needs further development of interoperable technologies.

The very existence of so many government telehealth programs is reflective of the industry itself, in that there are a number of providers operating on, in some cases, incompatible systems. In order to improve upon existing technologies and develop new ones, there is a need to continuously innovate and develop. In this instance public-private partnerships make sense. Development of a national health technology and information infrastructure requires the resources of both the private and the public sectors. The power of telecommunications can contribute significantly to an industry that is seeking to improve quality while at the same time contain costs. A more effective manner of delivering healthcare services is needed in order to respond to national emergencies in a manner that meets the expectations of the American people. Telehealth offers these opportunities. Due to the early stage of development of telehealth and the extent of disaggregation in the industry there is a need for a public partner.

Note

Certain commercial equipment, instruments, or materials are identified in this paper in order to specify the experimental procedure adequately. Such identification is not intended to imply recommendation or endorsement by the National Institute of Standards and Technology, nor is it intended to imply that the materials or equipment identified are necessarily the best available for the purpose.

Future of Intelligent and Extelligent Health Environment
R.G. Bushko (Ed.)
IOS Press, 2005

43

Present and Future Challenges in Medical Data Management: Economics, Ethics, and the Law

Salil H. PATEL
Johns Hopkins School of Medicine
Departments of Urology and Radiology
The Johns Hopkins Hospital, Baltimore, MD, USA

Abstract. Electronically-linked knowledge plays an increasingly central role in the delivery of health services worldwide. Medical data collection, archival, and analysis are all increasing in both rate and volume; large, cohesive collections of personal health information are emerging rapidly. Factors driving this integration include value-added methods of diagnosis and therapy, interest in evidence-based practices, safety concerns, and increased consumer demand for personalized, comprehensive medical services. Practitioners, businesses, patients, and the public at large would be well-served to develop and sustain a dialogue addressing these phenomena, including assessments their of economic, ethical, legal implications.

1. Introduction

Since Watson and Crick's elucidation of the structure of DNA in 1953, a revolutionary tide has swept across the fields of biology and chemistry, profoundly affecting the practice of clinical medical care. The era of the 1990's marked the inception of a second major shift in the practice of medicine: the informatics wave. Seminal developments in the domains of data collection, manipulation, and distribution have potentiated the spread of novel modalities for practice, treatment, and payment. Concomitantly, the pervasive adoption of an Internet infrastructure, underpinned by a host of standardized open protocols (e.g., TCP/IP, SSL, DICOM, and VPN), served as a means for convergence of these technologies. *Electronic medicine* generates economic activity on the order of hundreds of millions each year, at levels ranging from individual private practices to comprehensive provider networks. According to the 2002 American Medical Association Study on Physicians' Use of the World Wide Web, nearly 80% of American physicians use the Web as part of their practice. One-third of surveyed doctors are affiliated with a website for promotional or public-education purposes. The era of information has indeed altered the behaviors of individual consumers of medical goods and services, with nearly one-half of all adults in America using the Web as a source of healthcare information [1]. On larger scales, companies such as Healtheon have already begun to offer commercial solutions for patient data, prescription, and claims management [2]. The implementation of electronic patient record systems such as Siemens SIENET's MagicWeb, which claims a user-base of 25,000 clinicians, has increased the degree of enterprise-wide data aggregation and communication among care providers, diagnostic facilities, and insurers. Greater centralization of health information in databases, according to industry commentator Lawrence Gostin, is "already under way" and carries with it "an aura of inevitability." Although a monolithic, cross-industry and nationwide system might maximize the level of aggregation, it is perhaps more feasible that existing databases and information streams will interoperate by leveraging the current reach of open standards and Internet technologies. In light of these dramatic changes, it is possible to envision that the storage and manipulation of personal data such as medical histories, genetic profiles, and treatment delivery in novel paradigms, facilitated by information technology, may occur within a comprehensive electronic network established within our lifetimes. Such integration must proceed with careful consideration of issues such as economics, public health, and civil rights.

2. Economic Considerations

Linked information technology systems potentially bear a major impact upon the medical field in the realm of costs. Although the initial adoption of any new system entails some investment, in the long term, the savings to the health care system over a prolonged deployment period may be significant. In terms of startup expenditures, the major areas for investment will include software and hardware development and installation, as well as the creation of a robust services model to exploit fully the capabilities of the new system. The latter may entail changes in medical and consumer education methods, as well as training of *librarians* and *data custodians* to assist in data manipulation and storage. As Jones, *et al.* note, "Services are the most important factor in meeting organizational needs for knowledge-based information" [3]. The advantage of this early investment is a large projected return in terms of economic efficiency and effectiveness.

Inefficiencies in administration may be reduced through improved consistency in billing and data transfer practices. Such savings have already been demonstrated in the northeastern U.S., where the establishment of the New England Healthcare Electronic Data Interchange Network is currently reducing costs to care providers due to reduced administrative overhead and is forecasted to lead to annual savings on the order of 66 million dollars [4]. Furthermore, it is conceivable that an information-systems facilitated reduction in preventable medical errors, to be addressed shortly, and the employment of intelligent decision support systems may reduce exposure to malpractice suits, which have been partly responsible for dramatic increases in physician insurance premiums since 1999 [5]. In addition, the establishment of a "computerized decision support model" which analyzes care efficacy and alerts providers to treatment alternatives has been demonstrated empirically to reduce total expenditures and to decrease the length of hospital stays [6]. Even these models, however, must account for changes in the final "product" of quality of care delivered, as initial parameters of the treatment process are altered. Witness the enactment of an 80 hour workweek limitations for residents in accredited training programs at U.S. hospitals, a response to claims that fatigued residents are more likely to commit errors. One consequence of these regulations is that the care of a patient may be passed among several separate care teams within an initial span of 24–48 hours; the demands of multiple transfers of recent patient information may lead to altered content, granularity, and quality of these findings, and unintentionally compromised quality of care. Retrospective studies and randomized controlled trials are especially indicated in order to assess the response of the healthcare delivery system to such perturbations.

Tele-health services, involving remote diagnosis and supervision of care, may facilitate cost savings by increasing access and decreasing utilization of inpatient services [7]. The potential of using the nascent Internet II, with its high-bandwidth infrastructure, combined Quality of Service assurances and high network availability, for orthopaedic and cardiac telesurgery, promises to improve care efficiency even further [8]. Although cost-effectiveness for telemedicine has yet to be established [9], associated shifts in resource allocation may still improve overall efficiency of healthcare delivery in selected settings, such as rural areas [10] and public schools [11]. It has been proposed that a reimbursable-time or "billable hours" model, similar to that used by the legal profession, might be used to encourage physicians and allied health care professionals to incorporate electronic resources into busy clinical practices [12]. Finally, implications for cost reduction may reach across domestic borders and encourage developing countries to make use of a "leapfrog" model of healthcare development – *i.e.*, the directed and proactive integration of current information technology in nascent public health systems. This same leapfrogging process has already been demonstrated in the telephony sector in countries such as China, India, and the former Soviet Republics, where high-capacity wireless cellular services in some areas are being deployed in lieu of traditional land-lines [13]. Thus, cost savings issues may provide an impetus for the adoption of electronic medicine internationally.

3. Ensuring Public Health

The convergence of personal data and delivery systems presents myriad potential boons and challenges to the health of both the individual and population levels. Hospitals are already recognizing the utility of electronic systems for preventing iatrogenic injury [14], in domains ranging from drug dispensation, dosage errors, and interactions, to the prevention of idiosyncratic allergic reactions and dose-related toxicity. Online medical information empowers patients to become more informed and engaged in their treatment process, and may encourage utilization of preventative educational services. In fact, 95% of patients in a representative clinical study "strongly preferred" electronic education pre-operatively over the conventional physician-mediated consent process; this was attributed in part to reduced patient levels of anxiety and intimidation [15]. In the realm of prescription drugs, the World Wide Web is increasingly being used by pharmaceutical companies to provide marketing materials and prescription information directly to physicians and consumers. At the same time, independent organizations are releasing cost-effectiveness data and clinical practice guidelines as part of publicly-accessible therapeutics databases. Medical indices and journals are widely available online though public systems sponsored by the National Library of Medicine. Other types of medical data are now accessible to the public as well, including the release of physician malpractice and disciplinary records by state boards of certification, as well as morbidity and mortality results for practicing individuals, albeit in limited cases [16]. Electronic mail, bulletin boards, and directed broadcast systems may be vital facets of future coordinated responses of care providers during times of medical emergencies. Enthusiasm of such widespread dissemination of medical information must be tempered with caution, however. With the flood of drug data available online, the reports of "off-label" uses by patient group websites, and the increase in direct-to-consumer marketing, inefficient utilization patterns may quickly emerge [17]. Even more significantly, judicious audits have revealed a wide range in the accuracy and completeness of online databases, presenting the potential for public confusion and misinformation [18,19]. In response to these challenges, Stone, *et al.* suggest the following standards in particular for all websites which profile physicians: disclosure statements about data sources and compensation, explanations for blank or missing records, reports of database size and scope, and an indication of the timeliness of each data field [16].

In the domain of public health, informatics may play a key role in the evaluation of populations as well as the prevention and treatment of disease. For instance, under an electronic system liked to established health authorities, the dissemination of reportable disease information may become rapid, accurate, and automatic (privacy concerns notwithstanding). For instance, Dr. John Bartlett, chief of Division of Infectious Diseases at the Johns Hopkins School of Medicine, established an e-mail broadcast system in response to the anthrax attacks of October 2001, with an estimated 18 thousand subscribers to the service one year later. Commercially, Oracle Corp. is marketing its Lightweight Epidemiology Advanced Detection and Emergency Response System for centralized outbreak monitoring and coordinated resource allocation.

Clinical measures studies of large databases will allow for greater efficacy assessment across a wide population, help to identify dangerous interactions or reactions to prescription pharmaccuticals post-FDA-approval, and aid public hcalth planncrs in idcntifying populations with the greatest disease burden using objective and quantifiable metrics. The European Effective Health Care Bulletins and systematic reviews of the international Cochrane Collaboration, all available online, attempt to synthesize the current state of medical care and compare relative treatment efficacies in an attempt to promote evidence-based, cost-aware healthcare practices. In the U.S., the Federal Agency for Healthcare Research and Quality has sponsored studies correlating clinical practices and outcomes for several years [20], although current limitations in dataset size and structure still are significant. Variable granularity, or specificity of information fields, is a limiting characteristic of current records, making cross-datatype and cross-database comparisons difficult. Implementation of methods gleaned from the disciplines of knowledge engineering, complex systems, nonlinear analysis, biostatistics, and predictive analytics will all be necessary in order to fully exploit a large and accessible database of health measures and outcomes. Research teams at IBM [21] and SAS [22] have proposed a methodology grounded in these premises, termed Unstructured Data Mining, that may be particularly well-suited to the task of sifting through arrays of disparate patient datasets. In fact, many retail corporations already use data mining techniques in sales trends analysis and consumer profiling [23].

Regardless of the power of sampling methods, it is still a daunting task to extract information about poorly-characterized or multifactorial disease syndromes with the current predominance of relatively decentralized or disconnected independent patient records. One controversial solution to this problem has been pursued by deCODE Genetics, a private entity contracting with the government of Iceland. The company has managed to secure full and proprietary access to the health and family history of all Icelandic citizens [24]. In less than two years, the company has reportedly identified putative genes for susceptibility to complex conditions such as late-onset Parkinson's Disease, Alzheimer's Disease, Type II diabetes, and obesity [25,26]. The products of basic research, such as gene sequence and homology, as well as related clinical and pathophysiological data, are also correlated using open-access initiatives such as Online Mendelian Inheritance in Man.

4. Health Databases and Issues of Rights

4.1. Assessments of Personal Liberty

In addition to the above considerations, convergence of the Internet and medical practice has itself occurred at the nexus of practical implementation and the boundaries of civil liberties. Is privacy a moral imperative? Regardless, there are implicit constitutional protections, as outlined by the classical "penumbra" established within the U.S. Bill of Rights, which protect reasonable expectations of personal privacy; comments Supreme Court Justice William Brennan (1977):

"The central storage and easy accessibility of computerized data vastly increase the potential for abuse of that information, and I am not prepared to say that future development will not demonstrate the necessity of some curb on such technology." [27]

One unanswered and contentious issue cannot be ignored: who actually owns increasingly commoditized patient data? In most local jurisdictions, it is actually the creator of the record, not the patient, who has primacy over the use of database, although individual privacy rights in fact supercede authorship rights in selected instances [28]. When databases span states and even countries, which nations' laws apply and in what circumstances? When data becomes stripped of specific individual identifiers, dis-aggregated, completely de-identified, or compounded, at what point do individuals whose data is part of this new set abrogate their rights to the derivative work? Furthermore, in what circumstances does the government justify the appropriation of personal health data for the public interest? One may view tension between public health and individual autonomy as delineating the boundaries of personal liberty. The U.S. Supreme Court, in *Jacobson v. Massachusetts* (1905), ruled that mandatory vaccination is justified to protect public welfare, notes that "The Constitution of the United States... does not import an absolute right in each person to be, at all times and in all circumstances, wholly freed from restraint. There are manifold restraints to which every person is necessarily subject for the common good." These emerging issues, clearly beyond the scope of the federal Health Insurance Portability and Accountability Act of 1996 (HIPAA), will soon demand legislative attention and the establishment of common standards for privacy. In the case of deCODE Genetics, for instance, individuals may opt-out of the private database if desired, although the process is cumbersome [1]. In some countries, such as the Republic of Singapore, a system of unique medical identifiers is already in place nationwide.

I would like to propose the application of the assessment of the ethical validity of the use of personal data in research, using archetypical, universal, and simple criteria outlined such as those by Emanuel, Wendler, and Grady, summarized in Table 1 [29]. Adherence to models such as these should be given consideration as integral components of any comprehensive medical data management infrastructure.

4.2. Government and Corporations

To what extent may a republic exercise powers of "eminent domain" over public health data? Collated and mined datasets bear heightened utility in times of crisis such as a looming threat of bioterror. In such an environment, how is the appropriation of personal information justified? It may be useful to consider three concerns regarding decisions made by leadership bodies in times of crisis: first, such decisions, by necessity, are rapidly made; second, is the opportunity and danger of over-generalization; third, discrimination and judgment may defer to "herd mentality" and hysteria. The most natural counterbalance to each of these tendencies is strong policy, formulated well in advance of a crisis, that is both flexible and powerful, and granted legitimacy by support from both the government and the populace.

Table 1. Requirements for assessing the ethics of research on human subjects.

1	Social and scientific value of protocol
2	Scientific validity
3	Unbiased subject selection
4	Clear risk-to-benefit proposition
5	Independent review of protocol and reasoning
6	Informed consent of participants
7	Respect for autonomy and welfare of subjects

Emanuel, et al. (1999)

In addition, significant pitfalls emerge from the research process. Before research may be conducted, to what extent may informed consent be a part of the process? Despite the relaxing of some draft provisions of HIPAA pertaining to data access allowed to providers and researchers [30], HIPAA still incorporates the Security Final Rule as well as privacy provisions, and as electronic informed consent systems are under rapid development [15], their use will soon be a practical necessity.

Finally, where do the rights of corporate entities intersect with those of individuals in a world of highly connected data-flow? For instance, under present law, the Learned Intermediary Rule shields drug marketing companies from direct civil litigation, since information is often funneled first through physicians. How will the increasing popularity of direct marketing, facilitated by the Internet and other electronic media, change this balance of power between individuals, corporations, and providers? Furthermore, which groups and individuals, specifically, should have access to personal health information? Will access-licensure boards be required to grant and review privileges? These issues are becoming increasing relevant with the rise of "computational medicine," which correlates drug reactions and efficacy with specific patient populations. Using data from patient records and clinical trials, Compugen Corp. has contracted with HMOs to obtain access to millions of patient records for the purpose of such data mining [31].

4.3. Safeguards

In the realm of individual electronic patient records, how will patients be able to audit and ensure the accuracy of their personal data? Perhaps, in a "clearinghouse" model similar to that used by credit agencies, consumers can be afforded legal protections to view their files and contest inaccuracies. The provisions of HIPAA allow for consumers to request changes to their personal health records if they believe that an error is extant, with the responsible provider having a maximum of 90 days to review the request. Given the complexity and possible subjective nature of some elements of the health history, the effectiveness of the clearinghouse approach is yet untested.

Also, in legal malpractice cases, will lawyers be given access to records during the evidence discovery process? Cost/benefit analysis may also be conducted from the springboard of the *precautionary principle*, as proposed by David Kreibel; namely, that one must take preventative action in uncertain times, that the proponents of an activity bear the burden of proof, that alternative actions must be explored, and that public participation is key in the decision-making process [32]. This model is particularly germane to both clinical research and public health research contexts.

In addressing issues of privacy protections, the nature of implementation of disclosure policies for large-scale databases is a key issue. One consideration is the method of software and hardware development. As sound security infrastructure is required in order to safeguard civil liberties, the first major task to be addressed is a complete assessment of the scope of the problem (Table 2). What levels of protection are necessary? Is version control and tracking of records required? What degree of data archival and access logging is desired? In many situations, rapid deployment can begin by enabling secure, peer-reviewed technologies such as public key cryptography, redundancy, distributed systems, relational and regenerative databases that have been previously deployed in other service industries.

5. Complexity and Information Security

For collections of individual records assembled in databases, which themselves are linked in various ways, the topology of the network formed at each level attains particular importance. Yook, *et al.* have modeled the structure of Internet connections, and proposed that

Table 2. Goals for a comprehensive electronic patient record and order-entry system.

	Primary objective: Archival of patient personal health data
1	Histories and summary dictati
2	Diagnostic imaging requisitions and reports
3	Laboratory and pathology results
4	Treatments administered and problem list
5	Follow-up reports
	Specific Endpoints:
1	Facilitation of fault-tolerant, highly-available datastreams
2	Electronic prescription and impatient ordering capability
3	Assured data integrity through hashing and checksums
4	Physical security safeguards to access and modification
5	Crytographically-secure delivery of datastreams
6	Access auditing
7	Integration with billing processes and insurance claims
8	Dynamic assessment of eligibility for clinical trial enrollment and provision of value-added services
9	Links to external references (drug formularies, patient education literature, best-practice guidelines, and literature reviews)
10	Record of patient consent and support for electronic signature capture
11	Support for telemedicine (health care worker present at point-of-service) and cybermedicine (without end-location physician) providers
12	Incorporation of intelligent models to highlight gathering epidemics and nosocomial outbreaks

such a network may be classified as *scale-free* [33]; namely, a relatively small number of central nodes are responsible for a disproportionate level of the connectivity within the system [34]. The implications of identifying such a structure are important for several reasons: first, they offer an insight into the underlying communications load that various elements of the system must bear. Second, the central nodes are those which generally subserve critical functions (*i.e.*, house data which is of particular utility). The random failure of such a node may be a rare event, but a coordinated attack upon several nodes may be catastrophic for the system [35]. A given health-care network, much like the Internet, is a system with connectivity directed by human parsing, that relies heavily upon centralized data-centers for specific information such as patient identification numbers, allergies, and prior history. This implies that, to ensure robustness of a health care network, the most important nodes should be identified and the majority of available resources should be directed towards protecting these centers against failure.

Routine audits of software are key in maintaining effectiveness and security [36]. As software is developed, linking existing database structures into an interoperable continuum, secure practices should be a key element of design and implementation. This might be facilitated through freely-viewable source code to be inspected by the community at large. This transparency will allow for the implementers to be confident in the integrity of the middleware code – *cf.* the Unix community's experience with the OpenBSD operating system, which emphasizes security through open source development and open audits. Through the use of continuous auditing processes [36], and the payment of reward bounties for reported security exploits, both the private and public sector may be able to cooperate in developing a secure and reliable data services infrastructure for medical practice, education, and research. Finally, as the criminal assault on personal data grows [37], the development of hardware and software must be paralleled by legal protections against cybercrime and electronic terrorism. The potential for theft and abuse by legitimate providers will only rise as perceived value of personal medical records increases.

6. Issues for Future Consideration

Despite the aforementioned hazards, several positive ethical ramifications of records and treatment computerization should be noted. The Institute of Medicine (IOM), in a highly-publicized report entitled "Unequal Medicine," documented racial disparities in the administration of American mental health services, medication dispensation, and surgical procedures. One path to closing the divide, the IOM recommends, is the careful correlation of patient and doctor racial and ethnic demography in order to identify the roots and possible solutions to the problem [38]. Even this pathway is not without controversy, however, as racial profiling and correlation may itself be a violation of individual human rights. Furthermore, information reform may be one possible path to tort reform, as changes in data storage, diagnosis, and treatment modalities may force a re-thinking of liability assessment strategies [39]. For instance, as doctors from multiple regions all collaborate to treat a patient, and as doctors, managed care organizations, and pharmacists build closer relationships, previous protections and delineations of accountability become blurred and new models must be developed for quality control, restitution, and risk assessment in medical practice [20]. In this way, the Internet revolution may perhaps provide a basis for moving toward a more egalitarian, patient-centered, "no-fault" model of medical practice. Finally, the establishment of a broader records-based system may open a door for cross-sector and even trans-national coordination and cooperation in terms of deployment and maintenance of records systems, while preventing an imbalance in favor of governmental or corporate interests. Lessons gleaned from the governance mechanism of the World Wide Web itself, namely the non-governmental Internet Corp. for Assigned Names and Numbers, show that private officials, elected at large to represent a diverse community, have the capability to set strong standards, in concert with industry groups. It is precisely this adoption of open and consensus-based standards that has allowed the Web to flourish as an economic and academic entity, and perhaps this model can be reprised by the creation of a "health board," charged with the responsibility of establishing consistent guidelines for technological interoperability and access across all medical data networks.

Thus, the potential for a bright future for public health and the public welfare is indeed promising, but only in the context of pro-active engagement by government entities, healthcare providers, industry leaders, scientists, and the citizenry at large.

References

[1] eHealth Traffic Critically Dependent on Search Engines and Portals. *Harris Interactive Health Care News* April 23, 2001, 1–3.

[2] Nicolas Terry. Legal pitfalls of cybermedicine. *Lahey Clinical Medical Ethics Newsletter*. Winter ed., 2000.

[3] Christine Jones and Terrie Wheeler. The Role of Knowledge-Based Information. *SEA Currents* 1994 12(5).

[4] Karen Kaplan. E-Business: Meeting the Technology Challenge; Health care network gets big payoff from a simple solution. *Los Angeles Times* April 2, 2001, 1U.

[5] Joseph B Treaster. Doctors Face a Big Jump in Insurance. *New York Times* March 22, 2002.

[6] David W Bates. Commentary: Quality, Costs, Privacy, and Electronic Medical Data. *Journal of Law, Medicine, & Ethics* 1997 25(2–3):111–12.

[7] Richard Powelson. Telemedicine: A Way to Trim Medicare Costs? *Pittsburgh Post-Gazette* September 19, 2000, F5.

[8] Tom Arnold. Robots to improve surgery. *Ottawa Citizen* March 6, 2002, A12.

[9] Pamela S Whitten, Frances S Mair, Alan Haycox, Carl R May, Tracy L Williams, Seth Hellmich. Systematic review of cost effectiveness studies of telemedicine interventions. *BMJ* June 15, 2002, 324(7351):1434–7.

[10] N Maglaveras, V Koutkias, I Chouvarda, DG Goulis, A Avramides, D Adamidis, G Louridas, EA Balas. Home care delivery through the mobile telecommunications platform: the Citizen Health System perspective. *International Journal of Medical Informatics* 2002, 68:99–111.

[11] Gary C Doolittle, Art R Williams, David J Cook. An estimation of costs of a pediatric telemedicine practice in public schools. *Medical Care* January 2003, 41(1):100–9.

[12] Daniel R Masys. Effects Of Current And Future Information Technologies On The Health Care Workforce. *Health Affairs* 2002 21(5):33–41.

[13] Miriam Cu-Uy-Gam. Giving Cellular the Hard Sell: Technology ideal infrastructure fro developing nations. *The Financial Post* November 24, 1992, 24.

[14] Jeff Tieman. Technology's Rip Van Winkles: Hospitals are waking up, slowly, to the need to embrace computers and automation. *Modern Healthcare* July 16, 2001, 30.

[15] Joe Manning. Informed consent via the Web: Medical College pursues an Internet method of educating patients. *Milwaukee Journal Sentinel* September 10, 2001, 3D.

[16] Elliot M Stone, Jerilyn W Heinold, Lydia M Ewing, Stephen V Schoenbaum. Accessing Physician Information on the Internet. Commonwealth Fund, Field Report. Publication 503. January 2002, 1–38.

[17] Kristen Green. Marketing Health Care Product on the Internet: A Proposal for Updates Federal Regulation. *American Journal of Law & Medicine* 1998 24(2–3):365–86

[18] J Sybil Biermann, Gregory J Golladay, Mary Lou VH Greenfield, Laurence H Baker. Evaluation of Cancer Information on the Internet. Cancer 1999 86(3):381–90.

[19] Gretchen K Berland, Marc N Elliott, Leo S Morales, Jeffrey I Algazy, Richard L Kravitz, Michael S Broder, David E Kanouse, Jorge A Muñoz, Juan-Antonio Puyol, Marielena Lara, Katherine E Watkins, Hannah Yang, Elizabeth A McGlynn. Health Information on the Internet: Accessibility, Quality, and Readability in English and Spanish. *Journal of the American Medical Association* 2001 285(20):2612–1621.

[20] Deborah Haas-Wilson. Arrow and the information Market Failure in Health Care: The Changing Content and Sources of Health Care Information. *Journal of Health Politics, Policy, and Law* 2001 26(5):1031–44.

[21] Victor D Chase. Made to Order: IBM makes sense of unstructured data. *Think Research News*, March 8, 2002.

[22] Dennis Callahan. SAS Digging Into Unstructured Data. *EWeek*, January 28, 2002.

[23] Andrea M Singh. Using Data to Keep Tabs on Customers. *Newsday* March 26, 2001, C8.

[24] DeCODE Genetics. *Biotech Week* March 29, 2000, 28.

[25] Brower, Vicki. DeCODE, Roche map Arthritis gene, plan diagnostics and therapies. *Biotechnology Newswatch* December 17, 2001, 1.

[26] Parkinson Disease: First Gene Linked to Late-Onset Disease Located. *Genomics & Genetics Weekly* November 23, 2001, 6.

[27] William Brennan. *Whalen v Roe*, 1977, 589, 97 S. Ct. 869; 51 L. Ed. 2d 64, 607.

[28] William L Manning. Privacy and Confidentiality in Clinical Data Management Systems: Why You Should Guard the Safe. *Clinical Data Management* 1995 Summer ed.

[29] Ezekiel Emanuel, David Wendler, Christine Grady. What Makes Clinical Research Ethical? *Journal of the American Medical Association* 2000 283(20):2701–11.

[30] Robert Pear. Bush Acts to Drop Core Privacy Rule on Medical Data. *New York Times* March 22, 2002.

[31] Russell John. HMOs Begin Mining Patient Records. *Bio-IT World* July 11, 2002.

[32] David Kriebel and Joel Ticker. Reenergizing Public Health Through Precaution. *American Journal of Public Health* 2001 91(9):1351–1355.

[33] S-H Yook, Hawoong Jeong, Albert-Lászlo Barabasi. Modeling the Internet's large-scale topology. *Proceedings of the National Academy of Sciences* 2002 99:13382–6.

[34] Yuri I Wolf, Georgy Karev, Eugene V Koonin. Scale-free networks in biology: new insights into the fundamentals of evolution? *Bioessays* 2002 24:105–09.

[35] Reka Albert, Hawoong Jeong, Albert-Lászlo Barabasi. Attack and error tolerance of complex networks. *Nature* 2000 406:378 (2000).

[36] Software Quality Audit Session Breakout Session Summary. FDA Software Policy Workshop, September 1996. http://www.fda.gov/cdrh/ost/sqasumm.html (Accessed March 2004).

[37] Noel C Paul. Identity heist. *Christian Science Monitor* February 19, 2002, 17.

[38] Steve Sternberg. Study: Racial disparities persist in medicine. *USA Today* March 21, 2002, 6D.

[39] Patricia C Kuszler. Telemedicine and Integrated Health Care Delivery: Compounding Malpractice Liability. *American Journal of Law & Medicine* 1999 25:297–326.

Healthons Era –
Technology on Our Body, in Our Body
and All Around Us

Future of Intelligent and Extelligent Health Environment
R.G. Bushko (Ed.)
IOS Press, 2005

Healthwear:
Medical Technology Becomes Wearable

Alex PENTLAND, Ph.D.
Professor of Media Arts and Sciences & Director, Human Dynamics Research Group
MIT Media Laboratory, Cambridge, MA, US

Abstract. Widespread adoption of sensors that monitor the wearer's vital signs and other indicators promises to improve care for the aged and chronically ill while amassing a database that can enhance treatment and reduce medical costs.

1. Introduction

The concept of computing is rapidly expanding from simply using a desktop PC, where people sit and type for a small part of the day. Every day, more than one billion people carry around portable computation devices that have sensors and Internetcapable connections—but we call them cell phones rather than computers.

The most recent cell phones go far beyond telephony: They are truly wearable computers. These location-aware devices have sensors for detecting sounds, images, body motion, and ambient light level, have a secure Internet connection, and can download and upload programs as well as audio and image files. They also can serve as a situation aware intelligent assistant, whether as personal agents that use the digital equivalent of 3M's Post-it notes to augment reality or as a means of forming tight-knit intellectual collectives in which people can supercharge their social networks.

As part of this change in the way we use computers, my research group at the MIT Media Lab (http://hd.media.mit.edu) has been developing *healthwear*, wearable systems with sensors that can continuously monitor the user's vital signs, motor activity, social Interactions, sleep patterns, and other health indicators. The system's software can use the data from these sensors to build a personalized profile of the user's physical performance and nervous system activation throughout the entire day—providing a truly personal medical record that can, we believe, revolutionize healthcare.

2. Healthwear Overview

Until recently, researchers have had little success in extending healthcare into the home environment, yet there clearly is a huge demand for this service. Americans currently spend $27 billion on healthcare outside the formal medical establishment because they find it difficult to access, expensive, and painful (www.rwjf.org). A clear demand for better integrating the home into the healthcare environment exists. Not only that, but a dramatic shift in the composition of the US population makes it absolutely necessary to develop such distributed systems.

2.1. Caregiver Shortage

Although the US had 25 caregivers for each disabled person in 1970, the success of our healthcare system will lower the ratio of caregivers to at-home disabled to 6 to 1 by 2030 (www.agingstats.gov). How will those six people care for a disabled person? Certainly, a centralized system of visiting nurses is not an option for providing this care—such a system would leave too few individuals working at other jobs in the economy to support it.

Thus, a more highly distributed system is not only desirable, but absolutely necessary. These statistics provide the driving force behind the development of healthwear. This concept offers an unobtrusive method for acquiring in-depth knowledge about the body that could help manage chronic medical conditions such as cancer, diabetes, degenerative disorders of the nervous system, or chronic pain. Perhaps just as importantly, the deployment of continuous monitoring devices provides an excellent opportunity to fully inform medical providers about a patient's condition, thus helping the patient obtain the best treatment possible.

Already, health-conscious individuals are wearing small digital pedometers and exercise monitors. Indeed, some companies such as Nissan in Japan give such devices to employees to heighten health awareness and decrease medical insurance costs. In the future, people who dress for success may also wear a healthwear personal trainer that helps keep them active, knowledgeable, and involved.

2.2. Opportunities and Concerns

As new sensor, computing, and communication technology becomes available, healthcare professionals will be able to organize huge medical databases for use in tracking every test taken and medicine prescribed over an individual's lifetime. In addition to helping drive down healthcare costs, this data can provide powerful epidemiological information for use in improving our knowledge about keeping society healthy. For example, today because the huge expense of clinical trials limits the size and sensitivity of drug testing, harmful interactions are often detected only months or years after a drug is introduced to the general populace. Continuous, quantitative behavior logging has the potential to generate enough data so that researchers could discover these interactions more quickly.

Another application that is potentially even more important is the early detection of epidemics like SARS or biological weapons attacks. Today, reports of the treatment of an unusual number of patients with similar symptomatology at a medical facility often provide the first warning of a potential epidemic. Widespread continuous monitoring could detect such outbreaks much sooner by noticing when unusual numbers of people are behaving lethargically or staying home from work.

However, creating such an information architecture requires safeguards to maintain individual privacy. Indeed, we believe that this issue demands immediate, thoughtful attention and public debate, perhaps beginning with the current concern about using cell phone signals to track people. The current forces for creating huge databases and big medicine are powerful and all too successful. The potential solution is to place control and ownership of as much personal information as possible in the hands of the individual user, sharing only information cleansed of identifying features. This power-to-the-people approach favors using wearable sensing devices rather than sensors in the surrounding environment because the information starts out in the control of the individual, and the legal tradition in the US is that individuals own the data collected from their bodies.

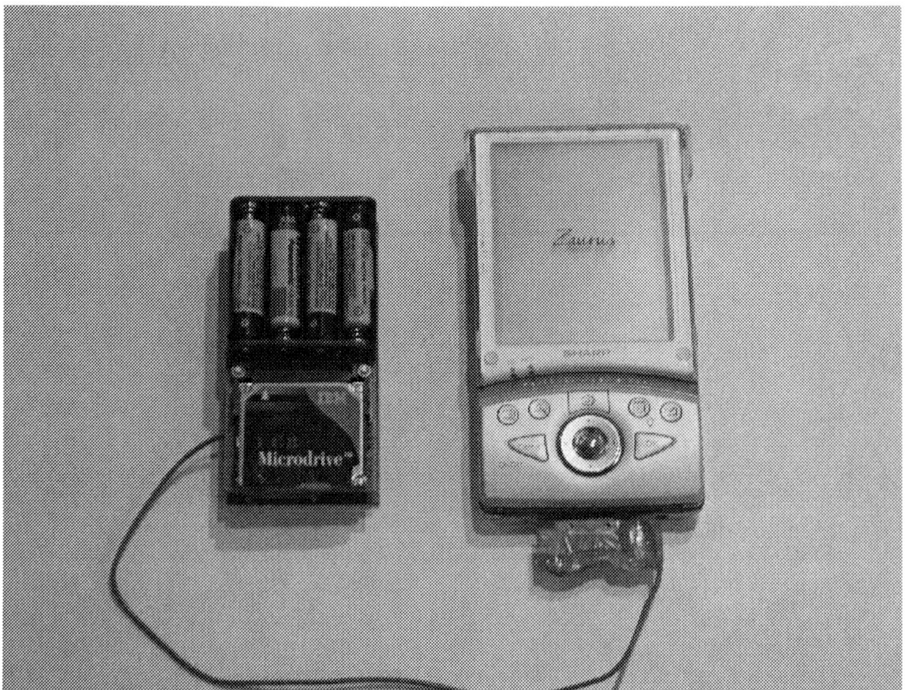

Figure 1. MIThril system. Plugging the biosensor hub into a cell phone or wireless PDA provides a system that offers input, output, and general computation functions and can support a wide range of physiological measurements.

3. MIThril

In J.R.R. Tolkien's Middle Earth stories, *mithril* is a precious metal used to craft armor with properties that protect its wearer from evil. The term thus seems an apt name for the technology that provides the basis for healthwear. Highly flexible, the MIThril architecture provides a modular system tied together by wireless networking protocols and a unified multiwired-protocol power and data bus for sensors and peripherals [1].

3.1. Hardware Components

Figure 1 shows the MIThril system. Designed for use with either a modern programmable cell phone or a wireless personal digital assistant (PDA), MIThril offers input, output, and general computation functions and can support a wide range of physiological measurements [1,2]. The MIThril hardware architecture is designed to be modular and easily configurable so that it can handle a variety of sensors and tasks. The software architecture supports using the ad hoc, on-the-fly combination of sensor signals from multiple users to control signaling and outputs.

A sensor hub interfaces with the MIThril body bus, which combines the Philips I2C multiple device serial protocol and power lines. The sensor hub provides a bridge to the sensor data, enabling data acquisition, buffering, and sequencing, and it can be used as a stand-alone data-acquisition system [2]. This is particularly useful for large-group applications that do not require real-time processing, wireless communication between users, or complex user interaction and thus do not require a cell phone or wireless PDA to be part of the system.

Currently supported devices include accelerometers for motion detection, IR active-tag readers for location and proximity detection, audio input and output devices, battery monitors, GPS, analog two-channel EKG/EMG, two-channel galvanic skin response sensors, and skin-temperature sensors. MIThril uses an RS-232 interface to communicate with a wide range of commercially available sensors for monitoring pulse oximetry, respiration, blood pressure, EEG, blood sugar, and CO2 levels.

3.2. Software Architecture

The core MIThril software components include the Enchantment Whiteboard, the Enchantment Signal system, and the MIThril Real-Time Context Engine. These tools provide the foundation for developing modular, distributed, context-aware wearable and ubiquitous computing applications. The Enchantment Whiteboard implements an interprocess communications system suitable for distributed, lightweight, embedded applications. Unlike traditional interprocess communications systems such as RMI and Unix/BSD sockets—which are based on point-to-point communications—the Enchantment Whiteboard uses a client-server model in which clients post and read structured information on a whiteboard server.

This architecture lets any client exchange information with any other client without the attendant complexity in negotiating direct client-to-client communication. These exchanges can take place without the client knowing anything at all about the other clients. Clients can subscribe to portions of the Enchantment Whiteboard, automatically receiving updates when changes occur. Further, clients can lock a portion of the whiteboard so that only the locking client can post updates. It also supports symbolic links across servers, letting whiteboards transparently refer to other whiteboards across a network.

Intended to act as a streaming database, the Enchantment Whiteboard captures the current state of some system, person, or group. On modest embedded hardware, the board can support many simultaneous clients distributed across a network while making hundreds of updates a second. We have used the Enchantment Whiteboard with the Enchantment Signal system for bandwidth-intensive voice-over-IP-style audio communications between teams of up to 50 users.

4. Life Patterns

The MIThril system provides a modular framework for real-time understanding of sensor data. The results of this process can be used locally for reminders and wearer feedback, or they can be broadcast to other users to enable smart-group communications and increased awareness of other members' health and activity levels. Pattern recognition techniques are the basis for modeling and interpreting the output of the wearable sensors. The standard pattern-recognition approach breaks this process into four stages:

- *Sensing.* A digital sensing device measures something in the real world, resulting in a digital signal of sampled values. For example, a microphone sensor converts continuous fluctuations in air pressure—sound—into discrete sampled values with a specified resolution, encoding, and sampling rate.
- *Feature extraction.* A raw sensor signal is transformed into a feature signal more suitable for a particular modeling task. For example, the feature extraction stage for a speaker-identification-classification task might involve converting a sound signal into a power-spectrum feature signal.

- *Modeling.* A generative or discriminative statistical model—such as a Gaussian mixture model, Support Vector Machine hyperplane classifier, or hidden Markov model—classifies a feature signal in real time. For example, a Gaussian mixture model could be used to classify accelerometer spectral features as walking, running, sitting, and so on.
- *Inference.* The results of the modeling stage, possibly combined with other information, are fed into a Bayesian inference system for complex interpretation and decision making.

We use machine-learning techniques to record raw sensor measurements and create statistical models of users' behavior and the surrounding context. Most commonly, we use hidden Markov models—which are also the basis of speech recognition systems—for behavior modeling. We have used this approach to build systems that use sensor measurements of hand motions to perform real-time recognition of American Sign Language and even to teach simple T'ai Chi movements [3]. Typically, these systems have vocabularies of 25 to 50 gestures and a recognition accuracy greater than 95 percent. We have also applied this same basic approach to audio and video to accurately identify the setting in which conversations take place—in a restaurant, in a vehicle, and so on—and even to classify the type of conversations a user engages in during the day [4,5].

Once we model the behavior and situation, we can classify incoming sensor data to build a model of the user's normal behavior. We can then use this model to monitor health, trigger reminders, or even notify caregivers. Information about the wearer's social interactions is particularly interesting. Understanding face-to-face encounters is critical to developing interfaces that respect and support the wearer's social life. Social interactions are also very sensitive indicators of mental health. Thus, an important challenge for our behavior modeling technology is to build computational models that we can use to predict the dynamics of individuals and their interactions.

The number of parameters is a significant factor in a model's learnability and interpretability. The requirement for minimal parameterization motivated our development of coupled hidden Markov models (CHMM) to describe interactions between two people, where the interaction parameters are limited to the inner products of the individual Markov chains [6]. As a practical matter, a CHMM is limited to the interactions between two people. We have therefore begun using a generalization of this idea, called the "influence model," which describes the connections between many Markov chains as a network of convex combinations of the chains [7]. This allows a simple parameterization in terms of the "influence" each chain has on the others, and we can use it to analyze complex phenomena involving interactions between large numbers of chains.

To apply the influence model to human networks, we have extended the original formulation to include hidden states and to develop a mechanism for learning the model's parameters from observations [8]. Modeling human behavior this way allows a simple parameterization of group dynamics in terms of the influence each person has on the others, and we have found that it provides a sensitive measure of social interactions.

5. Healthwear Application

Several ongoing projects hint at the capabilities healthwear will offer. These applications include medical monitoring and feedback systems for those with chronic medical conditions, monitoring social networking to reinforce healthy behavior, and mental monitoring to detect the symptoms of depression or dementia.

5.1. Medical Monitoring and Feedback

Healthwear promises to be especially effective for monitoring medical treatments.

Currently, doctors prescribe medications based on population averages rather than individual characteristics, and they check the appropriateness of the medication levels only occasionally—and expensively. With such a data-poor system, it is not surprising that medication doses are frequently over- or underestimated and that unforeseen drug interactions occur. Stratifying the population into phenotypes using genetic typing can improve the problem, but only to a degree. Continuous monitoring of motor activity, metabolism, and so on can be extremely effective in tailoring medications to the individual.

For example, consider Parkinson's patients. For them to function at their best, their medications must be optimally adjusted to the diurnal variation of symptoms. For this to occur, the managing clinician must have an accurate picture of how the patient's combined lack of normal movement (hypokinesia) and disruptive movements (dyskinesia) fluctuates throughout a typical day's activities. To achieve this, we combined the MIThril system's wearable accelerometers with standard statistical algorithms to classify the movement states of Parkinson's patients and provide a timeline of how those movements fluctuate throughout the day.

Two pilot studies were performed, consisting of seven patients, with the goal of assessing the ability to classify hypokinesia, dyskinesia, and bradykinesia (slow movement) based on accelerometer data, clinical observation, and videotaping. Using the patient's diary as the gold standard, the result was highly accurate identification of bradykinesia and hypokinesia. In addition, the studies classified the two most important clinical problems—predicting when the patient "feels off" or is about to experience troublesome dyskinesia—perfectly [9].

5.2. Memory Glasses

Regardless of age, we've all had our moments of forgetfulness. We accept such memory lapses as human fallibility, but we would be grateful if researchers could find a way to cue our natural memory and help us overcome these lapses. Perhaps such a device also could, for example, help improve an elderly person's memory or provide critical cues for emergency medical technicians, doctors, or firefighters in a nondistracting way.

Toward this end, we are developing *memory glasses* that might someday help people with challenges ranging from complex memory loss to simple absent-mindedness.

Figure 2 shows a prototype of this wearable, proactive, context-aware memory aid based on the MIThril platform and wearable sensors [10]. Memory glasses function like a reliable human assistant, storing reminder requests and delivering them under appropriate circumstances. Such a system differs qualitatively from a passive reminder system such as a paper organizer, or a context-blind reminder system such as a modern PDA, which records and structures reminder requests but which cannot know the user's context.

Perhaps the major obstacle to this vision is that people resist being reminded to exercise, take their medicine, or skip that extra helping of dessert. Subliminal memory aids—visual and audio reminders that lie just below the user's threshold of perception—may offer one way around this problem. Our research shows that under the right conditions, subliminal text or audio cues can jog the memory much like overt cues *even though the person receiving the cues is not aware of them.* In one experiment, for example, subliminal text cues improved performance on a name-recall task by 50 percent compared to the uncued control [11]. Perhaps more important than this positive effect, our research suggests that incorrect or misleading subliminal cues do not interfere with memory recall. This contrasts starkly with the effect of overt miscues, which have a significant misleading effect.

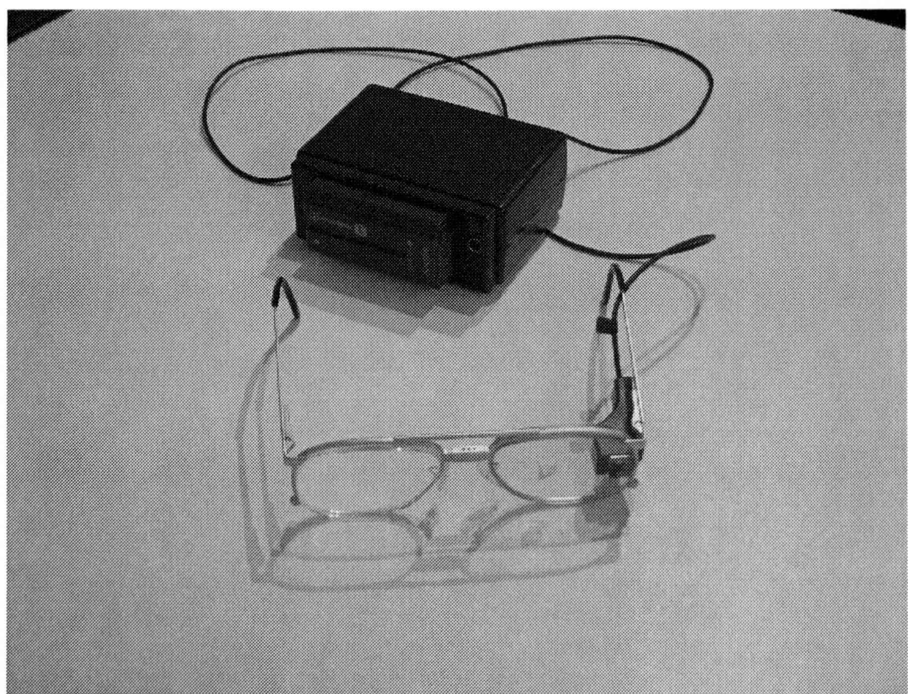

Figure 2. Memory glasses. A wearable, proactive, context aware memory aid, the memory glasses system combines the MIThril platform with wearable sensors to provide a device that functions like a human assistant, storing reminder requests and delivering them under appropriate circumstances.

A practical system might use a Bluetooth connection between cell phones to obtain the names of nearby friends. Similarly, a combination of information about location, proximity to others, time, and surrounding sounds could assist in situation recognition. The system could then use this context information to trigger the appropriate prompt, which would flash across the user's glasses or be communicated through an earpiece. If the system presented the prompt subliminally, users would not consciously process the reminder and so would be unaware that the prompt was jogging their memory. Thus, the subliminal prompts that the memory glasses provide would not interrupt a user's daily routines.

6. Social Networking

Reinforcing an individual's social support system may be the most effective way to encourage adopting more healthy behavior patterns. Thus, one aspect of healthwear's core functionality is interpersonal communications supported by continuous biomedical sensing [12].

6.1. Embedded Social Networking

Healthwear's social networking capabilities answer broad and immediate needs. For example, aging parents now commonly live far away from their families. Healthwear can help in such a situation by promoting communication between family members when it senses a suspicious change in an elder member's behavior. In one version, healthwear occasionally but continuously leaves phone messages reminding grown children to call their parents and vice versa. However, when a marked change in behavior occurs—such as decreased food consumption, socializing, or sleeping—healthwear increases the frequency of these reminders. The system would not tell people something is specifically wrong or describe why it left a particular message, nor would it call the doctor except in extreme circumstances, because doing so could violate people's privacy and might actually interfere with proper medical support. Instead, healthwear strengthens the social support network when the need is likely to be most significant.

6.2. DiaBetNet

Children also need social support networks, and they tend to be extremely sensitive to social context. We focused on this tendency when we created DiaBetNet, a computer game for young diabetics that uses belt-worn motion sensors, a wireless Internet connection, and a standard PDA for an interface [13]. DiaBetNet capitalizes on their passion for social games to encourage children with diabetes to keep track of their food intake, activity, and blood sugar level.

A typical day in the life of a diabetic child using DiaBetNet would unfold as follows. In the morning, the child clips his wireless accelerometer and DiaBetNet case—with wireless Internet connection, PDA, glucose meter, and wireless receiver for the accelerometer—onto his belt and goes off to school. Throughout the day, the PDA records his activity from the accelerometer, data from measuring glucose and injecting insulin from the glucose meter, and user-entered information about food consumption.

At any time, the user can see a graph on the PDA that summarizes the day's activity, carbohydrate consumption, and glucose data. From time to time, a wireless Internet connection sends this data to a secure central server.

DiaBetNet is a group gaming environment that requires guessing blood-sugar levels based on information that wearable sensors collect: The more accurate the answers, the higher the score. For example, imagine that a user named Tom begins to play DiaBetNet with others on the wireless network. Transformed into his cherished alias, Dr. T. Tom finds that his fellow players were all within 30 milligrams per deciliter of guessing their blood sugar levels correctly, but his guess was closer than anyone else's. Tom challenges a DiaBetNet player called Wizard and looks through Wizard's data. Although Wizard was euglycemic in the morning, he ate a late lunch. Therefore, Tom decides that Wizard's glucose level would be high and guesses 150 mg per dl. Wizard guesses his glucose to be 180 mg per dl. Tom wins again and grabs five more points. He shoots a brief conciliatory message to his vanquished foe and signs off.

In clinical trials, 93 percent of DiaBetNet participants successfully transmitted their data wirelessly to the server. The Game Group transmitted significantly more glucose values than the Control Group. The Game Group also had significantly less hyperglycemia—glucose 250 mg per dl—than the Control Group. Youth in the Game Group displayed a significant increase in diabetes knowledge over the four-week trial. Finally, more youth in the Game Group monitored their hemoglobin levels [14].

6.3. Mental Monitoring

Healthwear technology also can assist in the early detection of psychological disorders such as depression. Even though they are quite treatable, mental diseases rank among the top health problems worldwide in terms of cost to society. Major depression, for instance, is perhaps the leading cause of disability in established market economies [15].

Researchers have long known that speech activity can be affected in pathological states such as depression or mania. Thus, they have used audio features such as fundamental frequency, amplitude modulation, formant structure, and power distribution to distinguish between the speech of normal, depressed, and schizophrenic subjects [16]. Similarly, movement velocity, range, and frequency have been shown to correlate with depressed mood [17].

In the past, performing such measurements outside the laboratory was difficult given the required equipment's size and ambient noise. However, today even common cell phones have the computational power needed to monitor these correlates of mental state. We also can use the same methodology for more sophisticated inferences, such as the quantitative characterization of social interactions. The ability to use inexpensive, pervasive computational platforms such as cell phones to monitor these sensitive indicators of psychological state offers the dramatic possibility of early detection of mental problems.

Perhaps the most sensitive measure of mental function is social interaction, which clearly reveals attitudes, emotions, and cognitive function [18]. To investigate this idea, we are using a MIThril-based device dubbed the *sociometer* to collect data about daily Interactions with family, friends, and strangers such as:

- How frequent are the interactions?
- Are the interactions energetic or lethargic?
- Are the interactions appropriate without long gaps or frequent interruptions?

Using these sociometers we collected almost 1,700 hours of interaction data from 23 subjects. Participants in this study also filled out a daily survey that provided a list of their interactions with others. The sociometer and conversation-detection algorithms classified 87.5 percent of the conversations as greater or equal to one minute, a far greater accuracy than achieved using the survey method.

The few conversations that the automatic sociometer method missed typically took place in high-nise,multiple-speaker situations [19]. Once collected, researchers can use the *influence model*, a statistical framework that is a generalization of the hidden Markov models commonly used in speech recognition, to model the interaction data. Modeling spoken behavior this way allows a simple parameterization of group dynamics in terms of the influence each person has on the others. Our initial experiments show that these influence parameters are effective indicators of status within a social network and the degree of coupling to the social network [20].

7. Summary

Judging from the adoption rates of advanced cell phones and wearable health tools such as pedometers, within this decade much of the US population will likely have access to continuous, quantitative monitoring of its behavioral health status, coupled with easily accessible biosignals. How will this change our lives and our society?

An exciting possibility is that with the widespread adoption of healthwear, researchers could, for the first time, obtain enough data to really understand health at a societal level. For example, correlating a continuous, rich source of medication data from millions of people could make drug therapies more effective and help medical professionals detect drug interactions more quickly. If correlated with medical conditions, the data could illuminate the etiology and preconditions of disease far more powerfully than is possible today and, further, serve as an early warning system for epidemic diseases like SARS.

Comparing the medical data with genomic and protonomic data from different population samples could provide a powerful method for understanding complex gene and environment interactions. However, when considering the effects of healthwear systems, we would be wise to recall Marshall McLuhan's dictum that "the medium is the message." The way in which a new technology changes our lifestyle may well be more important than the information it conveys. Healthwear will likely be considered more personal and intimate than traditional health tools because it will form a constant part of a user's physical presence. Psychological studies have shown that clothes do indeed make the man.

Thus, healthwear will not only be part of what the user wears but part of who that user *is*. Body-worn technology will likely change our self-perception and self-confidence in ways that are today unpredictable. While it could be more effective at promoting healthy behavior than traditional approaches, healthwear also could be more seriously abused.

However, with more than one billion cell phones already being worn every day, there is no escape from being absorbed into this far more intimately connected new world. Our goal now should be to design this technology to make that world a very human place to live.

Acknowledgements

An earlier version of this article was published in the May 2004 IEEE Computer magazine, and is reprinted here by permission.

References

[1] R. DeVaul et al., "MIThril 2003: Applications and Architecture," *Proc. 7th Int'l Symp. Wearable Computers*, IEEE Press, 2003, pp. 4–11; www.media.mit.edu/wearables.

[2] V. Gerasimov, *Every Sign of Life*, doctoral dissertation, Dept. Media Arts and Sciences, MIT, 2003.

[3] T. Starner, J. Weaver, and A. Pentland, "Real-Time American Sign Language Recognition Using Desk and Wearable Computer-Based Video, Hidden Markov Models," *IEEE Trans. Pattern Analysis and Machine Vision*, Dec. 1998, pp. 1371–1375.

[4] A. Pentland, "Smart Rooms, Smart Clothes," *Scientific Am.*, Apr. 1996, pp. 68–76.

[5] S. Basu, *Conversational Scene Analysis*, doctoral dissertation, Dept. of Electrical Engineering and Computer Science, MIT, 2002.

[6] N. Oliver, B. Rosario, and A. Pentland, "A Bayesian Computer Vision System for Modeling Human Interactions," *IEEE Trans. Pattern Analysis and Machine Intelligence*, Aug. 2000, pp. 831–843.

[7] C. Asavathiratham, *The Influence Model: A TractableRepresentation for the Dynamics of Networked Markov Chains*, doctoral dissertation, Dept. of Electrical Eng. and Computer Science, MIT, 2000.

[8] T. Choudhury et al., "Learning Communities: Connectivity and Dynamics of Interactive Agents," *Proc. Int'l Joint Conf. Neural Networks, Special Session on Autonomus Mental Development*, IEEE Press, 2003, pp. 2797–2802; http://hd.media.mit.edu.

[9] D. Klapper, *Use of a Wearable Ambulatory Monitor in the Classification of Movement States in Parkinson's Disease*, master's thesis, Harvard-MIT Health Sciences and Technology Program, 2003.

[10] R. DeVaul, *Memory Glasses: Wearable Computing for Just-In-Time Memory Support*, doctoral dissertation, Dept. of Media Arts and Sciences, MIT, 2004.

[11] R. DeVaul, V. Corey, and A. Pentland, "The Memory Glasses: Subliminal vs. Overt Memory Support with Imperfect Information," *Proc. 7th Int'l Symp. Wearable Computers*, IEEE Press, 2003, pp. 146–153; www.media.mit.edu/wearables.

[12] M. Sung and A. Pentland, "LiveNet: Health and Lifestyle Networking through Distributed Mobile Devices," tech. report TR 575, MIT Media Lab, 2003; http://hd.media.mit.edu.

[13] V. Kumar et al., "DiaBetNet: Learning and Predicting Blood Glucose Results to Optimize Glycemic Control," poster exhibit, 4th Ann. Diabetes Technology Meeting, Atlanta, 2002; www.diabetestechnology.org.

[14] V. Kumar, *The Design and Testing of a Personal Health System to Motivate Adherence to Intensive Diabetes Management*, master's thesis, Harvard-MIT Health Sciences and Technology Program, 2004.

[15] C.L.J. Murray and A.D. Lopez, *The Global Burden of Disease*, Harvard Univ. Press, 1996.

[16] D.J. France et al., "Acoustical Properties of Speech as Indicators of Depression and Suicidal Risk," *IEEE Trans. Biomedical Eng.*, July 2000, pp. 829–837.

[17] M.H. Teicher, "Actigraphy and Motion Analysis: New Tools for Psychiatry," *Harvard Rev. Psychiatry*, 1995, vol. 3, pp. 18–35.

[18] P. Franks, T.L. Campbell, and C.G. Shields, "Social Relationships and Health: The Relative Roles of Family Functioning and Social Support," *Social Science & Medicine*, Apr. 1992, pp. 779–788.

[19] T. Choudhury and A. Pentland, "Modeling Face-to-Face Communication Using the Sociometer," W9 Workshop, *Proc. Int'l Conf. Ubiquitous Computing,* IEEE Press, 2003, pp. 3–8; http://hd.media.mit.edu.

[20] T. Choudhury, *Sensing and Modeling Human Networks*, doctoral dissertation, Dept. of Media Arts and Sciences, MIT, 2003.

Future of Intelligent and Extelligent Health Environment
R.G. Bushko (Ed.)
IOS Press, 2005

Interfacing Biology and Computing for Health: The Future of Home Diagnostics

Benjamin L. MILLER, Ph.D.
Department of Dermatology and the Center for Future Health
University of Rochester, Rochester, NY, USA

Abstract. Major advances in science and technology are converging to enable the development of a broad range of diagnostic aids for use in the home. These range from devices designed to diagnose infectious disease, to real-time continuous monitoring of endogenous biomarkers for cancer, cardiovascular health, and the like. This chapter briefly reviews some of the technical, biological, and social challenges associated with home diagnostic aids. In addition to providing several scenarios of how such devices might be used, we describe our own efforts in this area.

1. Introduction – Our Health Model Today

We live in an age of reactive, centralized health care. Most of us only come into contact with sophisticated medical instrumentation when something has gone seriously wrong with us, or if we've gone to a doctor's office or other centralized facility to undergo some sort of test. Medicine is probably the only area of our lives where we tolerate this lack of control; in entertainment, for example, we no longer rely on the concert schedule and theater tickets, but instead have home libraries (and on-demand online access) to more options than would have been conceivable even ten years ago. What differentiates home entertainment from home healthcare is threefold. First, knowledge (in the broadest sense): our understanding of the *science* behind healthcare is changing constantly. Second, knowledge (at an individual level): even young children are able to operate a television with enough facility to obtain an immediate benefit, while medical doctors require years of schooling, specialization, and practice to treat a patient. Third, technology: most medical diagnostic equipment today is large, cumbersome, complicated, and extraordinarily expensive. In order to gain greater control over our health, we must move health care towards the home, and to do so we must address both the knowledge and technology problems.

We can convert some of the knowledge issues into technology issues, if we fold the "individual knowledge" problem into a "user interface" issue. As diagnostic devices become more self-contained, and able to provide feedback to the user in common-language terms (or at least communicate with a centralized medical system or M.D. without user intervention), it will become more likely that individuals lacking a medical education (the vast majority of us) will be willing to use them. In the remainder of this chapter, we discuss the technical advances currently happening – and those that still need to happen – that will enable a broad array of home diagnostic and health-monitoring devices.

2. The Future: My Body, My Peripheral

What scenarios might we envision for the future of home diagnostics? In many respects, this is only limited by our imaginations; but here are some possibilities:

Home-based diagnosis of infectious disease. Sally came home from school with a nasty cough, and a stuffed-up nose. "We'd better check and make sure that's not the flu", Sally's mother thought. Taking one of the dozens of discarded tissues Sally had used to blow her nose, Sally's mother put the tissue into a small box attached to one of the family's PCs. After a short five-minute wait, a chime sounded and a window popped up on the computer: "Rhinovirus – common cold", it said, easing Sally's mother's worry.

Screening for genetic markers of cancer. Every morning, while Bill shaved in front of the bathroom mirror, the mirror was always busy with more than just reflecting his 58 year-old face back at him. For the past ten years, every morning, it had constructed a full three-dimensional image of Bill, and was able to compare each image to those that went before it using extraordinarily fast pattern-recognition algorithms. Over the past week, the mirror had noticed that a mole on Bill's neck had grown a fraction larger. "Bill, hold still a minute please, would you?" the mirror said through a nearby speaker. "There's something I want to check out in a bit more detail." With that, the mirror activated a wall-mounted infrared laser scanner and Raman spectrograph, zeroing in on the mole. "Just as I thought. Your thimidine dimer levels are high in that area, and there are some other spectroscopic indicators I don't like. I think you should have that checked out. Would you like me to upload the information to your dermatologist, and check with your scheduling program so you can set up an appointment?"

Continuous monitoring of a protein system. In her late 40's, Liza became concerned about her risk for cardiovascular disease. Not that she'd had any problems herself; she'd always been active and in fact still ran the occasional 5k race. Her father had passed away after his second heart attack, though, and Liza's grandmother had succumbed to congestive heart failure, leaving Liza with the feeling that she needed to do something to make sure she stayed in good health. So recently, Liza had gone into her doctor's office to have a Cardioguide™ implanted. The Cardioguide™ was new technology, able to continuously monitor levels of proteins involved in blood coagulation, as well as serum cholesterol and triglycerides. Every time Liza walked by her TV, it sensed the presence of the Cardioguide™ and uploaded the latest data from it. Liza didn't have to worry about any of this, however; the only time the system would alert her would be if any levels went outside an established "normal" range.

We're familiar (and comfortable) with the idea of hooking fax-printers, iPods, and video game controllers up to our home PCs for exchanging information and enabling certain functions on which we rely. In some respects, home diagnostics are about enabling the technology to interface our own bodies with the PC: my body, my peripheral. These examples above, and others like them, may sound today like science fiction. Indeed, we are a long way away from having some of these capabilities (particularly in the simple, autonomous format in which they've been described). However, efforts are underway at the labs around the world to address the feasibility of the scenarios described above. At the Center for Future Health at the University of Rochester [1], several research groups including that of the author work together to build the scientific and technological underpinnings of novel home diagnostic devices.

In some respects, developing diagnostics for disease (infections) is an easier task than monitoring endogenous biomarkers for health (such as in the second two examples above). First, infectious organisms typically provide a more clear-cut indication of a problem: if a sensor detects the presence of the SARS virus in a person, regardless of the amount, we know that person should seek treatment. Conversely, in many cases we do not yet have enough fundamental knowledge about human biochemistry to translate the detection of a particular protein (or quantity of that protein) to a disease state. Second, pathogens are most commonly found in easy-to-sample body fluids, while cancer markers and other potential targets are more difficult to find. Finally, there is considerable variation across the human species in what constitutes "normal", complicating analysis still further. This means that significant effort will need to be expended in establishing what "normal" is for each individual.

3. Three Revolutions: *-omics, Smart Materials, and Pervasive Computing*

Three rapidly advancing areas of science and technology are helping to make the approaching paradigm shift in home diagnosis possible – or at least enabling us to at least think about what remains to be done: "*-omics*", *smart materials*, and *pervasive computing*.

"*-omics*": Medical diagnostic devices rely on the ability to detect the presence, and quantity of, a molecule or set of molecules characteristic of a disease state. This can be as simple as a DNA sequence corresponding to a virus, or as complex as a protein signaling network. In the past, identifying such molecules has been a laborious process, requiring teams of researchers to isolate and characterize each individual molecule. That situation has changed dramatically in the past ten years. Characterized most famously by the human genome project, and the parallel efforts in industry by Celera and Human Genome Sciences, high-throughput methods have been developed allowing for explosive growth in the amount of information about the biochemical infrastructure of the human body, and other species including disease-causing organisms. Divided into the three key classes of biologically relevant molecules, such efforts are now characterized as *genomics*, for the study of the complete genomes (genetic sequences) of organisms, *proteomics*, for the study of the complete set of proteins making up that organism, and *metabolomics*, for the study of the complete set of small-molecule metabolites. Importantly, for the detection of pathogens in a diagnostic application, it is not even necessary to know the function of a target molecule; thus, by knowing that a DNA sequence is derived from a particular drug-resistant type of *Staphylococcus*, for example, one has made a positive identification of that organism assuming the sequence is unique. Full genomic (DNA) sequences are now available in public databases [2] for several pathogens, with the rate of sequencing accelerating (Table 1). Applications of various "-omics" in understanding human biochemistry and human health are more complicated, however, since one must understand not only what the sequence of a gene or protein *is*, but also what it *does*, and how that affects health. We'll discuss this more below.

Table 1. Selected complete genomes.

Organism	Reference
Homo sapiens	[3,4]
Plasmodium falciparum	[5]
Anopheles gambiae	[6]
Drosophila melanogaster	[6]
SARS coronavirus	[7]
Rubella virus	[8]
E. coli O157:H7	[9]
Haemophilus influenzae	[10]
Methicillin-resistant Staph	[11]

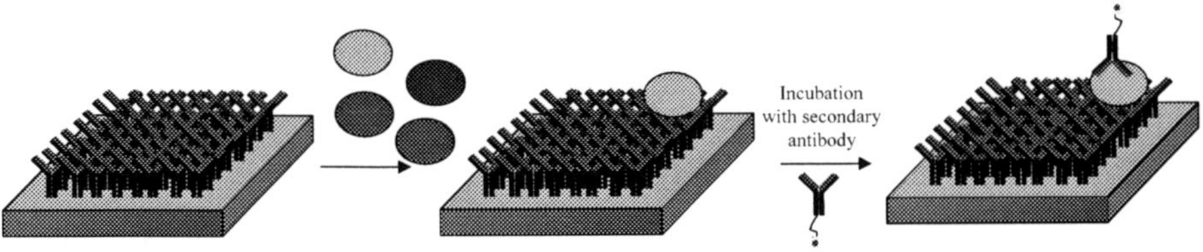

Figure 1. Operation of most current diagnostic materials. A surface coated with a capture molecule (for example, an antibody) is brought into contact with a clinical sample. After selected materials bind to the diagnostic chip, further incubation with a labeled secondary antibody is required for visualization.

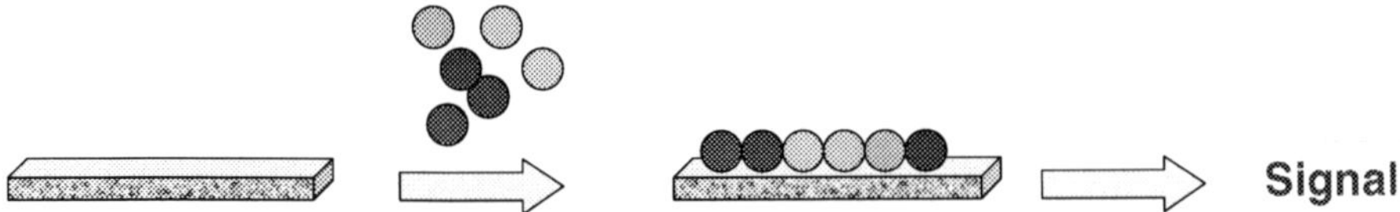

Figure 2. *Smart, responsive materials.* In contrast to the sensor shown in Fig. 1, this material directly produces a detectable signal when target molecules bind. No additional reagents are required for visualization.

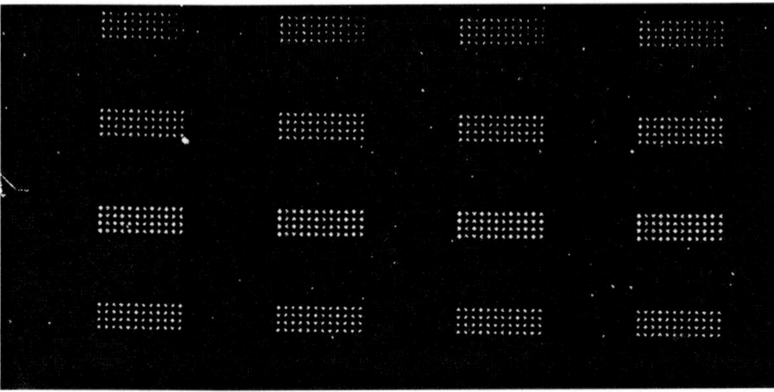

Figure 3. Microarray slide. Each spot represents an individual probe area, and is approximately 100 μm in diameter (image courtesy Brian R. McNaughton).

Smart materials and arrays refers to work being done on the sensor materials themselves. Current laboratory diagnostic methods rely on the addition of external reagents (chemicals) in order for a signal to be produced by a target molecule (Fig. 1). In a home diagnostic or biosensing situation, this is unwieldy, as well as an unnecessary added cost. New materials and analytical methodologies are becoming available that provide a signal *directly*, without added reagents, when a target molecule binds (Fig. 2). Since this is a major area of research in our laboratory, we'll give a few examples of these materials below. Along with these new materials, researchers are using the power of microarrays (chips with many sensor spots; Fig. 3) to allow for the development of sensors targeting large numbers of pathogens or biomarkers.

Pervasive computing is the revolution that probably needs the least explanation to the average reader. Within the last two decades, we have moved from ownership of a home computer being the provenance of "early adopters" and well-funded technophiles, to network-capable computers in an ever-increasing proportion of homes. The vast majority of appliances in modern homes are equipped with at least rudimentary computing power.

Critically, children in today's world have grown so accustomed to the ubiquity of computers that most cannot imagine a world without them. From the perspective of home medical diagnostics, this is important in two ways. First, it signals that computing technology is constantly becoming more capable and less expensive; at some point (whether this point has been reached or not may be arguable) computational performance and cost will be at a level sufficient to support the applications described herein at a price point consumers (or insurance companies) will be willing to support. Of course, it's also quite possible that companies will employ a "razors and razorblades" model to diagnostics, charging consumers very little for the base technology. Second, this comfort level with computing devices means that today's 20- and 30-year olds will be significantly more likely to accept computers updating them on their health (and potentially asking them for sample material).

4. What Research Needs To Be Done Now to Enable This Vision?

4.1. Convert Raw -omics Data into Useful Predictors of Health

As discussed earlier, we are still in the very early stages of the "omics" revolution. Except in instances where long-term biochemical and biomedical studies have provided indications of which genetic, protein, and small-molecule targets are effective markers (or predictors) of health, we still know very little about the relationship of individual biomolecules (or systems of biomolecules) to good health. Likewise, we don't yet know which genetic or protein markers need to be monitored with what frequency to make a difference in health outcome. In many cases, specific individual health markers and their use remain controversial for years after their initial discovery. For example, there is now general agreement in the scientific literature that levels of prostate serum antigen (PSA) are an important indicator of the probability of a patient developing prostate cancer. However, the specific application of information derived from PSA tests remains controversial, and it is unlikely that more frequent monitoring of PSA would be clinically useful [12,13]. Certainly, we can anticipate a similar level of controversy for other biomarkers – perhaps more so, given the number of variables involved and the fact that they will all interact with one another.

4.2. Acquisition of Baseline Data: What Is "Healthy", Anyhow?

Likewise, significant research remains to be done in order to define what "normal" is for most biochemical systems. We have a good idea of what a "normal" heart rate and blood pressure range is, but what is a typical level for a system of proteins? One possibility is that it will be necessary to collect some of this data for each individual; monitored over time, the monitoring system could produce both an indication of what constituted normal variation, and what would need to be considered as a potential indication of trouble. A model for this might be provided by some voice recognition software, which requires a "training period" before being able to respond to detailed user commands. Sticking with the voice recognition analogy, simple devices (such as cellular phones) exist that are able to respond to simple commands without any prior training. Likewise, once a sufficient body of biochemical knowledge has been developed for a particular biomedical system, devices may become available that can provide information based on complex networks of biochemical markers without any user-specific "training" period.

4.3. Device Operational Modes: Ambient, Contact, Sampling, Implanted

Ideally, the diagnostic devices we envision could be completely non-invasive, unobtrusive, and require no user attention…characteristics of the best household appliances! Devices of this type will likely fall into one of two categories: those based on ambient monitoring, and devices that can be implanted for long-term use. For ambient monitoring, this may be as simple as a device attached to the home HVAC system for monitoring the amount of allergens (or viruses, or other organisms) in the air. Alternatively, one can also imagine laser scanners that image exposed skin on a house's occupants, looking for spectroscopically detectable signs of cancer. An example of a device of this type is the VivaScope, a portable confocal laser system manufactured by the Lucid company. Although still at a level of cost and complexity well beyond what would be suitable for home use, the VivaScope has nevertheless demonstrated utility for diagnosing skin cancer, among other things [14].

Ambient monitoring devices also include wearable sensors that are used for monitoring heart rate, temperature, and respiration. In relation to the other devices we describe (and propose) herein, such systems are inherently "low tech", but they can nonetheless provide important information about the health of a wearer. The "Life Shirt" produced by VivoMetrics [15], is an example of this sort of "low tech" monitoring.

On the other end of the spectrum is the implanted diagnostic device. Implanted medical devices such as the pacemaker and the insulin pump have been in use for quite some time, and have provided substantial improvements in longevity and quality of life for large numbers of people. However, such devices are "one-way", in the sense that they go in, and no information comes out. Implanted devices that can exchange information with the outside world are an area of active research, primarily in the field of cybernetics. One example of this that has received wide media exposure is the work of Kevin Warwick at the University of Reading, UK. In a series of experiments, Warwick has implanted chips in his arm allowing limited two-way communication between himself and a computer [16]. More recently, passive RFID devices manufactured by VeriChip [17] have been approved by the FDA for implantation in humans. Capable of carrying a bearer's identity, these chips have been touted as a way to assist with the identification of kidnap victims. Importantly, such chips can also carry medical history, potentially allowing hospital emergency-room personnel to scan a nonresponsive patient for pre-existing medical conditions prior to providing treatment. Also importantly, the existence of these devices has been seen as a sign of the apocalypse by fringe religious groups, and has been the object of considerable discussion by conspiracy theorists. These kinds of responses cannot be dismissed out of hand, as there are clearly a number of privacy concerns raised by the existence of such devices.

In the middle of the spectrum are devices that sample body fluids. These include "smart toilets"; a staple of science fiction for some time, prototype devices from a number of manufacturers are now in development that are able to track blood sugar, serum albumin, and other biochemical markers. Sweat and saliva are also readily available fluids that might contain biomarkers of interest, and several clinical (and home) diagnostic devices that make use of these are currently available.

For the near-term future, it is likely that the largest number of useful molecular markers for human health will come from blood. None of us relishes the idea of having to periodically (or frequently) stick ourselves with a sharp object to obtain a blood sample, and therefore compliance will likely remain an important issue in this area. However, returning to the example of diabetes, it is clear that people can be convinced to do this if a significant health benefit is demonstrated.

5. Behavioral and Fiscal Challenges

Even with all of the potential advantages promised by the advent of rapid home diagnostics and continuous health monitoring, the greatest challenge remaining will be that of finding effective motivators for modifying human behavior. The biggest causes of mortality in the developed world today – heart disease, obesity, and cancer – are at least partially (if not primarily) self-induced. Will having continuously updated information about mutation load and other cancer risk-factors help smokers quit? Will a constantly updated readout of cholesterol and cardiovascular-related protein concentrations help an obese person modify eating patterns and stick to an exercise program? Clearly this will be a challenge. The availability of glucose monitoring devices is perhaps in some respects a model for other diagnostics. Prior to the advent of portable, inexpensive glucose meters and associated test strips, insulin regulation was largely a "hit and miss" affair. However, carefully controlled clinical studies have demonstrated that frequent monitoring of blood glucose through the course of a day can result in a significant improvement in overall health [18]. This in turn was sufficient to cause those with diabetes to change their behavior, self-monitoring glucose levels frequently throughout the day. We can anticipate that other home diagnostics will cause a similar behavior shift, if a sufficient benefit is demonstrated.

Of course, a major challenge to the development of home-based diagnostic devices and sensors will be the question of paying for them. Ideally, costs can be kept low enough, and a sufficiently large benefit shown, that consumers will want to buy these devices for themselves. An attractive model for distribution will be one analogous to that adopted by cable television, since technological improvements (likely to occur frequently as more information about useful biomarkers is uncovered) and quality control will necessitate frequent updates to installed equipment. Because of the intimate relationship new home diagnostic technologies will have with personal computers, it is also possible that computer hardware/software companies will participate in the development, manufacturing, and marketing of devices and consumables. What if consumers don't want to pay? In that case, the situation becomes significantly more complicated, and is realistically beyond the scope of this chapter.

Other Challenges: Who will develop standards for data acquisition, storage, and analysis?

Because we are at the very early stages in the development of home diagnostic and health-monitoring technologies, it may seem premature to worry about issues related to formats and standardization. However, establishing a set of recognized data formats and standards from the outset will significantly improve device interoperability and increase the likelihood of consumer acceptance. The proteomics and genomics fields have already been forced to face this issue, because of the immense quantities of data generated by microarray experiments [19]. One of the primary lessons from their experience is that solving the data storage and data standards problem early is essential.

6. Our Contribution: Research at the Center for Future Health at the University of Rochester

Our own work thus far has centered on developing new methods for the detection of biological molecules. We've focused on targets from pathogenic (disease-causing) organisms, but in principle the methods we've developed can be extended beyond detecting bacteria and viruses, to detection and quantitation of endogenous markers of health. Since it's likely that several different technologies will be needed for enabling home diagnostics and health monitoring, three methods developed in our laboratories will be described. All are based on

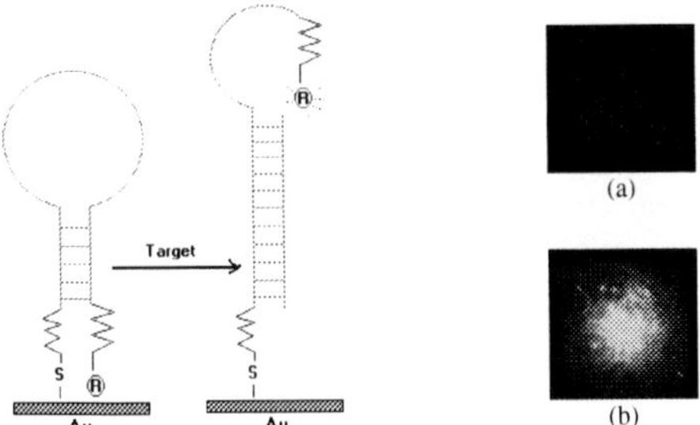

Figure 4. Operation of a gold-immobilized molecular beacon. Right: (a) CCD image pre-hybridization; (b) CCD image post-hybridization.

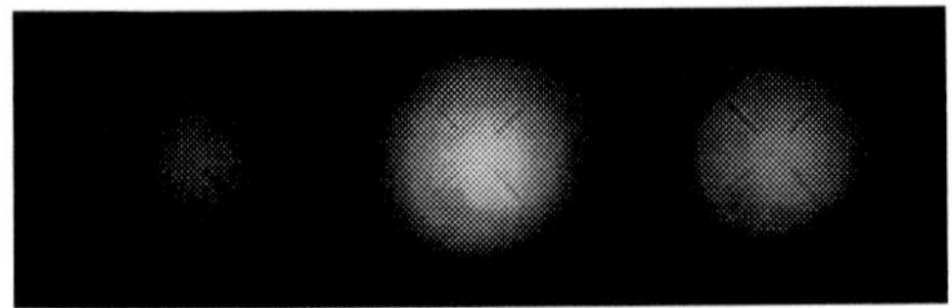

Figure 5. Digital photos demonstrating the sensitivity of the microarray. Left: post-immobilization of probe DNA. Center: post-treatment with 1.38 µM target DNA (synthetic antibiotic-resistant *Staphylococcus aureus*). Right: Post-treatment with 48.1 µM (oligonucleotide concentration) salmon sperm DNA.

the fundamental goal of having "reagentless" detection; that is, unlike current laboratory-scale diagnostic equipment, our goal is to provide devices that require no attention from the user other than application of a sample.

6.1. Molecular Beacons: Making Light of Nucleic Acids [20]

Our first technique takes advantage of the vast amount of information available from genomics efforts, described above. Termed an *immobilized molecular beacon* sensor, this method relies on our ability to design DNA probe molecules that fold back on themselves, in a "hairpin" structure (Fig. 4). One end of the DNA probe is chemically attached to a fluorescent molecule; the other end is attached to a thin gold film deposited on a flat surface such as a glass slide or microchip. In the absence of the target DNA or RNA sequence, the probe DNA remains folded over on itself, and the fluorescent molecule is quenched (the optical equivalent of short-circuiting) by the gold surface. If DNA or RNA from the target organism is encountered, however, it binds to the immobilized DNA probe causing it to straighten and removing the fluorescent molecule from the surface of the chip. This results in a brightly fluorescent "on" signal.

Most of our efforts thus far with the immobilized molecular beacon technique have focused on "proof of concept" experiments using synthetic DNA targets. However, we have already seen that we can readily detect sequences corresponding to antibiotic-resistant strains of *Staphylococcus aureus*, and sequences corresponding to the Anthrax bacterium. Importantly, the immobilized molecular beacon method allows for highly selective detection of the target nucleic acid sequence, in part because of the inherent selectivity of DNA base pairing (the fidelity of which is the fundamental reason DNA and RNA are such effective information-storage molecules for biological organisms), and in part because of the format of the device. For example, we can readily tell the difference between the target *Staph. aureus* DNA sequences, and a large excess of salmon sperm DNA (Fig. 5). Signal

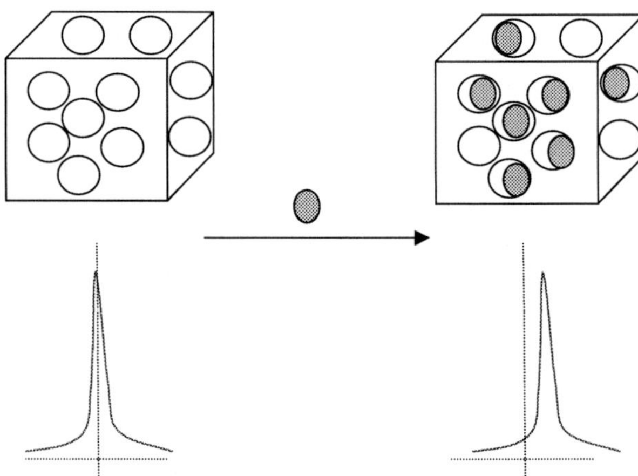

Figure 6. Operating principle of the porous silicon biosensor.

generation is fast, allowing for a "yes" or "no" answer within five minutes of the application of a sample.

The other two techniques we have explored are based on the optical properties of silicon substrates, modified in specific ways. Silicon is an ideal base material for biosensing, because of its long history in the microelectronics industry. This means that considerable infrastructure already exists for its manufacture and manipulation, and also that it's relatively inexpensive. Furthermore, silicon is biocompatible and nontoxic: several researchers have shown that silicon-based materials can be implanted in a host without ill effects. As we eventually move towards implantable, continuous-operation sensors, this will be a particularly important factor.

6.2. Porous Silicon Biosensors [21,22]

If a silicon wafer is subjected to an electrochemical etching process, it becomes porous. Porous silicon has unique optical properties that depend on the refractive index, which in turn is dependent on the size and density of the pores, and the material within them. Careful control of the electrochemical etching procedure allows for the production of complex multilayer mirror structures within the porous silicon, providing sharply defined reflectivity (or sometimes luminescence) spectra. Attachment of a probe molecule – a DNA strand, polypeptide, or small molecule – provides a porous silicon chip with an optical spectrum centered on a particular color. If a target biomolecule binds to the probe, this causes a change in the refractive index of the chip, which in turn causes a shift in the optical spectrum (Fig. 6).

In initial studies, we demonstrated that porous silicon could serve as an effective sensor for synthetic DNA strands, and for a simple virus. First, we chemically attached a DNA sequence to the surface of the porous silicon. This provided a sensor with an optical response shown by the top line in Fig. 7. Next, we treated the sensor with a solution containing DNA from lambda bacteriophage (a virus that infects bacteria). After a 30 minute incubation period, the solution was removed, and the chip was rinsed and dried. Because the lambda bacteriophage bound to the immobilized DNA sequence, this added to the material contained within the pores of the device, altering the refractive index of the sensor and shifting the luminescence spectrum (center and bottom lines, Fig. 7).

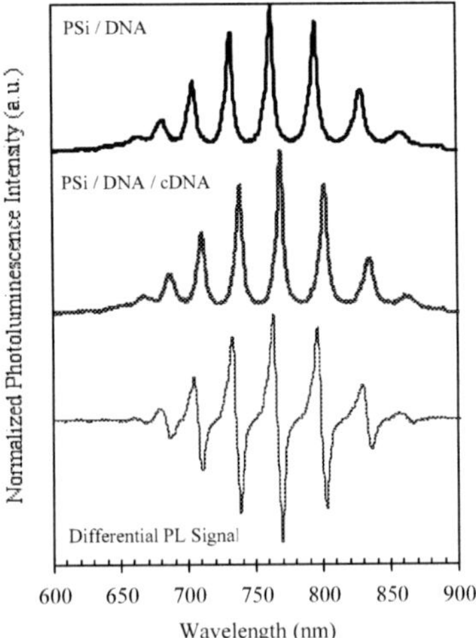

Figure 7. Detection of lambda-bacteriophage DNA using a porous silicon microcavity biosensor.

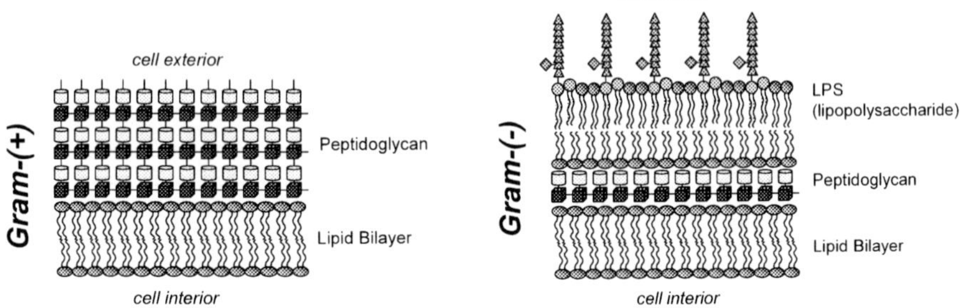

Figure 8. Gram-(+) and Gram-(−) bacterial cell membranes.

Next, we developed a sensor for Gram-(−) bacteria. The Gram stain is a basic procedure in microbiology, developed in the late 1800s by Hans Joachim Gram, a Dutch physician. Bacteria are divided into two broad classes (Gram-(+) and Gram-(−)) based on whether or not they acquire a violet color when stained by a specific dye. This test works because Gram-(+) bacteria have cell membranes containing a complex molecule called peptidoglycan. However, Gram-(−) bacteria also have a characteristic molecule in their cell membranes, called lipopolysaccharide (Fig. 8). We believed that by using a porous silicon sensor derivatized with a synthetic receptor designed to capture the "head group" of lipopolysaccharide, we could effectively detect Gram-(−) bacteria. In fact, this turned out to work quite well. Treating one of the sensors with Gram-(+) bacteria produces no signal, because the molecules that make up that type of bacteria don't bind to the designed receptor. However, Gram-(−) bacteria, with their lipopolysaccharide molecules, produce a strong signal when incubated with the sensor (Fig. 9).

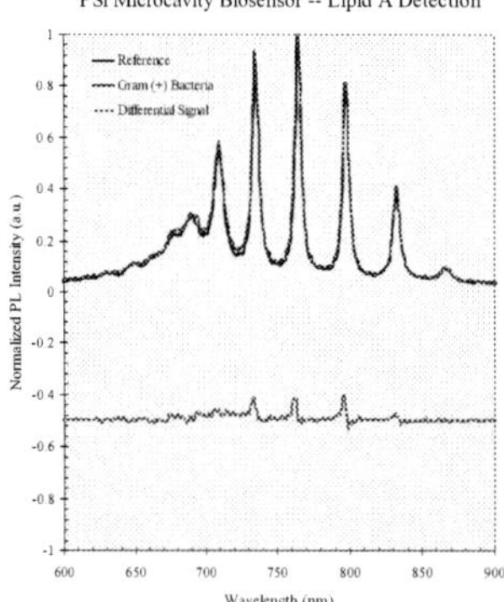
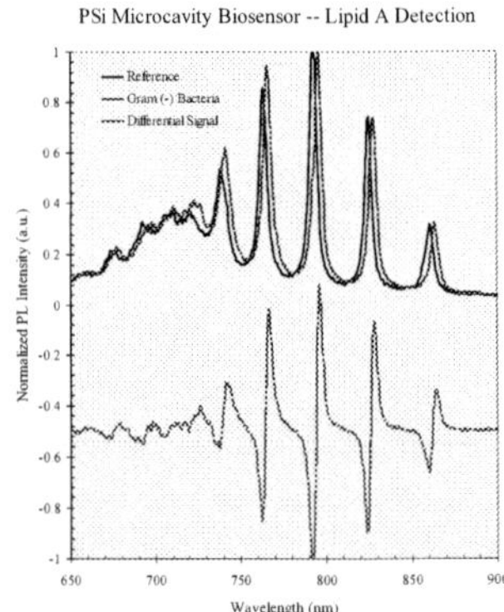

Figure 9. Detection of Gram-(–) bacteria with porous silicon microcavity biosensors. Left: Application of Gram-(+) bacteria produces no signal. Right: A signal is observed in the presence of Gram-(–) bacteria. From Reference [21].

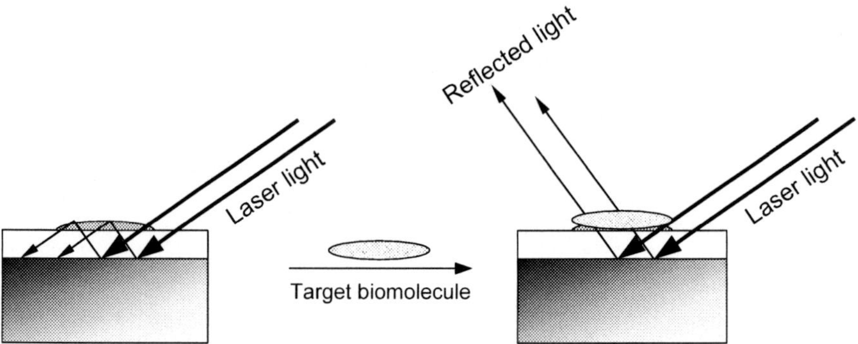

Figure 10. Principle of the Reflective Interferometry (RI) technique.

6.3. Reflective Interferometry [23]

The third technology under development in our labs is also based on silicon, but unlike the porous silicon sensors just described, *reflective interferometry* (RI) relies on changes on the surface of a silicon chip. In the RI system, a silicon chip is prepared with a surface layer of silicon dioxide. This silicon dioxide layer can be functionalized with probe molecules for a variety of targets, and is precisely calibrated such that polarized light of a specific wavelength interacting with the layer at a precise angle generates destructive interference. This destructive interference results in no light reflecting off the surface of the chip (Fig. 10). When a targeted molecule (or microorganism) binds to the probe molecule on the chip, this changes the thickness of the layer sufficiently that the destructive interference condition no longer holds, and light is reflected.

Simple in concept, RI turns out to work quite well as a detection technique. In initial experiments, we successfully employed RI chips derivatized with DNA sequences for the specific detection of complementary DNAs from *variola* (smallpox) virus (Fig. 11). Current work is focusing on the application of the technique to the detection of enteropathogenic *E. coli* (a causative agent of severe food poisoning), and several human proteins. With these latter applications, we hope to provide the first indications of whether tech-

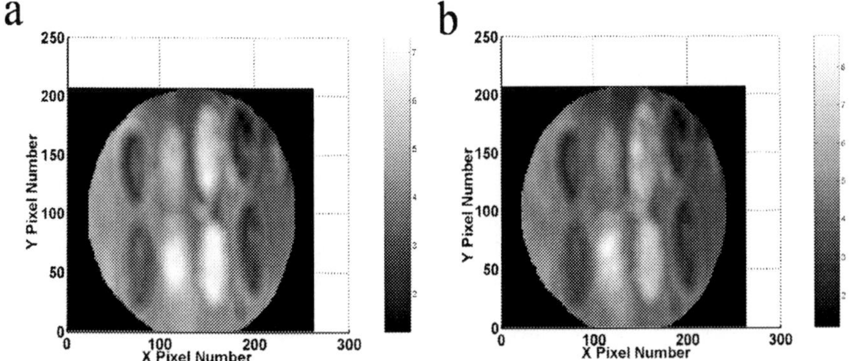

Figure 11. Detection of DNA by Reflective Interferometry. Lighter spots in the 4 x 2 arrays indicate heightened reflectivity due to the presence of DNA. From Reference [23].

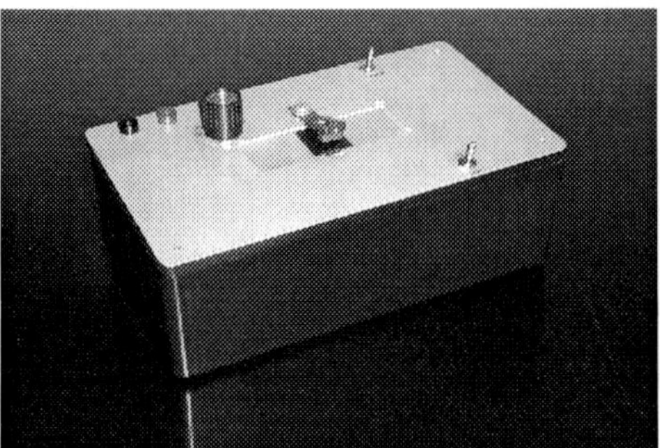

Figure 12. Prototypical hand-held RI sensor.

niques like RI can be useful in monitoring cardiovascular health and the behavior of the human immune system.

All three of the techniques described above are still at the laboratory stage; significant research and development remains to be done to bring them to a sufficient level of versatility and robust performance for use in the home. We have already made significant strides towards reducing the size of these devices to a manageable level; for example, a prototype handheld RI sensor is quite capable of detecting pathogens (Fig. 12).

7. Conclusions

A significant amount of research remains to be done to translate the early-stage laboratory successes described here (and those in other labs) into consumer products. Software-related issues will become particularly important as the technology begins to mature, and the problem of converting basic biochemical data into a suggested course of action for the user needs to be addressed. However, we can say with confidence that the sophistication and level of health benefit provided by home diagnostics will grow rapidly in the coming years – as we learn new information-rich methods of interfacing ourselves and our environment with technology.

References

[1] http://www.centerforfuturehealth.org.
[2] An excellent source for the most up-to-date listing of available genomic data is the National Center for Biotechnology Information (NCBI) website: http://www.ncbi.nlm.nih.gov/Genomes/index.html.
[3] International Human Genome Sequencing Consortium, *Nature* 2001, *409*, 860.
[4] Venter, C.J., et al. *Science* 2001, *291*, 1304.
[5] Gardner, M.J., et al. *Nature* 2002, *419*, 498.
[6] Zdobnov, E.M., et al. *Science* 2002, *298*, 149.
[7] Marra, M.A., et al. *Science* 2003, *300*, 1399.
[8] Dominguez, G.; Wang, C.Y.; Frey, T.K. *Virology* 1990, *177*, 225.
[9] Hayashi, T. et al. *DNA Res.* 2001, *8*, 11.
[10] Fleischmann, R.D., et al. *Science* 1995, *269*, 496.
[11] Holden, M.T.G., et al. *Proc. Natl. Acad. Sci. USA* 2004, *101*, 9786.
[12] Perron, L.; Moore, L.; Bairati, I.; Bernard, P.-M.; Meyer, F. *CMAJ*, 2002, *166*, 586.
[13] Coldman, A.J.; Phillips, N.; Pickels, T.A. *CMAJ* 2003, *168*, 31.
[14] Goldgeier, M.; Alessi-Fox, C.; Zavislan, J.M.; Harris, D.; Gonzalez, S. *Dermatol. Surg.* 2003, *29*, 1.
[15] http://www.vivometrics.com/site/system.html.
[16] Warwick, K.; Gasson, M. N. *Lecture Notes in Computer Science* 2004, *3058*, 7.
[17] http://www.4verichip.com/.
[18] Diabetes Control and Complications Trial Research Group, *New England Journal of Medicine* 1993, *329*, 977.
[19] Quackenbush, J. *Nat. Biotech.* 2004, *22*, 613.
[20] Du, K.; Disney, M.D.; Miller, B.L.; Krauss, T.D. *J. Am. Chem. Soc.* 2003, *125*, 4012.
[21] Chan, S.; Horner, S.R.; Miller, B.L.; Fauchet, P.M. *J. Am. Chem. Soc.* 2001, *123*, 11797.
[22] DeLouise, L.A.; Miller, B.L. *Anal. Chem.* 2004, *76*, 6915.
[23] Lu, J.; Strohsahl, C.M.; Miller, B.L.; Rothberg, L.J. *Anal. Chem.* 2004, *76*, 4416.

Future of Intelligent and Extelligent Health Environment
R.G. Bushko (Ed.)
IOS Press, 2005

Designing and Evaluating Home-Based, Just-in-Time Supportive Technology

Stephen S. INTILLE, Ph.D.[a] and Kent LARSON[b]
[a]*Technology Director, House_n Consortium, Department of Architecture,*
Massachusetts Institute of Technology, Cambridge, MA, USA
[b]*Director, House_n Consortium, Department of Architecture,*
Massachusetts Institute of Technology, Cambridge, MA, USA

Abstract. At MIT, a multi-disciplinary team of researchers is studying how to create pervasive computing environments for the home. We are developing technologies and design strategies that use context-aware sensing to empower people with information by presenting it at precisely the right time and place. Contrary to many visions of future home environments in the literature, we advocate an approach that uses technology to teach as opposed to using technology primarily for automated control. We have constructed a "living laboratory" that will provide a unique, flexible infrastructure for scientifically studying the power of pervasive computing for motivating learning and behavior change in the home. This facility, called the PlaceLab, is being used to study technology for creating homes that are supportive.

1. Changing Places of Living

People spend more time in their homes than in any other space. The home ideally provides a safe, comfortable environment in which to relax, communicate, learn, and be entertained. Increasingly, it is where people connect with friends and family, conduct business, manage resources, learn about the world, and maintain health and autonomy as they age. Unfortunately, technologies that are in the home are typically developed in isolation, and the general perception of homeowners is that computer devices are making life more complex and frustrating rather than easier and more relaxing. People are wary of the aesthetic, financial, and cognitive challenges of bringing new technologies into their homes.

Our multi-disciplinary research team at the Massachusetts Institute of Technology is investigating how the home and its related technologies, products, and services should evolve to better meet the opportunities and challenges of the future [1]. The "n" in House n represents a variable; we believe there is no single "home of the future." Our focus is on developing *design strategies* that meet the needs of multiple constituencies. In particular, we aim to create environments that are more flexible and that better meet the physical and cognitive needs of occupants than current environments. The spaces we envision seamlessly merge digital information with the physical environment. Four of the overarching goals of the House n project are to create supportive technologies that (1) help people create and customize environments and technologies that reflect their unique needs and values, (2) help people to live long and healthy lives in their homes, (3) help people reduce resource consumption, and (4) help people integrate learning into their everyday activity in the home.

Our research group is collectively asking the question, "How can we design spaces with technologies that are more than isolated gadgets, that are easier to use than today's technologies, and that provide real value to people in their homes over long periods of time?" Whenever possible, our team uses a participatory design approach, where we involve the stake holders in the design process. After discussions with physicians and patients interested in preventative health care, it became clear that the home of the future that would be of the most value is one that that does not use technology primarily to automatically control the environment but one that would help someone learn how to control the environment. This shift from the "controlling" home to the home that is supportive is the focus of this article.

A byproduct of this shift is that new tools are required to study technology in context of life in the home. Our team has constructed a "living laboratory" to support qualitative and quantitative studies investigating the relationships between spaces, the behaviors of people, and pervasive computing technologies. This facility, opened in summer 2004, is a single family residence with an integrated, ubiquitous sensor architecture. This architecture will be used by applications to acquire information about context, as is done in least one existing living lab (i.e. [2]). The laboratory infrastructure will also be used, however, for the quantitative measurement and qualitative study of the impact of new technologies on the behavior of people actually living in the environment.

2. Envisioning Homes of the Future

If one is to believe the majority of movies, television, and popular press articles that mention life in the homes of the future, our future homes will take care of our every need. Our homes will be so fully automated and "smart" that we will rarely have to think about everyday tasks at all. Nearly all of our time in the home will be spent engaged in leisure activities because digital and robotic agents will have taken over the mundane chores of day-to-day life.

Researchers and technologists are more cautious in their predictions, but a survey of ongoing work still shows a bias toward creating future home environments with the goal of eliminating the need to think about tasks such as controlling heating and lighting, going to the grocery store, cleaning, scheduling home appliances, and cooking.

Field interviews with medical professionals, educators, and homeowners have led our group in a different direction. Simplification or elimination of everyday tasks in the home may be in direct conflict with our goals of encouraging healthy lifestyles, resource conservation, and lifelong learning. On the contrary, medical professionals suggest that developing systems that *require* human effort in ways that keep people as mentally and physically engaged as possible as they age should be the goal. Although there are some instances in which we may want to use automation to allow people to accomplish tasks they can no longer perform on their own because of a disability or frailty, our primary vision is not one where computer technology is ubiquitously and proactively managing the details of the home.

Instead, the vision is one where computer technology is ever-present but in a more subtle way – tailored information is presented to people at precisely the time and the place when they need it so that they can learn how to take better care of themselves, learn how to conserve resources, or learn about topics that interest them. Medical experts tell us that the old adage, "use it or lose it," is applicable to both physical and mental health as we age. We want our pervasive technologies to empower people with information that helps them make decisions; we do not want to strip people of their sense of control, which has been shown to be psychologically and physically debilitating [3]. In short, we are designing pervasive computing environments that do not take over control of the environment for the home occupant as some previous systems have done (e.g. [4]) but rather help the home occupant to learn how to take control.

3. Control Versus Empowerment: An Example

To illustrate this shift in thinking, consider an example. Imagine our goal is to create an environment that uses pervasive computing technology to save energy by automatically controlling the heater-vent-air conditioning (HVAC) system. We assume that the environment has embedded sensors that can infer context such as where people are, what people are doing, and what the environmental conditions inside the home are. We also assume that the home contains computer-controlled HVAC appliances, windows, and blinds.

3.1. The Automated Home

One way to accomplish the goal of reducing resource consumption is to design a home environment that takes control of environmental conditions. The home uses a set of optimization algorithms to simultaneously maximize savings and comfort by automatically controlling the HVAC systems, windows, and blinds. For instance, on a day when the temperature is predicted to shift from warm to cool the home might determine the optimal cooling strategy is to shut down the AC and automatically open a set of blinds and windows to create an efficient cross breeze.

This scenario is relatively simple compared with other popular "smart home" visions. In practice, however, executing this scenario in an actual home setting is difficult. The situations in which the automatic system might succeed in optimizing temperature comfort yet fail in "doing the right thing" are many: something noisy is occurring outside, someone is smoking outside the window, someone in the home is allergic to pollen and the pollen count is high, it is raining outside, it is too quiet for a person reading when the hum of the air conditioner is off, someone did not want the blinds open because it throws glare on a computer screen, and so on. The system designer will be unable to program common-sense contingency plans for all possible contexts, and invariably the system will perform in unexpected, frustrating, and undesirable ways.

There is a fundamental problem: the more complexity the algorithms consider when making decisions the less transparent those decisions will be to the home owner [5]. The system will actually become less predictable as it acquires more expertise, and the success of the system some or most of the time will raise occupant expectations about what the system is capable of doing. Inevitably, the system will violate the occupant's high expectations given the unexplainable "intelligence" the system sometime shows when making these control decisions. Because the system is so complex, the occupant will be left feeling frustrated – helpless to understand the behavior. Why does it keep opening the windows when, clearly, the occupant wants and needs them closed? Other common scenarios for "smart" automatic control of the home suffer from identical problems.

3.2. The Home That Uses Subtle Reminders

Consider an alternative scenario. In this vision of the home of the future, the windows include a tiny light that is either embedded in the window frame (e.g. an LED) or that is projected on the window using pervasive computing display technology (e.g. an IBM Everywhere Display [6]). This home still has embedded sensors and optimization algorithms that compute a strategy for cooling the home by opening a particular set of windows. This home, however, does not proactively control the home to achieve the computed optimal settings. Instead, it uses pervasive technologies to *teach* the home occupant – in a non-obtrusive way – how to achieve the optimal settings.

For example, the light on the window will subtly illuminate. It does not interrupt the home occupant. When someone in the home notices it, that person knows the light indicates that, "it might be a good idea to open this window right now." The home thereby non-obtrusively informs the occupant of actions that the occupant might take to conserve energy or money. A similar approach can be taken when the goal is to improve health or introduce learning into everyday life.

This approach has several advantages over proactive control:

- Information can be presented that the occupant can react to without interrupting on-going activity in potentially irritating ways; this is especially true if information can be "augmented" onto the physical environment itself using projected light.
- Leaving the occupant in control of making decisions allows the home to present options based on partial information without confusing the occupant; the occupant will naturally consider contexts that the home has not and adjust his or her actions accordingly.
- Algorithms that make suggestions can degrade gracefully; algorithms that make decisions typically do not.
- Lack of control over aspects of life has been shown to diminish health [3]; this strategy empowers the home occupant.

The occupant ultimately makes the decision whether to open the window. Therefore, the task of interpreting the suggestion in context rests with the occupant: if it is noisy outside the occupant will simply decide not to open the window, realizing that this is not a good time. This is a pervasive computing application with an exceptionally simple user interface. Would a system with such a simple interface influence behavior? Yes. Controlled studies in homes show that using such a small, simple light on an AC unit can lead to 15% reductions in AC use [7].

3.3. The Teaching Home and Pervasive Information Display

The example above of the light on the AC may lead to some behavior change but it does so in a way that relies on the technology to be present. Fortunately, pervasive computing can be used to not only motivate the behavior but to *teach* at the moment when the behavior is being undertaken.

Systems that automatically make control decisions generally miss this opportunity. Occupants can become complacent if the system is functioning perfectly. Although a computer system might try to present the occupant with educational messages to explain the actions it is taking, to do this without interrupting and irritating the occupant is a challenge. The system must compute when a reasonable time to present the information might be. Even for relatively simple help applications this has proven to be difficult to do (e.g. ClipIt, the Microsoft Paperclip attempts just-in-time help but does so in ways that often requires the occupant to divert attention from the current task). On the other hand, if an occupant is unhappy with a control decision made by the home, the user is going to be in a state of annoyance and primarily interested in counteracting the home's actions – this is not the best time for the home to present explanatory information to promote learning.

A home that leaves the right amount of control to the occupant avoids the computational challenge of indirectly inferring occupant intent in order to determine the moment at which to teach. The extraordinary power of pervasive computing can come into play when an occupant decides to take an action such as opening the window. This is a "point of behavior" that can be easily identified by detecting a specific event (the opening of the window). The occupant has already made a decision to stop whatever he or she was doing to do a recommended task. The home can safely infer *directly from sensor data* that the occupant is opening the window and therefore is likely to be receptive to information that helps him or her determine how to do so. The occupant is also likely to be curious about why the home is making this recommendation. Finally, the occupant will have moved to the physical location of the object, which presents a good opportunity to teach by overlaying digital information on the physical space. In this scenario, at precisely the moment when the system determines that the occupant has decided to take action, information can be overlaid on the real world to educate the occupant about how to create the most effective cross breeze.

Even if the occupant does not have time to stop and study information, it is possible to present feedback that results in learning. For example, as the window is opened, information might be projected onto the nearby wall that estimates the magnitude of the breeze to be created. The person may notice that, counter-intuitively, opening the window further does not always result in a stronger cross breeze. The occupant's task has not been interrupted, so even if the occupant is completely uninterested in the information, no attentional disruption has been created. Immediately after the point of action the information could be removed.

It is the potential impact on behavior of this non-intrusive, "just-in-time" learning that our group is studying. We are interested in three points in time: the point of decision, the point of behavior, and point of consequence [8]. How can we use computers to educate people about how to take control of their environment by using sensors to automatically detect these specific (and sometimes fleeting) moments in time? In this particular example, as the occupant occasionally follows the recommendation of the home he or she will gradually learn how to efficiently control the temperature in the environment in sophisticated ways. Occupants will understand that the reason the lights appear on their windows is because it is cool enough outside to setup a cross breeze. They will also gradually learn how to create a cross breeze given the geometry of their house and the prevalent wind direction: using window inlets and outlets that maximize cooling through the home; understanding how to open window inlets and outlets to maximize air flow; understanding how long it will take for cooling to occur; understanding the best times and places to establish intake air; knowing how to use fans to facilitate cross-breeze cooling. These are things that most people do not know how to do because there is no one to instruct them on how to do it when they are in need of guidance at the point of behavior. Presentation of information at the point of behavior by a pervasive computing system can fill this need. The challenge then becomes to develop algorithms that can recognize the right time and select a presentation strategy suitable for the given context.

We have been conducting small user studies with mockup displays and are now implementing prototypes of some of the examples. Figure 1a shows a display that might appear on a wearable PDA or projected near the window at the moment a person is opening or closing a window: the "teachable moment." An open question that we plan to explore is how the way that information is presented and the current context influences the persuasive impact of educational messages.

An important consequence of using pervasive computing technology for just-in-time teaching rather than control is that the information people learn in that environment will transfer to other environments where there is no computer technology. Additionally, the just-in-time teaching scenario may still use automatic control of the windows but in a way that encourages people to use their physical abilities: a young healthy person would be encouraged (using pervasive computing messaging) to exercise muscles by opening the window, whereas a frail, elderly person who cannot lift the window would be encouraged to go to the window and push a real or virtual automatic button. We are also studying how to pre-

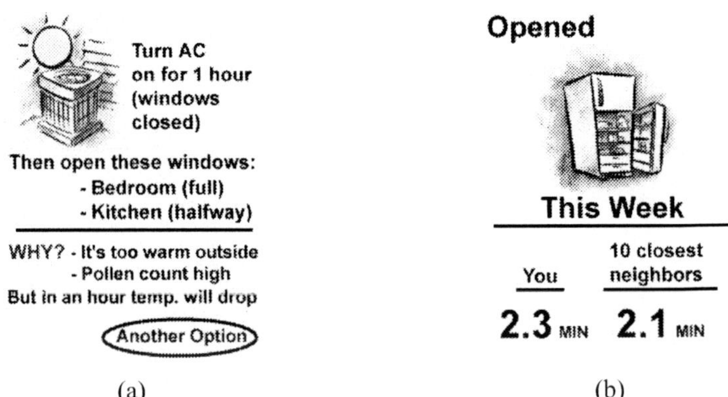

Figure 1. (a) This image shows a message that might be displayed within eyesight of a person just as that person opens a window in order to help that person learn how to conserve energy. (b) This message could be displayed on the refrigerator or on a wearable wrist computer just as someone closes the refrigerator door.

sent persuasive, pervasive messaging to motivate small behavior changes during everyday activities. For instance, Fig. 1b shows a message that could be displayed on a refrigerator door (or on a wearable wrist computer) just after the door has been closed to encourage awareness of energy conservation. People who are informed that their behavior is out of line with community standards will often naturally change their activity; in this case a greater awareness of the need to keep the door shut may result.

4. Design of the PlaceLab: A Living Laboratory

The shift in focus from creating automatic ("smart") environments to environments that help the occupant learn how to take self control impacts not only the type of technology we are designing but also our outlook on how we must conduct research to evaluate our work. We could construct a mockup space that simulates a home and then show that in particular situations the home can automatically control the physical and digital environments. Several of the pervasive computing environments built in the last several years have or are doing just that (e.g. [4,2,9]), and we have our own test environment.

However, pervasive environments that help people learn how to take to take control themselves cannot be evaluated independently of the people using them. We need to study the *people using the technology* in realistic, non-laboratory settings for long periods of time and then measure whether our interventions are leading to learning and behavior change.

To meet this need, we have designed and built an apartment-scale residential observational facility called the *PlaceLab*, an MIT and TIAX, LLC initiative. The PlaceLab serves as a "living laboratory" to study how people respond to new technologies. The facility is located a few blocks from MIT in a residential condominium building, and it opened in July 2004. The 1000 square foot lab consists of a living room, dining area, kitchen, small office, bedroom, full bath and half bath.

This facility serves two primary functions: (1) to provide an environment in which life in the home can be scientifically studied, and (2) to provide a means for evaluating whether new types of pervasive computing interventions have a long-term and meaningful impact on behavior in the home, especially behavior related to health and well-being.

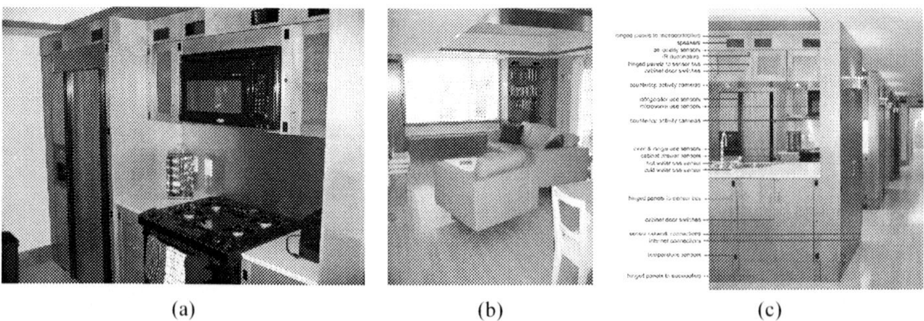

(a)   (b)   (c)

Figure 2. (a) Kitchen of the PlaceLab. Each cabinet contains a sensor infrastructure. (b) Living room of the PlaceLab. (c) Locations of some of the sensors built into a typical cabinet.

4.1. Ubiquitous Sensing

The PlaceLab uses a cabinet-based integrated interior infill system [10]. Despite ubiquitous sensing technology, the Place-Lab looks like a nicely designed home to the resident without any visible technologies other than standard home electronics.

Embedded within each cabinet in the PlaceLab is a suite of sensors, as marked on Fig. 2b. The sensors in the PlaceLab are used for two purposes: (1) the development of algorithms that infer what people are doing from sensor data, and (2) observation of activity in the space for research purposes. The PlaceLab is not intended to be a demonstration "home of the future." Instead it is a laboratory to study people in the home setting.

4.2. Using the PlaceLab

The PlaceLab is occupied by volunteer subjects who agree live in the home for periods of days, weeks, or months, depending upon the studies being run. While they occupy the facility, a rich dataset is collected on the behavior of the subjects. Researchers have the capability to monitor nearly every aspect of life in the home, particularly what people are doing and the interior and exterior environmental conditions in the space. Tools for the semi-automatic annotation and pruning of data aid researchers in studying the enormous amounts of data that are acquired daily by the laboratory. A suite of portable tools have also been developed that supplement the capabilities of the PlaceLab and permit studies where subjects are monitored in their own homes before and/or after they enter the PlaceLab, permitting studies that investigate pre- and post-occupancy behavior changes.

The facility is managed as a multi-disciplinary shared scientific tool in the tradition of other scientific facilities developed to study unique environments such as telescopes, microscopes, and undersea vessels. Researchers from many fields can submit proposals to a multi-disciplinary review board. These proposals are reviewed and ranked. High quality proposals are those that (1) can only be accomplished with the unique facilities of the PlaceLab, (2) will fundamentally increase scientific understanding of issues related to life in the home, and (3) consider the long-term implications of the technology, system, or architecture being studied and potential to create societal change. As in existing telescope facilities, complimentary and non-interfering studies are piggybacked to fill the facility calendar.

The PlaceLab is already being used to investigate questions such as, (1) What influences the behavior of people in their homes? (2) How can technology be effective in the home context for long time periods?, (3) Can technology and architectural design motivate life-extending behavior changes?, and (4) What new innovations for the home would most fundamentally alter the way we live our everyday lives? In summary, the PlaceLab is a multi-disciplinary, shared research facility for the study of people and their relationship with their living environments.

4.3. Studying Life in the Home and Physical/Digital Interactions

Relatively little research has been done on the relationship between the home and technology given the importance of the home in life [11]. We are using the PlaceLab's ubiquitous sensing for the quantitative and qualitative study of human behavior in the home – with and without new technologies. To do so, we are developing tools that will use the Place-Lab's sensing infrastructure to acquire and semi-automatically annotate data of interest to researchers.

The infrastructure of the PlaceLab has been designed so that video, audio, and appliance-level data can be continuously acquired from every part of the environment. For instance, the PlaceLab permits a researcher studying eating behaviors to make a request such as, "I'd like to see all the video and audio data of activity in rooms just before and after a subject opens a cabinet or appliance that relates to food storage or consumption." The researcher can collect and identify only the small subset of data relevant to that researcher's study. An algorithm developer can use the PlaceLab to acquire probabilistic data about the movement of people around environments throughout typical days. The lab provides an excellent resource with which to study how certain technologies disrupt activity in the home [5]. The combination of sensor data and audio-video recording (e.g. [12]) creates a powerful tool set for the researcher interested in evaluating technology designed for the home with people actually living in a home.

4.4. Measuring Effectiveness of Applications

The last function of the PlaceLab is to allow for the *evaluation* of certain types of pervasive computing applications. We are particularly interested in studying how context impacts the presentation and motivational impact of information presented in the home environment over long intervals of time.

The PlaceLab has being designed so that pervasive com-putting applications that present digital messages at the right time and place can be created without substantial amounts of system engineering. Our goal is not to develop new sensors for every situation but to investigate what can be accomplished with a given set of ubiquitous sensors that could be realistically retrofitted into existing living environments.

Our group consulted with researchers in a diverse set of fields as we developed the Placelab. Our goal has been to design a facility and infrastructure that leads to verifiable and quantifiable advances in understanding how to use pervasive computing in homes by measuring the impact of a set of implemented examples. Studies run in this lab have a limited sample size (i.e. one house and a small set of long-term occupants), and experimental problems such as the Hawthorne effect must be carefully addressed. However, our discussions with researchers in fields as disparate as preventative medicine and product development have led us to believe the PlaceLab will enable studies that can take place in no other way.

For instance, we have built a prototype system that uses a PDA device and context recognition (in this case location within the environment and proximity to large objects) to monitor for the onset of congestive heart failure (CHF) [13]. The software uses a Bayesian framework not only to integrate evidence for CHF onset but to select meaningful questions to ask a person in a home given the context. Cameras monitor the environment and detect contextual cues (e.g. in the kitchen, at the desk). A diagnosis system pools evidence acquired over the last month and, at any moment, can determine which question that is appropriate for the given context will yield the most valuable evidence. The home occupant carries a.PDA device. Whenever the person pulls it out to use it, a simple question may be displayed that is meaningful given the occupant's current context. The person quickly clicks one multiple-choice answer with almost no interruption to the intended task. Meanwhile, the system adds this new evidence to the preventative diagnosis information. If the system detects a progression towards CHF onset, the person or a medical monitoring service can be notified.

Will systems that present motivational information and ac-quire data for preventative diagnosis such as our CHF system work when placed in the complex environment of the home? Why or why not and to what degree? How does context impact the way the information is received and attended to? This is the type of investigation we, along with our other collaborators, foresee occurring in the PlaceLab. The experimental protocols that may be used differ based on the problems being studied. Our goal has been to design a tool that allows researchers from a variety of disciplines to design and execute studies that cannot be accomplished without the home's ubiquitous sensing infrastructure. One of the computer science challenges is to enhance the sensor infrastructure so it can support more advanced event detection over time.

5. Summary

We are interested in creating design strategies for environments that use pervasive displays and context-aware sensing to empower people with information presented at precisely the right time and place. Unlike many other visions for future home environments, we advocate an approach that uses technology primarily to teach as opposed to only for automated control. Therefore, we are developing new technologies but also new tools that permit us to evaluate our technology interventions in natural settings.

We have designed and built the PlaceLab, an MIT and TIAX, LLC initiative. The PlaceLab is a flexible, sensor-rich residential research facility that enables researchers to study how people respond to new technologies and design strategies. We invite researchers who may be interested in using this shared scientific tool in their own work to contact us.

Acknowledgements

The ideas presented here benefited greatly from discussions with Chuck Kukla and Dan Carlin. The PlaceLab is a collab-oration between MIT and TIAX, LLC.

References

[1] House_n, "Changing Places / House n: MIT Home of the Future Consor-tium," Access date: April 15 2002, http://architecture.mit.edu/house_n.

[2] C. Kidd, R. Orr, G. Abowd, C. Atkeson, I. Essa, B. MacIntyre, E. Mynatt, T. Starner, and W. Newstetter, "The Aware Home: A living laboratory for ubiquitous computing research," in *Proceedings of the Second International Workshop on Cooperative Buildings – CoBuild'99*, 1999.

[3] J. Rodin and E. Langer, "Long-term effects of a control-relevant intervention with the institutionalized aged," *Journal of Personality and Social Psychology*, vol. 35, no. 12, pp. 897–902, 1977.

[4] M. Mozer, "The Neural Network House: an environment that adapts to its inhabitants," in *Proceedings of the AAAI Spring Symposium on Intelligent Environments*, ser. Technical Report SS-98–02. Menlo Park, CA: AAAI Press, 1998, pp. 110–114.

[5] W. Edwards and R. Grinter, "At Home with Ubiquitous Computing: Seven Challenges," in *Proceedings of the Conference on Ubiquitous Computing*, 2001, pp. 256–272.

[6] C. Pinhanez, "The Everywhere Displays Projector: A device to create ubiquitous graphical interfaces," in *Proceedings of the Conference on Ubiquitous Computing*, ser. LNCS 2201, G. Abowd, B. Brumitt, and S. Shafer, Eds. Berlin Heidelberg: Springer-Verlag, 2001, pp. 315–331.

[7] C. Seligman, L. Becker, and J. Darley, "Behavioral approaches to residential energy conservation," *Energy and Building*, vol. 1, pp. 325–337, 1978.

[8] B. Fogg, "Persuasive technologies and netsmart devices," in *Information Appliances and Beyond*, E. Bergman, Ed., 2000, pp. 335–360.

[9] M. Coen, "Design principles for intelligent environments," in *Proceedings of the Fifteenth National Conference on Artificial Intelligence*. AAAI Press, 1998.

[10] K. Larson, "Places of Living: Integrated Components for Mass Customization," Massachusetts Institute of Technology," Changing Places Technical Report, March 2002.

[11] D. Hindus, "The importance of homes in technology research," in *Proceedings of the Second International Workshop on Cooperative Buildings- CoBuild'99*, V. Hartkopf, N. Streitz, J. Siegel, and S. Konomi, Eds., 1999.

[12] S. Intille, C. Kukla, and X. Ma, "Eliciting user preferences using image-based experience sampling and reflection," in *Proceedings of the CHI'02 Extended Abstracts on Human Factors in Computing Systems*. New York, NY: ACM Press, 2002, pp. 738–739.

[13] S. Intille, K. Larson, and C. Kukla, "Just-in-time context-sensitive questioning for preventative health care," in *Proceedings of the AAAI 2002 Workshop on Automation as Caregiver: The Role of Intelligent Technology in Elder Care*, ser. AAAI Technical Report WS-02-02. Menlo Park, CA: AAAI Press, 2002.

Future of Intelligent and Extelligent Health Environment
R.G. Bushko (Ed.)
IOS Press, 2005

Health. Care. Anywhere. Today

David ANDRE, Ph.D. and Astro TELLER, Ph.D.
Director of Informatics and CEO, respectively, BodyMedia, Inc, Pittsburgh, PA, USA

Abstract. What if clinical quality medical equipment were available to every consumer in a form factor that was inexpensive, accurate, and easy to use? What if this equipment provided information that previously was un-measurable or very difficult to measure? What if the physiological state of individuals, at resolutions measured in thousandths of a second instead of in visits per year, could be measured easily, making it possible to ascertain caloric intake and expenditure, patterns of sleep, contextual activities such as working-out and driving, even parameters of mental state and health. What aspect of healthcare wouldn't change? We present a system that is available today that enables this vision. This award-wining multi-channel wearable physiological monitor has enabled the collection of more than 90 million minutes of data in natural settings from thousands of subjects engaged in diverse activities. Data modeling efforts are resulting in applications that present meaningful and actionable information in real-time to users and their designated collaborators (physicians, family members, counselors, coaches, etc.) We describe the SenseWear system, its design, and a summary of validation studies, current commercial applications, and ongoing research. This discussion will show how the convergence of design for wearability, advances in machine learning, and improvements in wireless technology will manifest the future of health care as personal, ubiquitous, and collaborative.

1. Introduction

In 2005, the United States spent approximately 1.8 *trillion* dollars on healthcare. Of this, approximately 0.6 trillion can be attributed to diseases or conditions caused by the genetic makeup of the patients. Approximately 1.2 trillion is attributed to poor lifestyle choices – people not taking care of themselves. Despite this at most 9 *billion* (0.5% of the total) dollars were spent on helping people better manage their health. Why is this? Certainly, convincing people to change their behaviors is difficult, but a large part of the problem is that you can't manage what you can't measure. You wouldn't try to fly an airplane without instruments, but most people try to navigate their lives without a dashboard for their bodies.

Most traditional devices for measuring physiological signals are large, bulky, and expensive. Polysomnography machines [1] measure how well a patient sleeps, but require a (probably restless) night in a sleep clinic with many wires and electrodes glued to their bodies. Measuring energy expenditure requires an indirect calorimetry machine [2], and although some are becoming more portable, they require breathing into a tube and carting around heavy equipment for the analysis.

Surely, however, the advances in miniaturization and electronics can provide medical devices and computers that are smaller, cheaper, more sophisticated, and more personalized [3–5]. On the computing side, this push has culminated today in the explosion of handhelds (mobile phones, iPods, gameboys, digital cameras, PDAs, etc.) as the new computing platform—cheaper and more sophisticated enabling smaller and more personal interactions. On the medical side, similar advances have been made. Watches with ambient temperature sensors and glucose monitors, heart straps for joggers, pedometers for dieters, etc. [6–9]. There are clinical body monitors your doctor can prescribe and your nurse can administer such as holter monitors and ambulatory blood pressure cuffs. These devices are becoming wireless and less dependent on professionals for their application. More and more they are providing the means to transmit information back to caregivers quickly and seamlessly. So is that all that is required? No. The killer applications are just starting to emerge; applications from weight management to fitness to disease management. But the critical element in all of these areas is the interpretation and presentation of the data.

Wearable body monitoring goes from delivering potentially interesting data to delivering life altering information when it does enough of the data analysis to provide consumable, actionable nuggets of body knowledge automatically to wearers and their overseers. This is the difference between the sheet music and the violin concerto, the difference between the haystack and the needle. In that sense the future of wearable body monitoring will be a story about data and data analysis, as much as it will be a story about form factors and size reduction. The physical monitors are conduits to these distilled facts about our bodies, not the value in and of themselves, just as mobile phones are the conduits for wireless spoken communication between people. But even more than portability for mobile phones, wearability is a requirement for physiological sensors. If you can't stand wearing it, you won't wear it. And that means that the constraints of wearability in the most physical and practical sense, the constraints of where sensors can gather useful information on the human body, and the constraints of wearability, sociology and fashion all need be attended to for this vision to be realized. Fundamentally that means that the lines between design (industrial, mechanical, product, communication) and traditional engineering (e.g. electrical engineering, software engineering, biomedical sensing, and data modeling) will continue to blur as the ubiquitous, pervasive, and collaborative computing revolutions manifest a future of computing and healthcare that is wearable, personal, and sympathetic.

This chapter will discuss the design, current applications, and future of the SenseWear system. The first sections will describe the sensors, hardware, software and the design parameters and capabilities that enable the tracking of multiple channels of physiology at resolutions up to 32 Hz, in natural settings, for extended time periods, with high degrees of comfort. The sociological challenges of introducing physiological devices and new models of human health metrics to medical research and to consumers will be discussed. This will be followed by an introduction to the data-mining prediction and classification that underlie the utility of the SenseWear system, along with a discussion of the value of context for interpreting physiological measurements. Finally, a promising and diverse array of research findings and ongoing initiatives will be summarized.

2. The SenseWear System

As mentioned in the introduction, a device that can begin to transform health care must meet two difficult criteria. It must provide medically accurate data about a person's life but be designed well enough that it is unobtrusive and easy to wear. The system must be simple enough for the consumer but provide information useful to the healthcare professional. Although BodyMedia, Inc has several wearable body monitoring products, this chapter focuses on its SenseWear system, which includes a wearable armband that senses acceleration, heat flux, galvanic skin response, and temperature and records the data and derived measures over that data for later presentation to the user.

2.1. Designing a Physiological Computing Device for Everyday Use

The design of a wearable physiological computing device is an effort in finding the synergy among competing criteria ranging from physiological accuracy to comfort, and mechanical engineering to social acceptability. The design of a product that is to be in continuous contact with the human body twenty four hours a day is to design for an extreme environment. People carry all sorts of devices around with them every day, such as PDAs, cell phones, wallets, wrist watches, etc. BodyMedia first had to ask what makes people comfortable and then design all the electronics, sensors, and packaging around those human needs. Through the creation of a multi-channel, ergonomic and durable sensor hub, individuals who would otherwise be tethered to machines are being granted greater freedom. For others, they opt to wear the device, though they would never have been suffered the annoyance and cost of a lab device, because the device provides them benefits worth the effort to wear it. In the development of SenseWear, BodyMedia prototyped a number of devices ranging from chest straps to smart rings. These prototypes and the development of the design criteria were informed by studies on wearable computing and medical devices such as those used for sleep apnea research, actigraphy measurements, the accuracy of accelerometers for energy expenditure measurements, and on materials such as elastic straps [10–15]. The criteria for the SenseWear Armband included that it had to: accurately work for up to two weeks under continuous use (24/7); work during active athletic and work situations as well as during sleep; be easy to manufacture and robust enough to survive everyday use in low (0 °C) and high (45 °C) temperature environments; be small enough to keep the overall monitor height and footprint unobtrusive beneath clothing; be non-invasive and non-irritating to the skin and hypoallergenic; have extremely low power consumption; and be cost effective.

To meet these objectives the area of the body where the device would be worn had to be: similar in size and shape on men and women between the 5 and 95% size range; relatively large in surface area (at least 2 in. by 3 in.) to accommodate the required components, including batteries and electronics; low in mobility (non-bending or stretching even during high activity); and have a continuous circumference for easy attachment and detachment. Figure 1 shows how the upper arm meets many of these criteria. It is unoccupied 'real estate', gender-neutral, least obtrusive and low in the number of collisions, a relatively soft area where a device can be worn comfortably, and is generally concealed by clothing. On the upper arm it is also the case that device weight in this area does not induce fatigue and an adjustable strap accommodates a one size fits all design.

Many of the objectives were met through engineering novel design features. The symmetrical flexible wings (shown in Fig. 2) stabilize the device, accommodate diverse arm sizes, and create sufficient pressure for the sensors to function. A proprietary hypoallergenic and non-latex elastic strap was developed for appropriate tension and repeatable attachment. Iterative user testing was conducted with hospital patients, football players, factory workers, rescue workers, firefighters, and the general public.

The goal in making this wearable device was actually to make it as invisible to the user as possible. Very comfortable, very easy to use, something that blends into your life so you forget it is there. In a case study, a high school student wearing the monitor for two weeks said, "You kind of get used to it and don't even know you're wearing it." [16].

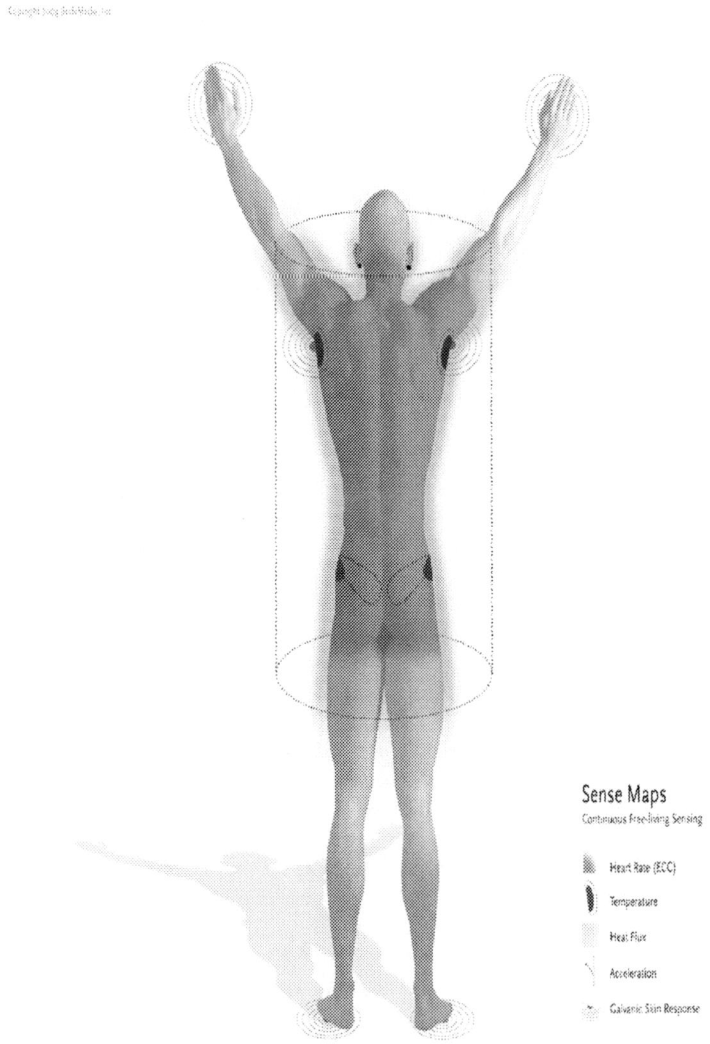

Figure 1. Wearability maps for heat flow, GSR, acceleration, heart rate, and temperature.

2.2. The SenseWear Pro2 Wearable Body Monitor

The SenseWear Pro2 Armband is a sensor hub worn on the back of the upper right arm (tricep area, Fig. 2) [17]. It enables continuous collection of low-level physiological vital sign streams and derives from those accurate statements of human body states and behaviors. The device contains five different sensors. A two-axis accelerometer tracks the movement of the upper arm and provides information about body position. A proprietary heat-flux sensor measures the amount of heat being dissipated by the body by measuring the heat loss along a thermally conductive path between the skin and a vent on the side of the armband. Skin temperature and near-armband temperature are also measured by sensitive thermistors. The armband also measures galvanic skin response (GSR – the conductivity of the wearer's skin) which varies due to sweating and emotional stimuli. The unit also contains a wireless

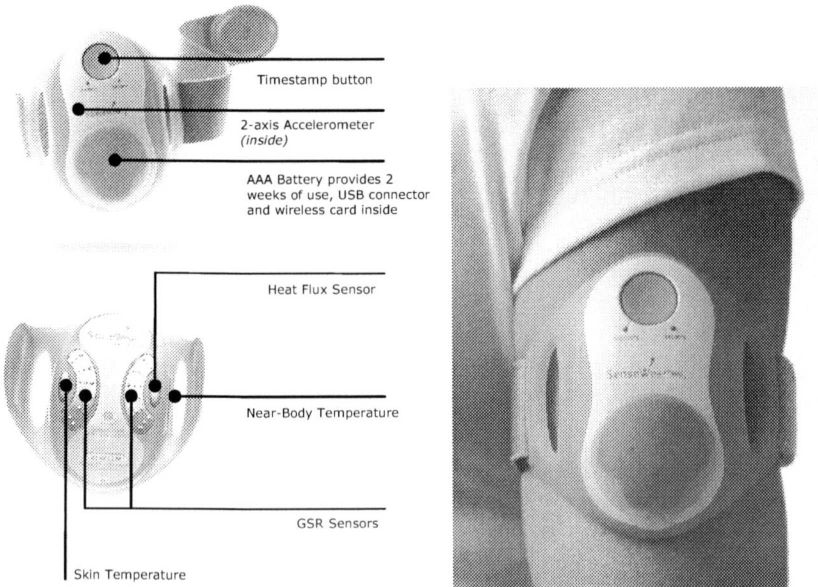

Figure 2. SenseWear Armband front with time stamp button, back showing sensor interface, and shown on arm.

chip and can communicate wirelessly with scales, blood pressure cuffs, and other medical systems. It can transmit collected sensor data with 916 MHz wireless body-LAN connectivity to a wireless communicator unit with <1 mW power output. The armband is made of flexible ABS, attaches with an elastic Velcro strap (custom designed to have stretch, air/water permeability, and hypoallergenic properties so as to mimic the skin to the greatest extent possible), weighs less than 3 oz., stores 14 days of continuous body data and has enough power for 14 days of continuous wear from a single AAA battery. Using a 4MHz MSP chip from Texas Instruments it transforms the raw physiological data such as movement, heat flux, skin temperature, near-body temperature, and galvanic skin response into snapshots of the user's life.

Each sensor is monitored 32 times per second, and data is tracked over a period of time (typically a minute but this can be adjusted through software). Currently, 41 different features of this multi-dimensional raw data stream are gathered as separate channels. For example, the variance of the heat flux is a channel, as is the average of the heat flux values. Some channels are fairly standard features (e.g. standard deviation) and others are complex proprietary algorithms. Then typically, these summary features for the epoch are stored and the raw data discarded to save memory. The raw data values can be retained (reducing the recording time, of course) through a simple software switch.

Enclosed in a shock and splash proof thermoplastic housing, the monitor straps to the user's right upper arm. At 0.8 in. tall by 3.4 in. long and 2.1 in. wide, the housing squeezes under all but the tightest shirtsleeves with barely a bulge. As it is wearable and unobtrusive, the Armband 'sees' people in the context of their natural daily activities rather than from the constrained viewpoint of a laboratory.

2.3. What SenseWear Senses Is Not What It Reports

Having multiple sensors is very important to the success of the armband and its ability to accurately monitor the physiological states of the wearers. Multiple sensors allow for the disambiguation of contexts that might confuse a single sensor. For example, if a wearer's motion is high, it might be due to exercising or to being in a moving vehicle. However, the signatures of temperature, sweat, and heat flux are typically quite different for exercise and being in a car. The algorithms in BodyMedia's software utilize the physiologic signals from all the sensors to first detect the wearer's context and then apply an appropriate formula to estimate energy expenditure from the sensor values. The armband can recognize many basic activities such as weight-lifting, walking, running, biking, resting, and riding in a car, bus, or train. Other activities are classified into combinations of these basic activities; for example, baseball could be broken down into a combination of mostly near-restful activity and running. Key to the armband's utility is that it can be worn comfortably during a person's normal life, and does not require any time in the laboratory for uncomfortable measurements.

The algorithms are all created using a proprietary algorithm development process that utilizes a data-driven machine learning approach. Data is first collected at clinical sites with laboratory equipment such as metabolic carts or metabolic chambers. Next, compressed channels are created from this raw data that can stored on the armband that are useful for determining both the wearer's activity as well as measures such as energy expenditure or sleep state. After this, context detectors are developed that classify the wearer's context. Finally, for each context, a specific algorithm is created using automated machine learning techniques to predict the measure of interest (such as energy expenditure). Section 5 describes the algorithm development process in more detail. At this point, accurate algorithms have been developed for energy expenditure, sleep, physical activity, and the set of activities mentioned above: weight-lifting, walking, running, biking, resting, and riding in a car, bus, or train.

2.4. Wireless Technology

The SenseWear system includes a 916 Mhz wireless technology that allows the armband to communicate securely and wirelessly with other devices including computing devices (PCs, PDAs), display devices (watches, kiosks), and other medical devices (blood glucose meters, weight scales, blood pressure cuffs, pulse oximetry meters). BodyMedia has enabled these devices with the SenseWear Transceiver (Fig. 3), allowing them to communicate with the armband. Users can take their measurements on these other devices, press the button on the armband, and the measurements are stored in the armband along with the data it records itself. All of the recorded data can then be transmitted to a PC via a wireless communicator (Fig. 4) that connects to USB port on the PC. Alternatively, the data can be uploaded to a web-server via a wireless gateway (Fig. 5) which contains either a standard or cellular modem, depending on the application.

This ability to communicate with different devices allows the user to receive feedback anywhere – whether on the go, at their home, or in their doctor's office. Furthermore, their trusted health advisors (e.g. friends, nurses, nutritionists, coaches, physicians) can look at the information on a printed report given to them by the user, online, or on their own PC. Figure 10 shows a representation of the entire system, with the armband serving as a hub for information that is reported to the web, to a PC, to a custom remote device (such as a baby monitor), to a cellular phone, or to a watch display.

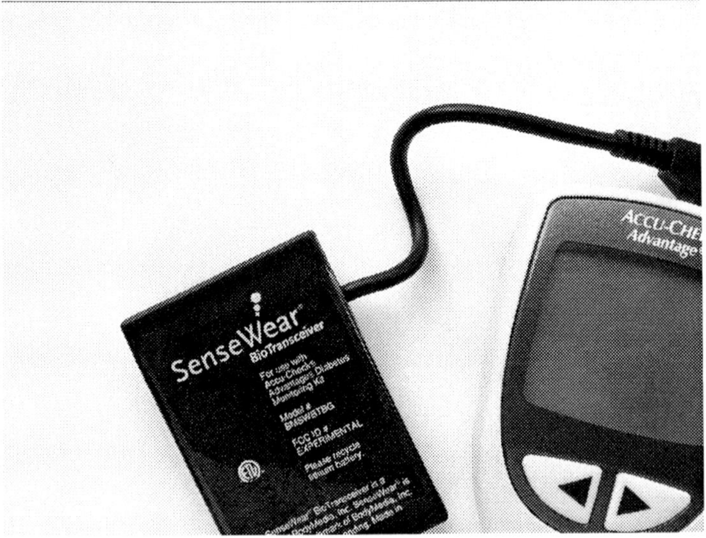

Figure 3. The SenseWear BioTransceiver that allows medical devices to communicate with the armband.

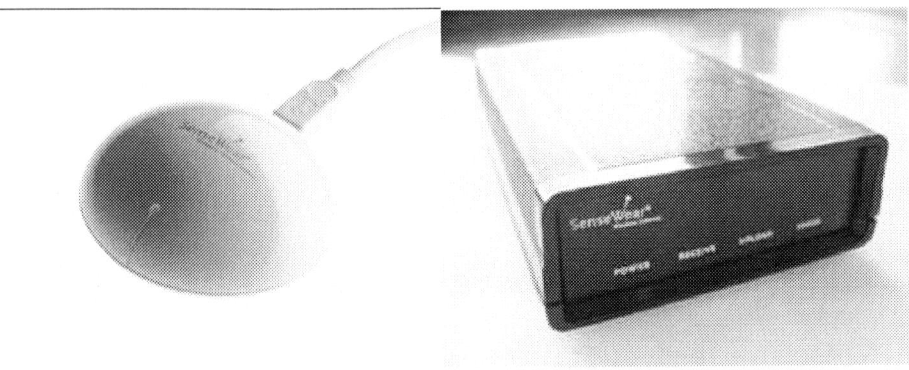

Figure 4. The SenseWear Wireless Communicator (left) and Wireless Gateway (right) allow communication with a PC or a web-server.

3. Current Applications of the SenseWear System

The thing that is really going to change society with respect to health care, wellness and fitness is the ability for people to start to learn about themselves. BodyMedia's design mantra is, 'make it fun and meaningful to see how you feel.' The BodyMedia platform creates a feedback loop: people want to manage their own health but until now, trying to do it was like dieting without a scale. The feedback loop is the presentation of actionable information that is otherwise unavailable to them (e.g. sleep/awake states each night down to a per minute basis if desired). This information allows people to assess progress toward their health goals. There are numerous applications that can be supported once data is being tracked. People could track elements of their health as closely as they track their financial portfolios. Having baseline data from an aggregate population and from individuals themselves, it is becoming possible to flag individual anomalies and detect potential health problems.

    D. Andre and A. Teller / Health. Care. Anywhere. Today

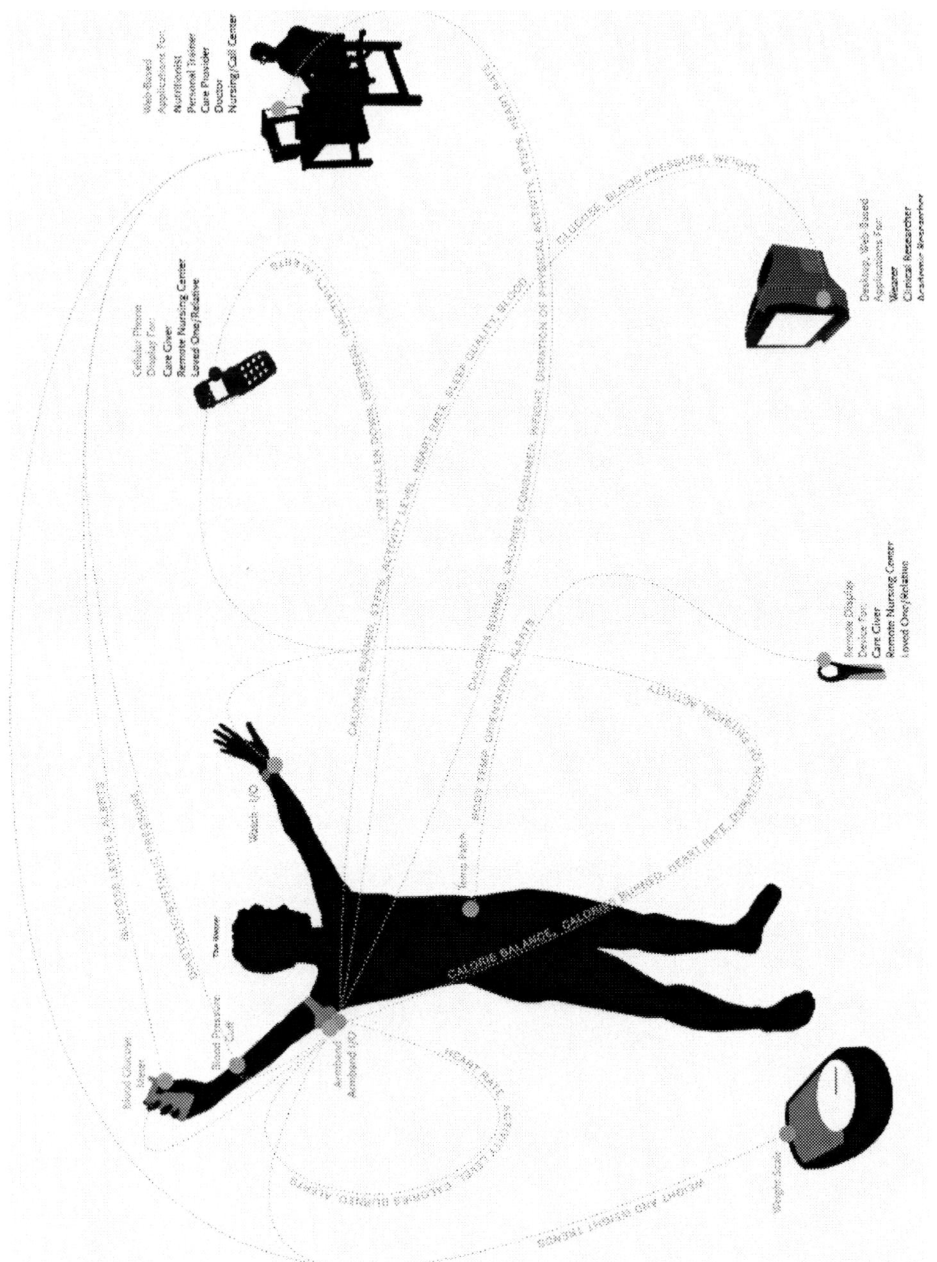

Figure 5. A platform for immediate and remote body monitoring.

The armband interface is highly customizable. It can be programmed to beep or vibrate when calorie-burn targets are met or as a reminder to take medicine. It is a communications 'hub' collecting and transmitting data from multiple devices worn on the body, all toward the goal of keeping the wearer alert to danger signals and mindful of health necessities. This system provides comprehensive, actionable feedback about a person's body and lifestyle that can be shared with researchers, physicians, dieticians and personal trainers via the Internet (Fig. 7). Internet applications can allow consumers to enter additional data such as calories consumed and body fat measurements to add further meaning to the body data gathered from their armbands. BodyMedia's goal is to help people become more aware of themselves in ways they have never done before and have a fun and engaging time doing that. One opportunity that has significant benefits is to employ a human relationship such as that with a physical fitness trainer. Similarly Debra Tate showed that the combination of online information and regular feedback from a coach along with the ability to self-monitor diet and calorie estimates resulted in preliminary successes [18].

The SenseWear system has been deployed in several applications to date. The first application was a research software package called the Innerview Research Software that was designed for researchers and clinicians to use. This piece of software offers the ability to customize the armband's recording rates as well as reports, summaries, and detailed information about the sensor values that were recorded. Figure 6 shows a report, with one screen showing totals, daily totals of energy expenditure, steps taken, amount of sleep, amount of lying down, and amount of physical activity. For example, you can see that David played soccer on Monday and went snowboarding on Friday from these graphs. The lower part of the figure shows the software's ability to display detailed information. You can see at the top of this part of the figure an auto-journaling of Friday and Saturday, showing when David was physically active, was motoring (in a moving vehicle), sleeping, sedentary, and lying down. The bottom of the graph shows a minute by minute plot of energy expenditure, heat flux, and skin temperature. The sensor values shown in the report are configurable in the software.

The Innerview Research Software has been used at thousands of sites for a variety of purposes. Some of these include to analyze exercise physiology data, serve as a measure for tracking medical conditions such as pain or physical activity during recovery from surgery, examine skin temperature in soldiers, build emotion-detecting algorithms from the data collected by the armband [19], analyze a person's reactions to architectural spaces [20], and as a variable in longitudinal studies of disease causation.

Other applications have included the study of sleep behaviors, competitive sailing, human computer interactions, and stress response in car and tank drivers. Groups studied range from professional athletes to the elderly to children. The products have survived intact in extreme environments such as Mt Everest, the North Pole, the South Pole, the highest lake in the world, the Pittsburgh Steelers training camp, and National Guard live firefighter training sessions inside burning planes.

A case study such as the following can help to illuminate the power of this kind of free-living body information. Using the Innerview Research Software, Perini et al. [21] investigated the relationship between physical activity estimates and energy expenditure estimates with the recovery of a subject with Sydenham's Chorea. Sydenham's Chorea is a childhood disease that causes rapid and frequent involuntary movements but is benign in that spontaneous recovery will occur in a few weeks. This subject was treated with antibiotics, steroids, and antiepileptic therapy. At the outset, the subject was burning 1910 kcals/day as measured by the armband, with frequent involuntary muscle movements. In the following few days, the subject burned fewer and fewer calories per day as measured by the armband and additionally scored lower on several indicies (TAS, flogosis) of the progression of the disease. After six days, the subject was nearly back to normal, with only minimal choreic movements in the limbs. Blood tests revealed normal TAS and flogosis levels and the armband showed only 1400 kcals/day expenditure. At day 10, energy expenditure as measured by the armband increased in conjunction with some reappearance of symptoms. The SenseWear system with the Innerview Research Software is being increasingly used in clinical situations in Europe.

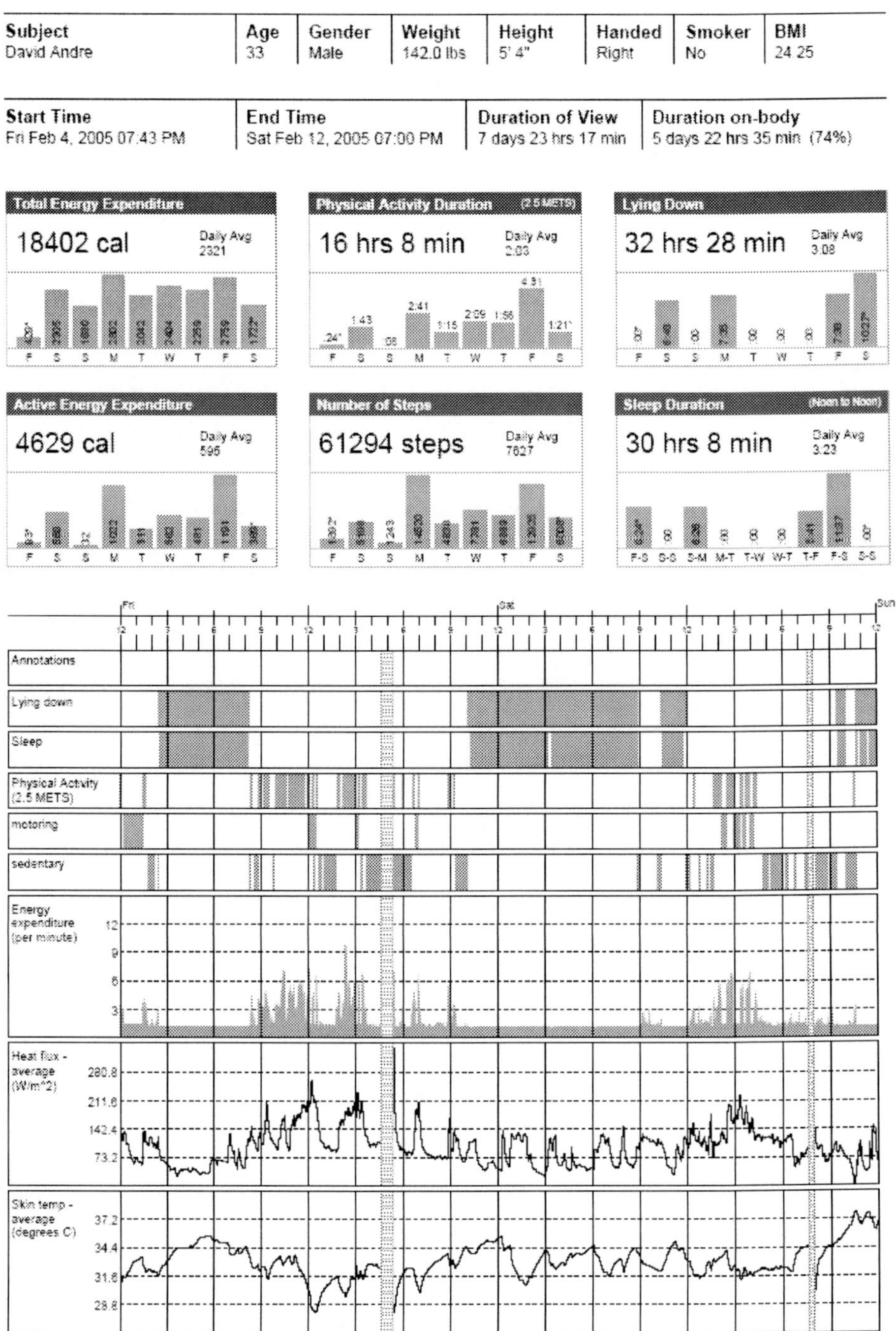

Figure 6. Reports from the Innerview Research Software.

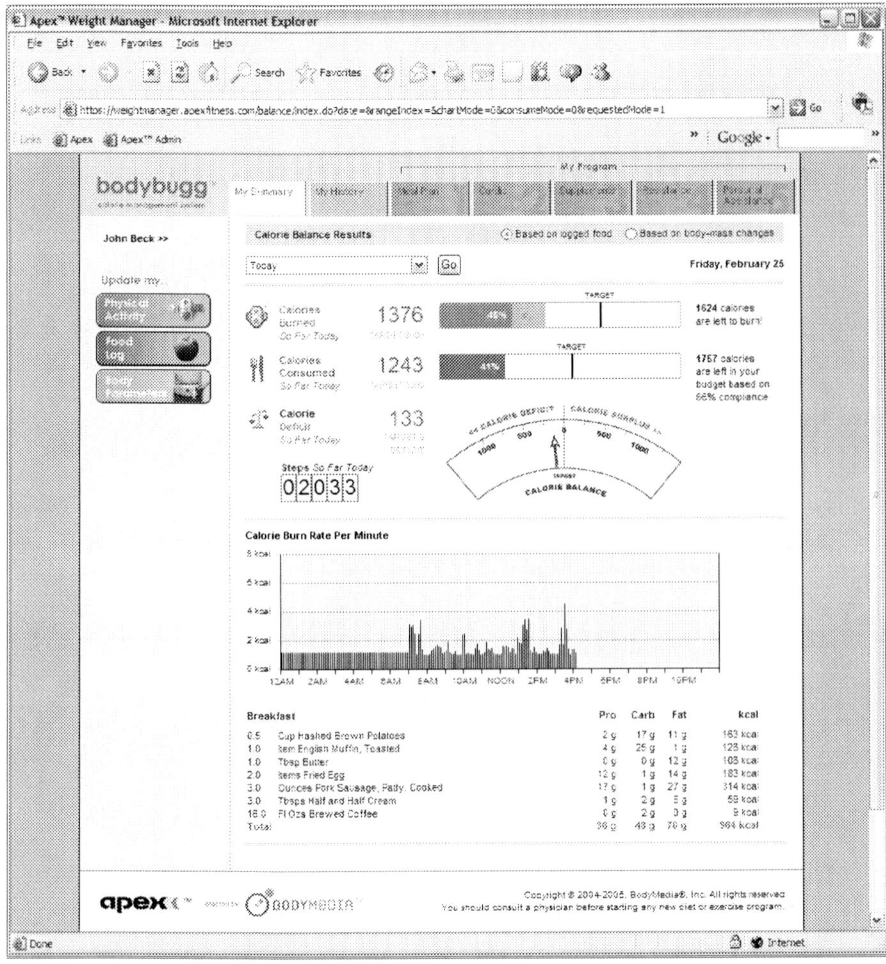

Figure 7. The bodybugg web application.

In addition to the Innerview Research software, the SenseWear system is utilized by several commercial web applications to address issues of wellness, weight-loss, and fitness. Apex Fitness and BodyMedia launched bodybugg (a private labeling of the BodyMedia technology) to the general public in the US at the start of 2005. On a daily basis, the body-bugg weight management system (the left side of Fig. 7) monitors and calculates a patient's caloric intake and expenditure and returns to both the patients and their care providers the difference between the two as the patient's day-by-day caloric balance. In providing this information, bodybugg is a weight management system that uses the continuous monitoring and collecting of physiological data to show the effect that lifestyle has on weight loss. Depicting calories burned, calories consumed, activity duration, and steps per day, the product strives to increase personal awareness of health and parameters of weight management. The ability for a third-party to view the data (in this case, the personal trainer or Fitness Professional) provides the user with a greater sense of integration and allows the third-party to give significantly better feedback. The bodybugg program (www.bodybugg.com) has thousands of users and is growing quickly.

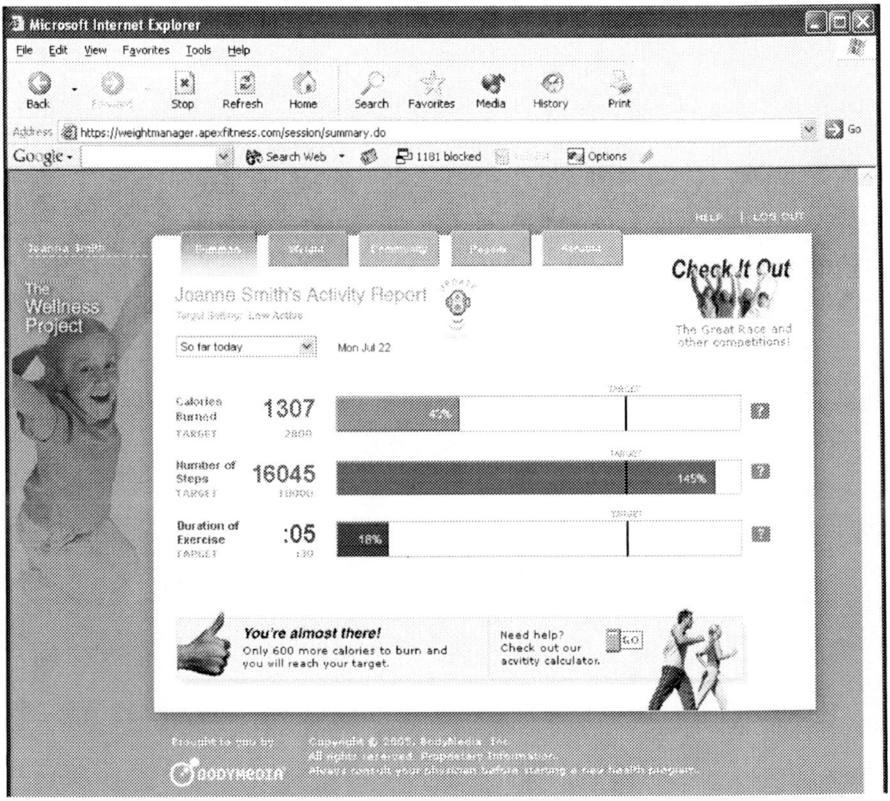

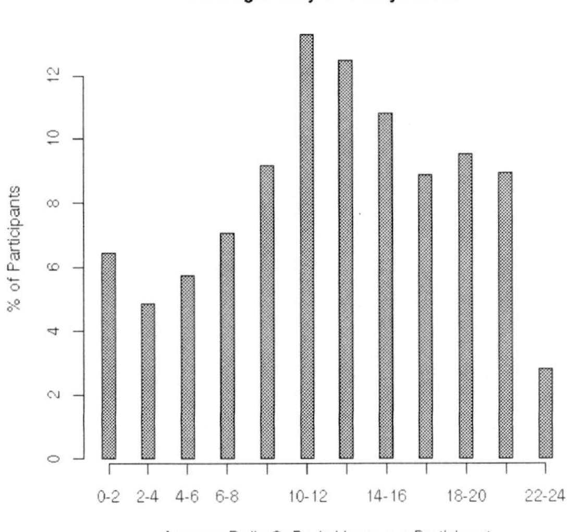

Figure 7a. The Wellness Project web application.

Average Daily OnBody Hours

Figure 7b. Daily use patterns from one of Bodymedia's commercial products.

Other variants of weight-management software have also been developed. One such system, designed for clinical weight management and diabetes management, has been piloted since 2003 with great results, with many subjects losing weight – even as much as 80 pounds. Another related application is The Wellness Project. This variant focuses on meeting calorie burn, step, and physical activity duration goals in the context of an online community setting. Groups can compete amongst their members or among different groups. The right side of Fig. 7 shows this web application.

One question many have when first encountering the armband is whether people will actually wear the armband over long periods of time. Figure 3 illustrates the amount of time users of the device actually wore it. That 83% of users wear it for more than 7 hours a day is a testament to the wearabilty of the device. To the extent that industry and commercial review is an indicator of reaching the goals for appropriate design, the SenseWear system has won both the Industrial Design Excellence Award and the Medical Device Excellence Award [22,23]. In fact, it is interesting that BodyMedia is the only company in the world ever to win top honors in both of these awards for the same product platform.

4. The Sociological Context of the Modeling of Human Health

Traditionally, models of human health have been models of how the human body works. That the previous sentence sounds like a tautology exposes how deep the bias goes that you cannot model human health without modeling how the human body works. This bias is understandable since until very recently there did not seem to be any alternative.

But the ability to put very small high performance computers on the human body in natural environments over long periods of time has opened a new avenue. That avenue is the modeling of human health through the modeling of the data given-off by the human body, often without any initial deep understanding of why that data is what it is. In Section 6, evidence will be presented that this method is accurate in powerful, valuable, and broad ways. But first, asks the skeptic, "Is this even good science?" "Should this even be allowed to count as a model of human health?"

Science is the making of models of the world and the testing of those models to show their predictive value. A model is nothing other than a simplification of the world, ideally reducing non-essential aspects of the world and retaining just those elements that are 'useful' (that are required for accurate predictions to be made). The 'models' or algorithms that BodyMedia constructs are mathematic simplifications of large amounts of raw data gathered with its devices, gathered in the presence of medical gold-standard lab equipment (such as metabolic carts (Fig. 8) or polysomnography machines) [2,1]. Ideally, these algorithms have captured the underlying trends in the data so that when worn by a person not in the presence of medical gold-standard equipment, the result a BodyMedia device returns accurately predicts what the medical gold-standard lab equipment would have returned in the same situation. So these are models of human health. They just happen to be models of what the body is doing rather than why it is doing it. These models are tested against the very same yardstick as classic models of human health: their ability to accurately predict what is happening to the body in question.

The next natural question, once the legitimacy of the method has been satisfied, is the real value of the method. There is a prevalent assumption, in both the medical industry and the general public, that any model built or 'learned' by a machine (as all statistical mathematical models are to some degree) could not possibly be as accurate, or as useful as a model built by a person. More specifically, there is often an unarticulated assumption that when these models are wrong they will be wrong in much larger or much more problematic ways than equivalent models built by a person. The first response to these concerns is that

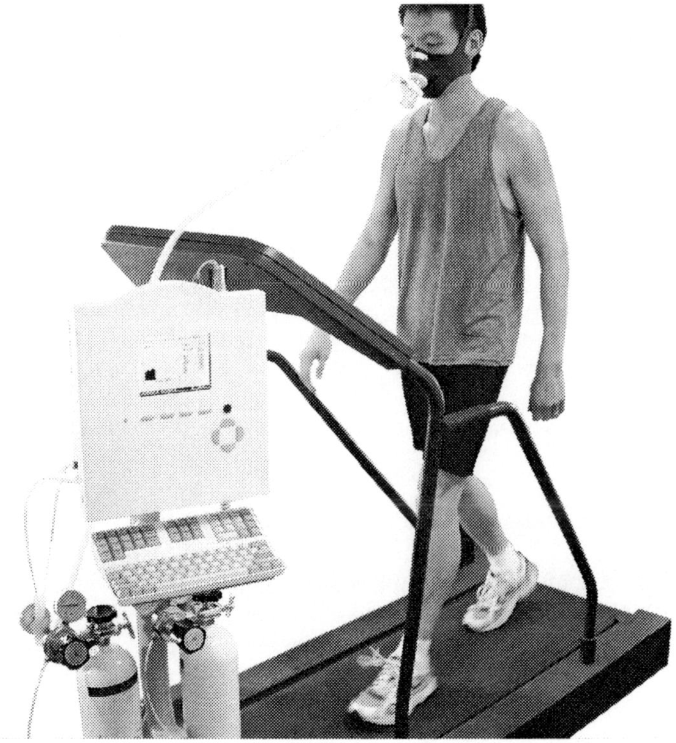

Figure 8. Metabolic cart in a lab setting.

real-time or long-term body monitoring in natural environments involves tens of thousands of times as much data as the current models of human health are built upon (periodic readings of blood pressure, cholesterol, bone density, etc.). Kuhn [24] describes the institutional adoption of new paradigms as a 25-year process; and it took the medical community the better part of a century to build a set of models of human health around this data. So waiting for a community, even one as smart and as dedicated as today's medical community, to build this next generation of models as we move, metaphorically, from physiologic snap shots to physiologic movies, is not realistic.

The second issue is that statistical mathematical models are built by trying to minimize some error function with respect to the predictions that connect the dependent axes (the inputs, which are in BodyMedia's case the raw data measured many times per second by the SenseWear Armband) to the independent axis (the output, the predicted value, in this case BodyMedia derived values such as sleep state, calories burned in the past day, body position, etc.). Assuming that the data has been properly collected (an assumption that is necessary for verification in all model building exercises) the people and situations on which these mathematical models are built and tested represent the conditions that happen the most often or are the most important to predict correctly. Models such as the ones built by BodyMedia are constructed explicitly to minimize these errors when applied to unseen subjects. This cannot honestly be said for more traditional models of human health because they have, as an additional constraint, that the model is understandable to the researcher building the model. The case can be made that special cases not seen during the training and testing phase of a statistical mathematical model may be predicted incorrectly in the real world. Of course, when these same special cases are withheld from human researchers building more classic models of human health, the same risk for a model that miss-predicts in these same situations exists.

5. Data Modeling, Data Mining and Sensor Fusion from Multi-Sensor Streams

'Bioinformatics,' is the intersection of life science and computer science. The SenseWear system allows for the gathering and interpreting of multiple streams of vital sign data which is then used to derive statements about the human body, such as calories burned, sleep, and activity type. The fundamental insight for BodyMedia is this—instead of monitoring individual parameters (symptoms) that healthcare institutions are used to looking at—blood pressure, pulse oximetry, cholesterol level and so on—BodyMedia monitors lower level vital signs many times a second, and then builds mathematical models of the data collected. These models are built in the context of the 'right answers' from medical gold standard equipment such as metabolic carts for energy expenditure or polysomnography for sleep states. This process of building mathematical models goes by several names in different disciplines, but is most commonly called supervised machine learning in the computer science community.

The process of supervised machine learning is the building of a model in some chosen representation (such as an artificial neural network, a decision tree, or a probabilistic network). Input signals are collected in the presence of the labels to be predicted by the model being learned. This set of input signals and labels is often referred to as the training set. These labels are usually either classifications (e.g. 'Astro was jogging between 2 and 3 pm') or regression values (e.g. 'Astro's level of energy expended in the past minute was 5.65 kcals'). These labels are treated as ground truth though in practice there is almost always some error in them. Statistical machine learning techniques (e.g. back propagation in the case of an artificial neural network) are then used to create, train, or 'learn' a model such that the model accurately relates the inputs to the known outputs (labels). These techniques often search through possible model frameworks to find the best one. The models are compared using methods such as statistical bootstrapping and cross-validation, which measure the ability of the model to generalize to unseen data. After the best model is selected, it is evaluated on a completely unseen set of data.

There is considerable science in picking from existing model representations or making a new representation when going through this supervised machine learning process. In addition, it is often the case (as it is with BodyMedia) that the predictions are not made by single classification or regression models, but by hierarchical or networked groups of these models. For example, for a stream of vital sign signals collected by the SenseWear Armband, a first model might attempt to classify the kind of activity represented by these signals (e.g. jogging, biking, resting, sleeping, etc.). Then, for each of these particular activities, a specialized model has been built that is particularly good at rating some prediction problem (e.g. energy expended per minute) for that particular kind of activity (e.g. biking). BodyMedia approaches the data modeling process through a variety of statistical methods including symbolic modeling where expert knowledge exists (e.g. Decision Trees, Production Systems, etc.), numeric modeling to fill in gaps in expert knowledge (e.g. Neural Networks, Bayesian Networks), state modeling for body states such as sleep states that shift in predictable ways (e.g. Hidden Markov Models, Partially Observable Markov Models), and clustering when all else fails or when labels are not available.

The bottom line, however, is that for real world problems, what generally makes the most difference is the quantity and quality of the training data available to the models being learned. To date the combined time that users, researchers, subjects, and customers have worn SenseWear Armbands amounts to over 300 million min over the past 5 years. Data

Armband Data by Time

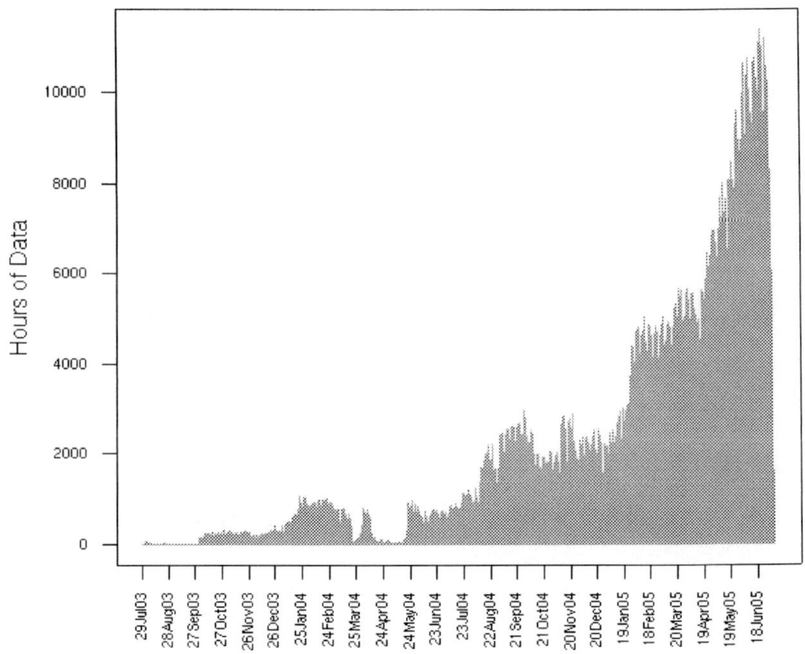

Figure 9. Hours of data uploaded to BodyMedia, by day.

from approximately 100 million minutes, from over 3000 individuals, have been collected by BodyMedia to form a corpus of physiological data. Of those 100 million minutes of physiological data (the inputs in our discussion above), around 10 million min of that data have been explicitly labeled as to their classification (e.g. 'lying in bed') or their level (e.g. stage 2 sleep according to the polysomnography machine). These 10 million min of streaming physiological data have been accrued from over 500 subjects with over 120 different labeled activity types.

Figure 9 shows the rate at which this data stream is increasing. The advantage of receiving all of this data is that even where the data is not annotated or explicitly labeled, the data can be used to improve the algorithms – both by helping in testing the algorithms but also through semi-supervised learning techniques. Exactly because this data improves the algorithms, users have some impetus to provide data, which can improve the information they themselves receive from the system. This creates a virtuous data cycle that encourages the use of the system and the contribution of data toward the general good.

The next question many ask is reasonably, 'Are all these different parameters really necessary?' The challenge in real world (i.e. out-of-the-hospital) body monitoring is that there are a lot of states of the human body that are ambiguous when seen from the perspective of a single sensor. By choosing sensors carefully, a higher dimensional space of streaming vital signs can disambiguate these human body states, dramatically increasing what a wearable device can determine; and increase the accuracy of any indirect measurements derived from the lower-level vital signs.

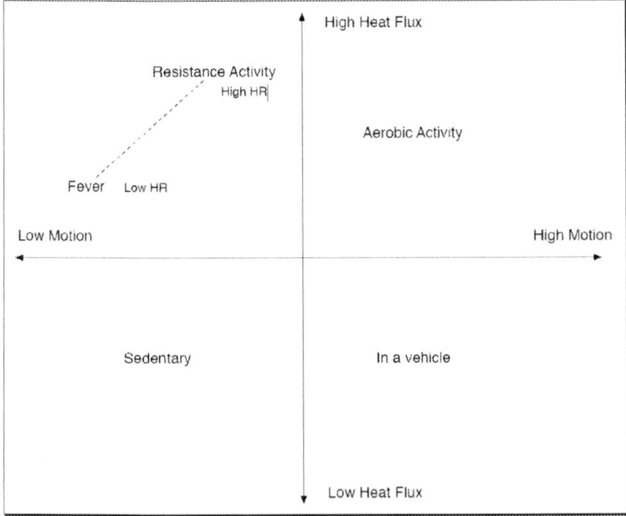

Figure 10. Activity and condition map: sedentary, vehicle, aerobic, resistance vs. fever characterized by heat, motion and heart rate.

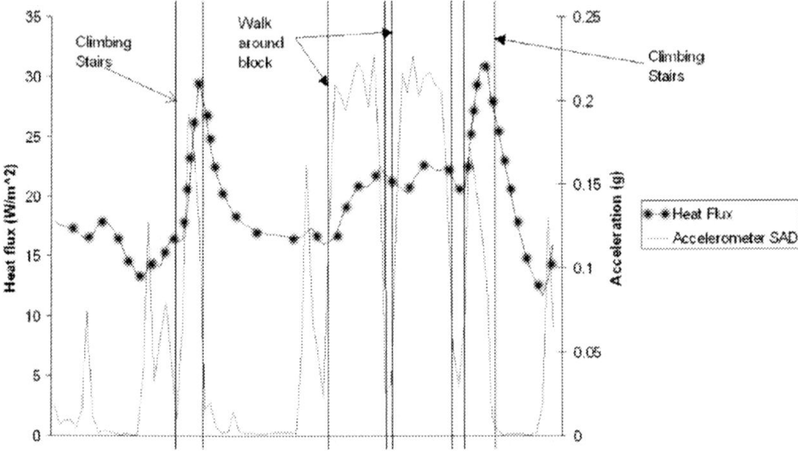

Figure 11. Sensor data from accelerometery and heat flux comparing flat walking and stair climbing.

Figure 10 shows a simplistic example of how multi-sensors can disambiguate human body states that would appear ambiguous to any single sensor. In this example, the challenge is to identify the type of state the human body is currently in. The use of multiple sensors can also help to more accurately capture the correct level from a particular category. For example in Fig. 11, a model that could see only the motion of a person would credit the person with a higher level of energy expended per minute during the 'walk around the block' activities rather than during the 'climbing stair' activities. This is, it turns out, generally false. And that can be seen by the model built by BodyMedia through the use of multiple sensors. Again in Fig. 11, we see that the rate the person is producing and releasing heat is higher during the stair climbing activities and the models can take advantage of this additional information to more closely approximate what a metabolic cart (one of the

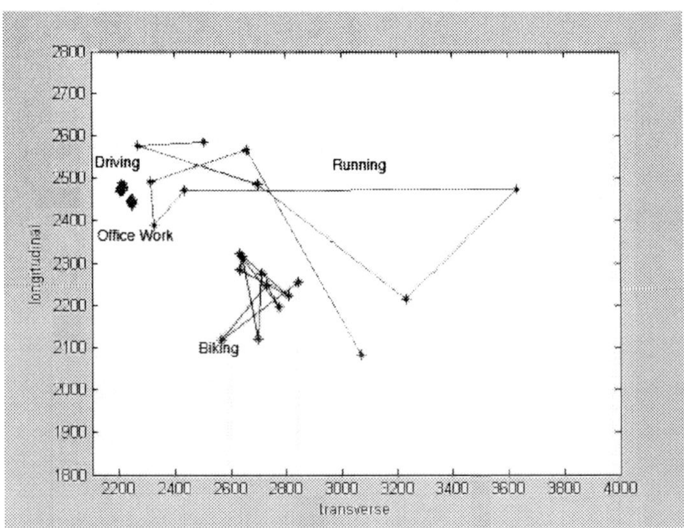

Figure 12. Longitudinal and transverse accelerometer data from the armband for biking, running, driving, and office conditions (in micrograms per millisecond).

medical gold standards on the subject of energy expenditure) would say under these same circumstances.

In practice, these examples do not capture the complexities the models must address. For example, it is possible that if during a period sensor A is increasing and sensor B is decreasing, or vice versa, then the output should be judged to be increasing, but if both or neither of the sensors is increasing, then the output should be judged to be decreasing. This sort of relationship cannot be captured by any first order statistical models as the correlations between A, B, and the output are all zero. This conceptual example highlights the demands on the models being learned to capture arbitrarily complex relationships in the data, not just linear trends. As an example of this, in Fig. 12, examples from four classes of human activity are shown. In all four cases, the two axes represent two orthogonal dimensions of motion and the points represent a trace in that two dimensional space over two seconds. What we see here are patterns that might be thought of as 'strange attractors' that help to identify and differentiate these different activities. These patterns are not just a matter of the amount of motion per minute, but the kinds or patterns of motion that occur in sequences over short (or even over long) periods of time.

What does all this amount to in the end? These learned models allows BodyMedia, with very high accuracy, to say to a new user who puts on a SenseWear Armband statements such as, "You burned 400 calories over the past hour" or "You were in bed for 8 hours last night, but you only slept for 5 hours and with frequent interruptions." The following table shows our current accuracies for a set of new vital signs we derive from the raw data.

Algorithm	Accuracy	Algorithm	Accuracy
Energy Expenditure	Error < 10%	Lying down duration	Error < 1%
Exercise Duration	Error < 3%	Sleep onset	Error < 3 minutes
Exercise type recognition	Error < 5%	Wake Time	Error < 3 minutes
Step count	Error < 2%	Sleep Duration	Error < 5%
Sedentary duration	Error < 3%	Motoring Duration	Error < 5%

Independent researchers have written many validation papers about the SenseWear system, especially with respect to comparing energy expenditure measurements from the system to estimates from gold-standard laboratory equipment. These include tests on normal individuals from 18 to 75 on a variety of exercise equipment comparing against indirect calorimetry, such as Jakicic et al. [25], Fruin and Rankin [26], Wadsworth et al. [27], and McClain et al. [28], all showing significant correlations. Several researchers have examined disease-specific populations, such as cardiac patients [29] and patients with chronic obstructive pulmonary disease [30], finding good results as well. In a very interesting preliminary study, Mignault et al. [31] compare the armband to doubly labeled water over a ten day period. The subjects were diabetics examined as part of a larger study. In these patients, the researchers noticed no significant differences between the doubly labeled water technique and the estimates from the armband. The correlations were extremely high (0.9696), with a technical error of measurement of only 104 kcal/day (less than 5%). The authors conclude: "... preliminary analyses suggest that the [...] Armband is an acceptable device to accurately measure total daily energy expenditure in type 2 diabetic patients over a 10-day period".

Human body data, when aggregated, also has tremendous value beyond the value of the individual statements to individual users. The revolution in the financial services industry over the past 30 years came as a direct result of the access to and real-time analysis of the world's minute-to-minute financial vital signs. Wearable physiological computing is just at the beginning of a similar revolution as a natural outcome of pulling additional meaning from the long-term, detailed, objective and accurate views of the physical states of large numbers of people and transforming these into meaningful, desirable, and actionable applications. We envision utilizing this data scientifically for data mining and commercially as a resource for creating and improving algorithms. It will be possible to compare a user's data with similar users, creating empirical definitions of what is the norm and what is abnormal. These data mining challenges and opportunities on large collections of group data are in their infancy, but an active area of effort for BodyMedia.

6. Research and Development Directions

While there are many exciting on-going applications discussed above, BodyMedia is engaging in continued refinements to the platform and the development of new body monitoring capabilities. These including the integration of new sensors and the ongoing development of data models to extract new physiological features and contextual activities. Some of the areas that BodyMedia is focusing on include: fine-grained sleep detail (e.g. Rapid Eye Movement); personal duress; fatigue, alertness, drowsiness; mental stress, anxiety; hydration, perfusion, homeostasis; surrogates for glucose level; calories consumed (when, and approximate quantity); biometric identification ('finger printing' based on personal biometrics); heart information taken solely on the upper arm; and core body temperature prediction. Efforts to make the device more unobtrusive are also underway.

For all of these areas, BodyMedia has collected some anecdotal data and discovered, in many cases, compelling signs that significant opportunities for armband-based monitoring exist. For example, in the case of measuring heart signals from the upper arm, BodyMedia has discovered a new, patent-pending, method of obtaining electrical signals from the heart solely from electrodes placed on the upper left arm continuously, and for extended periods of time. This latest BodyMedia innovation can record ECG data from the upper arm, as well as other locations on the human body previously considered impractical by conventional standards, without wires, adhesives, or other equipment. BodyMedia has integrated the technology into prototype versions of the armband using one non-adhesive electrode

                    D. Andre and A. Teller / Health. Care. Anywhere. Today

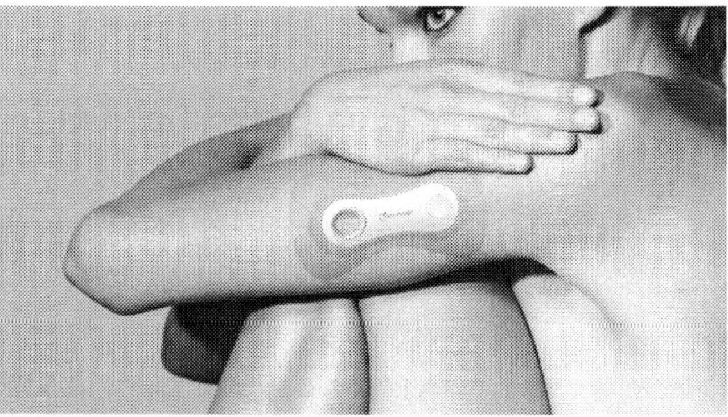

Figure 13. A prototype version of a future BodyMedia platform for ambient computing.

and one adhesive electrode. Production of a non-adhesive system is underway. Their invention is particularly noteworthy because it challenges conventional wisdom in electrocardiology that ECG can only be observed using electrodes spaced on "either side" of the heart. Al-Ahmad, Homer, and Wang [32] have presented preliminary results of validating these prototypes, showing that the armband measures heart rate and beat-to-beat variability comparably to a Holter monitor. Preliminary results in incorporating heart rate information into the equations for energy expenditure are supporting McClain et al's [28] finding that the incorporation of heart rate can reduce the error of the algorithms for certain activities. Figure 13 shows a prototype of a new version of the device that incorporates heart-rate electrodes in a patch version of the armband.

To accomplish many of these research goals for additional body state prediction, further additional sensors may need to be added to versions of the body monitors made by Body-Media. BodyMedia is experimenting with acoustic sensors; optical sensors, pressure and barometric sensors; GPS digital compass, and gyroscopic elements; ambulatory blood pressure; micro-needles for the administration of medication and sample collection; ambulatory pulse oximetry; bioimpedance [33], and near-body ambient air and environmental sensors. The potential to increase the understanding of human physiology in natural settings and humans' physiological interactions with their environment is substantial.

7. Conclusions

As many pundits have commented, the current state of healthcare is problematic. Costs are skyrocketing and the current institutions are breaking under the load. Consumers are getting saddled with more of the financial responsibility of their own healthcare. Dissatisfied with their options and their care, many patients fail to comply with the treatments and programs that can best help them. Patients and caregivers alike have a hard time managing that which they can't see – and it is exactly those things that go unmeasured that are costing us the most – 1.2 *trillion* dollars last year alone.

In attempting to address these problems, we must take into account several factors. First, healthcare will increasingly come to be ruled by consumers due to the power of the market. Second, consumers will need personal health care tools to help them manage their health and wellness through helping them manage the root causes of their health and wellness – their choices and behaviors. Nearly all of the tools that consumers end up using will require as inputs physiological information about their bodies. This will require wearable body monitoring that is simultaneously medical-grade and consumer-desirable.

BodyMedia is today addressing this need by following a few simple principles. We strive to find the new vital signs that resonate with consumers and the behaviors they wish to manage. In addition to incorporating our increasing knowledge of the human body, we also directly model the relationship between these new vital signs and the physiological signals we can measure from the body. A fundamental question for us is "how can we get accurate information from the body in a way users will love?" Given that users won't wear twenty different devices, we work to build a single system that delivers value on multiple fronts from the same piece of effort. Finally, we recognize that continuous body monitoring is providing data that science and medicine haven't seen before. We are working to build systems that take advantage of these increasingly large data streams both to better help the consumer and to increase our knowledge of health, physiology, and human behavior.

The SenseWear system and its applications are a first step toward a vision of the future of healthcare that enables users to manage their health and care for their bodies anywhere they choose to do so. The future of healthcare is happening today.

Acknowledgements

The authors would like to thank the many, many researchers who incorporate our products into their research and share their assessments with the world. We'd also like to acknowledge everyone at Bodymedia who created the products, systems, and concepts that make it all possible. Special thanks to Jong-Lin Yu, Chris Pacione, Max Crossley, Jonny Farringdon, Quang Tang for their assistance in creating this chapter.

References

[1] Van Bemmel, J.H., Musen, M.A. (Eds.), 1997. Handbook of Medical Informatics. Springer, New York.
[2] Timmermans, S., Berg, M., 2002. The Gold Standard: a Sociological Exploration of Evidence-Based Medicine and Standardization in Health Care. Temple University Press, Philadelphia, PA.
[3] Weisner, M., July 1996. Some Computer Science Issues in Ubiquitous Computing Communications of the ACM, July 1993. (Reprinted as Ubiquitous Computing. Nikkei Electronics, December 6, 1993, pp. 137–143).
[4] Weisner, M., Brown, J., 1996. The coming age of calm technology updated version of 'Designing Calm Technology'. PowerGrid Journal 1.01.
[5] Moore, G.E., April 19, 1965. Cramming more components onto integrated circuits Electronics. 38 (8). Retrieved on May 15th, 2004 from the World Wide Web: ftp://download.intel.com/research/silicon/moorespaper.pdf.
[6] Wilhelm, F.H., Roth, W.T., Sackner, M., 2004. The LifeShirt: an advanced system for ambulatory measurement of respiratory and cardiac function. Behavior Modification 2004; in press.
[7] Fitsense, 2004. Retrieved on May 15th, 2004 from the World Wide Web: http://www.fitsense.com.
[8] Polar USA, Heart Monitors, 2004. Retrieved on May 15th, 2004 from the World Wide Web: http://www.polarusa.com/.
[9] Glucon, 2005. Retrieved on March 13th, 2005 from the World Wide Web: http://www.glucon.com.
[10] Pittman, S.D., Pillar, G., Ayas, N.T., Suraiya, S., Malhorta, A., White, D.P., 2002. Can obstructive apnea be diagnosed in the home using a wrist-mounted device with automated analysis of peripheral arteral tonometry, pulse oximetry and actigraphy? Sleep 25, A42–A43.
[11] Surratt, P.M., Nikova, M., D'Andrea, L., 1996. Actigraphy measurements of sleep and activity during sleep in children with sleep disorder breathing. Sleep 25, A54–A55.
[12] Chun, S.H., 1999. Salutron Technology Evaluation Data Summary. Stanford Hospital, Fremont, CA.
[13] Jakicic, J.M., Winters, C., Lagally, K., Ho, J., Robertson, R.J., Wing, R.R., 1998. The accuracy of the TriTrac-R3d accelerometer to estimate energy expenditure. ACSM 1998.
[14] Gemperle, F., Kasabach, C., Stivoric, J., Bauer, M., Martin, R., 1998. Design for wearability. In: IEEE International Symposium on Wearable Computers, Pittsburgh, PA, USA.
[15] Forlizzi, J., McCormack, M., 2000. Case study: user research to inform the design and development of integrated wearable computers and web based services, Proceedings of the ACM Conference on Designing Interactive Systems 2000.

[16] Spohn, J., Sunday, May 2, 2004. Fitness challenge means steady monitoring; Post-Gazzett.com, Pittsburgh, PA.

[17] Teller, A., Stivoric, J., Kasabach, C., Pacione, C., Moss, J., Liden, C., McCormack, M., 2003. System For Monitoring Health, Wellness and Fitness patent, United States Patent No. 6,605,038.

[18] Tate, D.F., Wing, R.R., Winett, R.A., 2001. Using Internet technology to deliver a behavioral weight loss program. Journal of the American Medical Association 285, 1172–1177.

[19] Lisetti, C., Nasoz, F., LeRouge, C., Ozyer, O., Alvarez, K., 2004. Developing Multimodal Intelligent Affective Interfaces for Tele-Home Health Care.

[20] Work with Arup Engineering, cited on Bodymedia web page: http://landslide/research/customers.jsp.

[21] Perini, M., Fiocchi, A., Bollini, F., Lanfranchi, S., Zarcone, D., 2005 Relationship between Active Energy Expenditure in Sydenham's Chorea: A Clinical Case. May 2005.

[22] IDEA, 2002. Retrieved on May 15th, 2004 from the World Wide Web: http://new.idsa.org/idea/idea2002/medsci.htm.

[23] MEDA, April 2004. From Algo to Zassi: 2004. Winners Shine in Design, Medical Device and Diagnostic Industry. Retrieved on May 15th, 2004 from the World Wide Web: http://www.devicelink.com/mddi/archive/04/04/004.html.

[24] Kuhn, T., 1962. The Structure of Scientific Revolutions. University of Chicago Press, Chicago, IL.

[25] Jakicic, J.M., Marcus, M., Gallagher, K., Randall, C., Thomas, E., Goff, F.L., Robertson, R.J., 2004 Evaluation of the SenseWear Pro Armband® to Assess Energy Expenditure During Exercise. Medicine & Science in Sports & Exercise. 36(5):897–904.

[26] Fruin, M.L., Rankin, J.W., 2004 Validity of a Multi-Sensor Armband in Estimating Rest and Exercise Energy Expenditure. Medicine & Science in Sports & Exercise. 36(6):1063–1069.

[27] Wadsworth, D.D., Howard, T., Hallam, J.S., Blunt, G., A Validation Study Of A Continuous Body-monitoring Device: Assessing Energy Expenditure At Rest And During Exercise, Medicine & Science in Sports & Exercise: Volume 37(5) Supplement May 2005 p. S24.

[28] McClain, James J.1; Welk, Gregory J.2; Wickel, Eric E.2; Eisenmann, Joey C.2, Accuracy Of Energy Expenditure Estimates From The Bodymedia Sensewear® Pro 2 Armband, Medicine & Science in Sports & Exercise: Volume 37(5) Supplement May 2005 p. S116–S117.

[29] Cole, P.J., LeMura, L.M., Klinger, T.A., Strohecker, K, McConnell, T.R., 2004. Measure Energy Expenditure In Cardiat Patients Using The BodyMedia™ Armband Versus Indirect Calorimetry. A Validation Study. Journal of Sports Medicine and Physical Fitness.

[30] COPD, Patel, S.A., MD, MPH, Slivka, W.A., RPFT, Sciurba, F.C., MD, 2004. Validation Of A Wearable Body Monitoring Device In COPD. American Journal of Respiratory and Critical Care Medicine. University of Pittsburgh, Pittsburgh, PA.

[31] Mignault, D., St.-Onge, M., Karelis, A.D., Allison, D.B., Rabasa-Lhoret, R., 2005 Evaluation of the Portable HealthWear Armband. Diabetes Care January 2005 Article.

[32] Al-Ahmad, A., Homer, M., Wang, P., 2004. Accuracy and Utility of Multi-Sensor Armband ECG Signal Compared With Holter Monitoring. Cardiac Arrhythmia Service, Stanford University Medical Center, Stanford, CA New Arrhythmia Technologies Retreat in Chicago, IL.

[33] Grimnes, S., Martinsen, Ø., 2000. Bioimpedance and Bioelectricity Basics. Academic Press, New York. ISBN 0-12-3032601-1.

Future of Intelligent and Extelligent Health Environment
R.G. Bushko (Ed.)
IOS Press, 2005

How Do We Get the
Medical Intelligence Out?

Aaron OPPENHEIMER
Principal Product Behaviorist, Design Continuum Inc., Boston, MA, US

Abstract. Two factors are driving a new wave of medical products. The first is the use of technology to make products "intelligent" – that is, build them not only to measure a particular parameter, like blood glucose, but to help patients and caregivers *manage conditions*. This allows the users of these products focus less on the technical aspects of treating a condition (e.g. calculating the proper amount of insulin to treat a given level of blood glucose) and more on the overall management of the disease. The second development is the rapid movement of devices from the doctor's office to the home. Chain drugstores carry dozens of medical devices for home use by consumers. The challenge for manufacturers and designers is to present the medical device's intelligence in a way that is palatable to the consumer. One important theme is that medical product consumers are also consumers of everything else: home electronics, appliances, clothing, etc. These consumers are applying the same decision-making processes they use when buying a blender to the process of buying a medical device. It is therefore necessary for medical product manufacturers to create devices that interact with consumers in consumer-friendly ways. Putting intelligence into a product is one thing; helping the consumer utilize and appreciate it is quite another. This chapter covers some principles to keep in mind, and discusses a framework for better design of intelligent medical products that connect with consumers on emotional and functional levels beyond simple medical efficacy.

1. Understanding Product Intelligence

As a product designer, it seems to me that getting "intelligence" into a product is easy. Research effort aside, it just takes time, money, and the typical development activities required to make anything into a product. I find that the hard part is getting the intelligence *out*: designing the consumer's experience with the product so she can enjoy all of its intended benefit. An "intelligent" product tends to want to change the world somewhat: to alter the process someone goes through as they (for instance) manage a disease. However, if not done carefully, the new process won't be adopted, in which case the manufacturer needn't have bothered. A product that tries to force a change in process may be rejected outright by consumers set in their ways. And while a product that supplies added features on top of a currently existing use model may avoid summary rejection, the features may never be used (consider the percentage of features on your cell phone that you actually use regularly). When the gap between what the manufacturer envisions and what the consumer is equipped to receive can be very wide, results disappoint on both sides: the consumer doesn't get what he thought he was going to get; the manufacturer doesn't change the world the way he imagined (not to mention lackluster sales).

Consider the Palm Pilot as a supremely successful product that provided "intelligence" in a product category that had seen modest successes and dismal failures. Technology pundits often use the Palm Pilot as an example of a product that succeeded because it was so much "simpler" than those products that came before. But the Palm Pilot was not particularly simple; among other things, it required the consumer to learn an entirely new skill – modified handwriting as computer input – just to use it at all. The Palm Pilot succeeded by offering the right connection between the technology inside and the consumer outside, providing a mix of features, interactions, and physical embodiment that could be easily understood, internalized, and utilized.

Finding this connection is the real challenge in turning any technology into product, and making the product "intelligent" increases that challenge. Intelligent products are no longer just tools – they do not simply perform a single function, but rather go beyond and extend their roles, gathering information and making decisions. As such, they become more like other people: they're assistants, nurses, coaches. Designing products like these requires more than just smart algorithms and low cost – it requires the manufacturer to think about the product at a higher level; to understand how people relate to *each other* and to embody in a product some of the attributes that lend themselves to successful interpersonal communications.

In their book, The Media Equation,[1] Byron Reeves and Clifford Nass describe sociological experiments they performed to understand communication, not between people, but between people and media (computers, television, etc.). They found that people treat interactions with "intelligent" systems the same way they treat interactions with other people; we humans are wired to answer politeness with politeness, to spare feelings, to assume that anyone looking directly at us (even on TV) is talking directly to us. This shouldn't be tremendously surprising; after all, for most of human history, the only things in our environment with which we enjoyed social interactions were other people. It's only very recently that inanimate objects started beeping and flashing at us – on other words, being social with us. Since we evolved to understand social interaction as a human-to-human activity, it makes sense for us to apply our sense of how to socialize to the newcomers to our social circles, like TV and computers.

As products get more "intelligent," the social rules hardwired in our brains become more important for designers to understand and leverage. If a manufacturer intends to give a product the power to help make decisions, the product needs to be trustworthy and persuasive, among other human-like traits. This is not simple anthropomorphizing; the point is not to give a product a "human" face or voice just to be cute (see Microsoft Word's defunct "talking paperclip" assistant). The notion is that, to communicate intelligence to the user of the product, designers must understand what *communication* means in this context.

We've all known people who were undeniably intelligent – capable of nuanced thought and delicate decision-making – but who were nevertheless incapable of simple, easygoing communication with other people. In a person, this can be off-putting; in a product, it can be maddening. As designers, we must imbue our intelligent medical products with the ability to communicate effectively; we want users to form relationships with their products. If we fail, the product's intelligence is for naught.

2. Principles

The issues to consider when designing an intelligent medical product are both complex and complicated. Designing well requires deep understanding of the context of a product's use – who will use it, where, when, etc. And it requires a broad view of what's possible and what's realistic. But careful consideration of a few principles serves the designer well:

---

[1] Byron Reeves and Clifford Nass, *The Media Equation* (CSLI Publications, 1996).

1. Technology and Benefit Are Not the Same: the magic that makes a product run is not as important as what it enables for the end user.
2. Your Product Is Important, But Not That Important: a manufacturer's perspective on his product is different than that of the consumer.
3. Avoid the Lure of the Dubious: features that don't add value make a product worse, not better.
4. The Consumer Is, and Is Not, the Problem: "user error" is a reality, but that doesn't mean manufacturers can abdicate responsibility for making products manageable.
5. A Patient Is a Consumer: In the end, what matters in medical product design are the same things that matter in the design of any product: efficacy, of course, but also concepts like self-image and projected image.

These are simple principles, and may even seem obvious when out of the context of your project, but failure to understand these ideas results in products that are complicated, frustrating, and, in worst case, market failures.

2.1. Principle 1: Technology and Benefit Are Not the Same

Just handing over a piece of technology is not the same as magically imbuing benefit. Making it possible for a diabetes patient to connect his glucose meter to the internet for the purposes of uploading data into a web-based database, where it can be managed by an intelligent application that looks for trends and makes dietary and exercise recommendations via pager, doesn't mean the patient will ever see the value in it. And patients who do understand the value of such a system may never master the process for getting data into and out of the system.

It's often said that people hate technology, but that's not really true. What people hate is *dealing with* technology: setup, configuration, troubleshooting. People love technology that hides the "tech," delivering only the benefit – hence the popularity of automatic transmissions, auto-focus cameras, and microwave popcorn. These products are "higher tech," but they are also simpler to use, in that they take guesswork, burdensome decision-making, and grueling calculation out of the hands (and off the back) of consumers. The goals of an intelligent medical product (error reduction, improved communication, labor saving) are generally met the same way: by shifting some burden from the end user to the device. The designer's job is to understand what the burdens really are and to determine the proper way to shift them with a minimum amount of disruption. If an automatic transmission required a driver to manually enter the speeds at which it should shift, using a keypad, every time the car was started, it would be unpopular; in such a system, not enough of the burden has been shifted. And a transmission that makes decisions not only about shifting but also about how fast to go might be taking on too much of the driving task – at least for now. Such automatic driving systems are featured in countless science-fiction films, and real-world collision-avoidance systems are occasionally demonstrated in concept form by automobile manufacturers, but today's consumer may not be prepared to actually rely on one.

This is an interesting point: The definition of the "appropriate" level of burden to lift from the user changes as attitudes about what's important change. For example, what seems like an acceptable level of hassle to manage diabetes today may seem like an unacceptable millstone at some future date. Manufactures of medical devices must often play the dangerous game of predicting what will seem "normal" several years in the future when their device finally ships to consumers.

The point is simply that what's important to consumers is not the technology, but what it does for them.

2.2. Principle 2: Your Product Is Important, but Not That Important

To a manufacturer, his product is the most important thing in the world. Envisioning it, designing it, engineering, manufacturing, marketing, selling – those things are exciting, besides the fact that they put food on his table.

To the consumer, however, it's one product out of hundreds in her life. Think about the products that you use every day. Here's a list of just the gadgets I used this morning: alarm clock, baby monitor, television, cable box, stereo, toaster, stove, microwave, refrigerator, cell phone, computer (laptop connected to gateway connected to cable modem, with email and web browser), electric toothbrush, and space heater – all of this within the first hour of my day.

Even a product that makes a large impact tends to fade into the background fairly quickly, replaced front-of-mind by other products, or just daily life; each of the gizmos I used was a big deal when it first arrived, and is now just part of the landscape. It is tempting to say something like, "yes, but *my* device is life-changing (or life-supporting) and so will automatically be always front-of-mind" – but to do this is to lose sight of why we create these devices in the first place: to make the patient's life more "normal," which is to say, unencumbered. We *want* our devices to disappear. Consider this maxim: if the stage lighting for a play is ever mentioned in a review, it has failed. The same should be true of medical products, and manufacturers should strive to create devices that don't need to be front-of-mind.

The upshot is that intelligent devices need to be intelligent in their expectations of the consumer. For the same reasons that a child must be taught to say "excuse me" in order to get an adult's attention, devices must consider their place in a consumer's life. We are bombarded by messages from the products around us, and are very well versed in the art of filtering most of them out. Products must be smart in the ways they communicate with consumers; they can't assume full attention from the user. We only need look at the mobile phone market to get a feel for the issues. A typical mobile may light up, play an irritating tune, or vibrate – or do all at once – in order to get attention, and sometimes even that's not enough.

If a medical device is to grab attention from a consumer, it must insinuate itself into the user's *process* – it must make itself indispensable, and create a situation where the patient gives the product attention automatically.

2.3. Principle 3: Avoid the Lure of the Dubious

Don't add features unrelated to a device's function in an attempt to become "more important" to a consumer. Features only make sense in light of the overall personality and occupation of a product; adding a feature unrelated to these just makes the product more complicated. For example, a bedside medical device needn't include an alarm clock just because the consumer might travel with it to a hotel. Assuming consumers will learn to program yet another digital clock in their lives isn't doing them a service – most mobile phones have alarm clocks built into them, but how many of us bother to learn to use them? A medical device is there to provide medical benefit, and just because it happens to have a clock built in for logging purposes does not mean the consumer needs or wants another alarm clock.

This emphasizes one of the curses that go along with the blessing of cheap technology: if a device has any electronics in it at all, the incremental cost to add some more is generally small. When a device has a microprocessor inside, adding features can be just a matter of software. It's important for designers to keep the purpose of the product in mind, and fight the urge to "bulk up" a product by adding features just because it's inexpensive to do

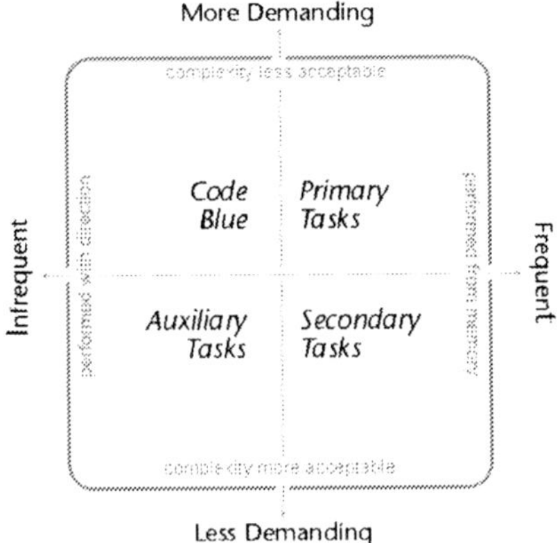

Figure 1. Frequency/Intensity Map.

so. Consumers have a better chance of building a relationship with straightforward products that are easy to learn and easy to use over time.

2.4. Principle 4: The Consumer Is, and Is Not, the Problem

At some point, everyone will fail in their attempts to use a product to perform a task. Whether it's cutting a finger while chopping an onion, getting into a fender-bender while driving a car, or misaddressing an irate email, Murphy's Law is always in effect: whatever can go wrong, will go wrong. Even with life-saving medical equipment, people are only human; according to a report on medical mistakes from the National Academy of Sciences' Institute of Medicine, as many as 98,000 Americans die each year due to medical errors.[2]

There's a temptation among manufacturers to call such events "user error," and to treat them as just part of the unpredictable consequences of putting technology and people together – and sometimes they are. But a product designer's job must include a certain amount of predicting what could go wrong, and designing the product to avoid the situation if possible, deal with it when it happens, and clean up the mess afterward.

Much of the design of product behavior consists of the equivalent of what engineers refer to as FMEA – Failure Mode and Effects Analysis. The process consists of examining a system, its subsystems, and their components, and trying to understand the failures that could occur, their effects, their causes, and how they can be detected and corrected, or redesigned for avoidance. For the behavior designer, this analysis is as high-level as "does the device get left home by accident?" and as detailed as "does the color of the text on screen make it less readable?"

One way to help avoid errors has already been discussed above: understanding the position a device holds in the consciousness of the end user, and designing the device to "live there." I need to consider what it will take to get the user's attention given what I know about how the user is relates to the device. If it's a back-of-mind, set-and-forget sort of product like an insulin pump, I may need to do something different than if it's a consult-every-five-minutes product like an anesthesiology device.

A commonly-used tool for analyzing product features to better understand the relationship between user and product is the Frequency/Intensity map [see Fig. 1].

A Frequency/Intensity map is a representation of when and how particular features are used. Each feature (or task to be done with a product) is rated along two axes: its frequency

---

[2] Institute of Medicine, "To Err Is Human: Building a Safer Health System" (2000).

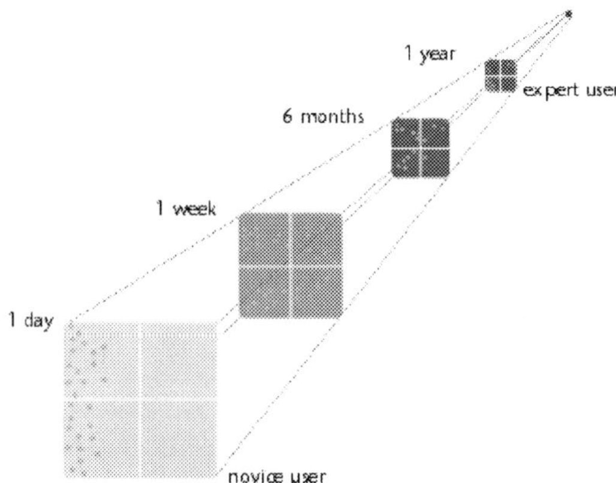

Figure 2. Changes in frequency/intensity over time.

(how often the job is performed) and its intensity (how much concentration is required by the end user).

For example, consider designing an intelligent, handheld product to assist a librarian in her daily tasks. Careful observation of a librarian would uncover a long list of things she does during her day; the question is, how best to support her? We could start by mapping each of her tasks:

- Helping people find stuff: this is high frequency, high intensity – a "primary task," one that is at the core of being a librarian.
- Shelving books: this is high frequency, but low intensity – it happens all the time, but it's rather mindless; a "secondary task"
- Pointing people to the bathroom: low frequency, low intensity – not really part of a librarian's job, it nonetheless occurs occasionally as an "auxiliary task."
- Transporting a Gutenberg Bible from the rare book room one part of the building to another – it doesn't happen often, but when it does, it requires careful concentration. This is what we might call a "code blue" task; this is hospital slang for "something really important is happening, so pay attention."

With this level of understanding of a librarian's day, we can start to make good choices when it comes to designing an assistant. Helping the librarian find stuff would be a good place to start. Building an automatic "this way to the bathroom" sign would be less useful. Deciding whether or not to build in a Gutenberg Transporter is probably a business decision more than a help-the-user decision; it might not happen regularly enough for the librarian to really care about a technological solution, but might be high profile enough that the device with such a feature could get some visibility in the marketplace.

We must add another layer of complexity to our frequency/intensity model by acknowledging that the relationship between user and product changes over time [see Fig. 2]. Let's say we've sold a many-featured medical product to a consumer. When he takes it out of the box and tries it for the first time, every feature is new – in effect, they are all low-frequency, and many are high-intensity. Over the next few days, as the patient figures out how to live with the product, the intensity of performing the basic functions will settle down, and as a rhythm develops, the frequency of some of the tasks will also drop. One year later, only a few functions may be regularly used, and the patient will be an expert at using them. Once in a while, though, something will pop up requiring extra attention. What we see is, though it is often suggested that a product have a "novice" mode and an "expert" mode, the reality is that people tend to be both at once for various uses of a product.

This sort of analysis is universally applicable: every component of every product or process can be mapped this way. As a first step in helping understand how to apply resources, design a product, or sell a product, this sort of model is invaluable.

Understanding which features and tasks happen frequently (and so may suffer from waning attention from the user, incurring errors) and which happen with high intensity (maybe requiring more careful error detection) helps keep Murphy's Law in its place.

2.5. Principle 5: A Patient Is a Consumer

Picture this: newly diagnosed with diabetes, a man goes into his local drug store to purchase a glucose meter. He finds a dozen choices, each priced about the same, each about the same size with a similar list of features. How does he choose a meter?

The answer to this question about a specific kind of patient choosing a specific medical product also happens to be the answer to a more general question: How does any consumer choose any product?

Efficacy is clearly important; consumers want products that do what they're supposed to do, and consumers of medical products are especially motivated to pay attention to this. But in most cases, there is more than one device that can fill the bill. And when the playing field is fairly level, two other questions assert themselves.

How Does Is Make Me Feel?

Think about a product that you own – anything – that you are particularly fond of. What do you like about it? How it works might be part of it, but probably not all – there are undoubtedly other products offering similar service. Do you like the design? Does it remind you of the time and place you got it? Is it an heirloom, or something you enjoy with others in your family?

Medical product designers have traditionally focused on creating products that work well, rather than products that consumers *like*. But as more medical devices and treatments are available for use in the home, it is becoming clear that consumers are bringing the same sensibilities to medical product purchases that they bring to every other purchase. The internet offers countless opportunities for a newly diagnosed patient to read device reviews and communicate directly with others people while shopping for products; consumers are trading not just facts, but their opinions.

How Does It Make Me Look?

The other important question consumers ask is externally focused, and it's really two questions. One is, does this product make me look good? The other is, does this product *not* make me look bad?

The "looking good" question is straightforward, and is in some sense an extension of the "how does it make me feel?" question. People obviously want to look to other people like they're smart, attractive, cool, etc. The second part, through, is trickier. We can't fault a manufacturer for being proud of its products, but from the consumer's perspective, a large corporate logo on a product may be broadcasting, "I have a medical condition." Just as we want our medical products to become an integral part of a patient's life and not stick out from a process perspective, patients don't want them to stick out to other people.

One of the best-selling glucose meters on the market is camouflaged as a mobile phone. Pediatricians can buy reflex hammers that look like funny animals instead of stainless steel mallets. These products offer the same functionality as competing products that look more "medical," but have been designed to put the patient at ease; this kind of differentiation offers consumers an added level of differentiation in a crowded field of competing products.

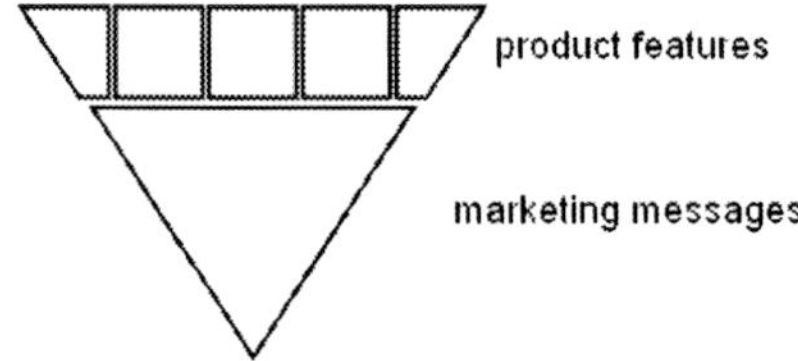

Figure 3. The "inverted pyramid" model resulting from a feature-centric view of a product.

3. The Product Analyst's Couch

Once we've all internalized these principles, what do we do? If technology shouldn't be the focus, what should? In our design consultancy practice, we've found a framework based around Product Psychology is useful to tease out the various levels at which people understand products and the interactions between people and things. What this framework tries to do is tease apart the features from the higher-level attributes of a product, so that the design team can have a better feel for what's important and how the end user will perceive the device, and so the marketing story and product features can be built together, resulting in a more cohesive product.

Product Psychology allows a manufacturer to consider a device as more than just a list of features. As we've discussed, consumers want more than features – they want benefits. And yet, when given the opportunity to describe the benefits of a product, manufacturers tend to resort to a bulleted list of features. For proof, go to any small-appliance store and view the side of most any box containing a blender – as a rule, you'll see a picture of the product and a bulleted list of features. No real reason why one blender is better than any other, and no particular order to the features.

Think about the feature-driven view of products as an inverted pyramid [see Fig. 3]. A list of individual features represent the broad "top" of the pyramid, supported by a marketing story designed to convince the consumer that these features are the ones to have, as in, "this glucose meter is the fastest on the market." The trouble is, as with all inverted pyramids, this is not a particularly stable model. As soon as another manufacturer comes out with a slightly faster model – and they always will – the product's support story is no longer relevant.

The Product Psychology framework gets away from thinking of a product as a list of individual selling points. It refers to those aspects of a product that communicate the personality, occupation, and abilities of a product to the consumer, and allows for a broader understanding of the benefits a product can deliver. Whether this or that glucose meter is the "fastest" matters less than how well it helps someone manage her diabetes, and that assistance is based on what the product can do, but also on how the product acts, how it treats the end user, and how she feels toward the product. To truly help manage a disease, for instance, a product must be trusted. "Trustworthiness" is a desired attribute of this product, but cannot be engineered in like typical product features. It is this sort of higher-level attribute that Product Psychology seeks to uncover.

4. Components of Product Psychology

The framework consists of three types of attributes that mirror the makeup of human beings. Products, like people, have a personality, an occupation, and a set of abilities. Thinking about it this way helps the design team to remember what Reeves and Nass found – people want to relate to their products the way they relate to people.

A product's set of "abilities" is the most commonly used aspect of how a product behaves: its features. When many device manufacturers describe their products, they simply list these abilities and hope that the list alone communicates the benefits of owning the product. But again, at the risk of repetition: manufacturers can do better by communicating at a higher level.

Product "occupation" is concerned directly with the style of user-device interaction. An intelligent device that acts like a "Doctor" might be designed to ask questions, form hypotheses, test them, and prescribe treatment. A device that acts like a "Best Friend" might suggest some ideas to try, help monitor the results, and work with the user to understand the results. A "Teacher"-style device might have a focus on education and just-in-time information that lets the user come to his own conclusions, with the best information possible.

Finally, a product's "personality" is its overall feel: is it a friendly product? Is it serious? Precise? Fun? Personalities might be described as being "task-oriented" vs. "emotion-oriented," or "directing" vs. "inviting." These descriptions help guide the overall feel of the product. Personality is the product's strong connection with the manufacturer's brand – the impression a company wants to make with its consumers is expressed in its products' personalities. In a real sense, a consumer interacting with a product is interacting with the company that made the product – if the company wants to be seen as "serious" or "fun" or "responsive," the product had better communicate exactly the same attributes.

5. Putting Product Psychology into Practice

Applying the Product Psychology framework is a simple matter of thinking about a product the same way we think about other people. For example, let's just consider me (it's all about me!), and how I describe myself to people.

I have a long list of "abilities," including good typing skills, computer programming, playing the ukulele, and speaking a little bit of French. If I relied solely on this list to describe myself, I would be hoping that one or more of these random bits of information would catch the attention of a prospective employer or friend – that it would stick. But my pyramid would be inverted – if those few abilities didn't happen to connect, an opportunity for a relationship might pass me by. So, if I described myself as a "ukulele-playing typist" I would miss out on relationships with people who might like me but don't happen to care about music or typing. Sounds silly, but that's precisely what a manufacturer is doing by listing product features on the side of the box.

Note that I don't apply those skills all at the same time, all the time – I don't usually play music at work, and I don't usually program a computer while entertaining my children. When describing myself, I pay careful attention to the goals of the person to whom I'm describing – is this a prospective employer? Someone who I can play music with? One of my kids? This is where the concept of "occupation" comes in – depending on what job I'm doing, I use different abilities. So someone looking to hire me will be interested in those things that make me a good product behavior designer: more about thinking skill and computer skills, and less about musicianship and tourist French. Someone looking to hire me to entertain at a party will want to know about my ukulele skills. When I add new skills to my repertoire, I think about how they will enable to me to perform one of my occupations better – or enable me to act in an entirely new capacity.

So instead of describing myself by just listing my skills, I can abstract a level and describe what I *do*. I can describe myself as a "musician" or "designer," and get the point across. And there's no need to get hung up on details; if a new friend plays the trombone, we can relate at an occupational level – as musicians – instead of missing out because of some trombone-ukulele mutual snobbery. Also, relying on this "occupational" view makes it easier for me to change the individual skills around – if I give up the ukulele for the accordion, I can still fulfill the job of entertainer.

Finally, anyone interested in me will want to know, overall, what I'm like – my "personality." Am I easygoing? Serious? Fun? Am I aggressive, or wait-and-see? Any of these might be appropriate for my different roles, but my prospective employer or band mate or playmate will want to know this bit of information most of all – if my personality is counter to theirs, it will be a bad fit.

6. Applying Psychology to a New Product

Imagine creating an advanced medical product – for example, a device that can measure blood glucose through the skin of a diabetes patient, calculate the appropriate amount of insulin he needs, and deliver the insulin through the skin without a needle. The patient simply holds the device against his skin, and it all happens in a couple of seconds.[3]

The abilities of such a product are easy to dream up; in fact, we just listed them:

- Takes a couple of seconds
- No needles
- Automatic measurement of glucose
- Does all the calculation
- Delivers insulin through the skin

What is the product's occupation? Maybe it's a…

- Doctor; it assesses the patient's medical condition and treats the problem directly, without much interaction
- Nurse Educator; it assesses the patient's medical condition and explains the ways in which the patient can live healthier, while making a treatment recommendation
- Assistant; it reports the patient's blood glucose to him and lets the patient decide what to do about it

There are pros and cons to each of these setups; for instance, the "doctor" model might be simplest for the consumer, but might face a difficult regulatory path. The "assistant" model might be an easier sell to the FDA, but might not take enough burden from the end user to be interesting.

What should the overall personality of a device like this be? It depends on who we're building it for. Is it a device for twenty-somethings, used to computers? Is it for elderly patients who are uncomfortable with technology? Or is it aimed at children, who want to be engaged and entertained, even by medical equipment? One size usually doesn't fit all, and since the personality sets the tone for the product, it is imperative that the design team, marketing team, and sales team be aligned around this aspect of the product.

7. Conclusion

Consumers have complex reasons for choosing the products they choose, and they develop complex relationships with those products. And even though medical consumers can have a more vested interest in choosing products for performance reasons than shoppers choosing something like a toaster, deep down, they are still consumers.

---

[3] This would be a great product, but unfortunately it's a little bit in the future.

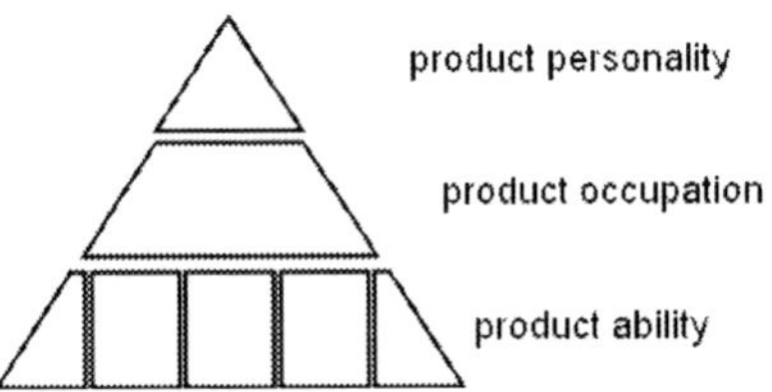

Figure 4. A better view of a product. The overriding personality and occupation are supported by individual features.

Manufacturers must focus on product benefits, not just features. A reliance on a list of features does not do a product justice and makes it difficult for consumers to understand what makes it better. And competitors need merely offer equivalent features to neutralize a marketing message based only on performance.

With a good "psychological profile" of a product in place, manufacturers can make decisions based on how proposed features support the personality and occupation of a product, instead of managing the design based on a list of features disconnected from the brand and high-level interactions between user and product. The "product psychology" framework inverts the pyramid [see Fig. 4] putting a broad range of abilities (features) at the base, with occupation and personality levels sitting on top. Individual features matter less, and can be changed around without disturbing the overall feel of the product, and the ways the product fits into the life of the consumer.

In the end, the principles and frameworks described here are simply reminders to keep perspective and consider every feature decision from the user's eyes. When business and design work together to deliver intelligent products, patients and manufacturers both benefit.

Cyborgs Era –
Implants, Merging Humans with Machines
and Caring Machines

Future of Intelligent and Extelligent Health Environment
R.G. Bushko (Ed.)
IOS Press, 2005

Future of Computer Implant Technology and Intelligent Human-Machine Systems

Kevin WARWICK, Ph.D.
Professor of Cybernetics, Department of Cybernetics, University of Reading, UK

Abstract. Linking the human nervous system and brain directly to a computer opens up innumerable possibilities, not only in the future world of medicine, but also as a potential way of technically evolving all humans. This, however, presents something of an ethical problem. Nevertheless, the only way to actually find out what is realistically possible and what is not is to carry out practical experimentation using implant technology and to witness the results. This chapter describes the most recent self-experimentation trials carried out by the author and his team.

1. Introduction

Technically, we are now in a position to make a useful direct connection between the human nervous system and computer technology. This has come about partly due to significant advances in the means of establishing a bond between biology and technology. The chances of a body rejecting technology or of infection setting in, although still not zero, can now be regarded as almost negligible if extreme care is taken. At the same time, the increased capabilities of computers, both in terms of computing power and networking, have opened up a whole new raft of possibilities.

As a result, we have, in recent years, witnessed a number of experiments involving animals, for example rat reward and punishment and maze following tests [1,2] and monkey remote signalling [3]. But where the trials are of considerably greater interest is where humans are involved. Various studies have involved the employment of implants to try and bring about some basic movement or control for those who are paralysed, however some of the most significant are those by Philip Kennedy [4] allowing stroke victims to control basic elements of their local environment simply by thinking about moving.

Using implant technology to help those who have a mental or physical problem, such as a paralysis, allowing them to do things that they would not ordinarily be able to do, is seen by most to be a good thing. However, the same technology can also potentially augment all humans, giving them abilities over and above those of other humans.

Clearly this presents something of an ethical issue as to whether the technology should be developed at all. Indeed it is, in itself, an intriguing question as to whether it is a good thing or a bad thing to 'evolve' humans in a technical, rather than a biological, way.

Reasons for wishing to consider extending human capabilities are manifold. Indeed it is part of human nature to try and do so. Nowadays, for example, all sorts of possibilities arise when the abilities of machine (computer) intelligence are compared with the finite, limited brain size of humans – clearly it can be seen that the two entities have distinctly different modes of operation and in a number of ways the machine exhibits distinct performance advantages.

Obvious examples are the mathematical, number crunching, abilities of a computer and the networked computer's memory base. These are both reasons why we use computers as we do now – simply because an individual human brain cannot compete. Nevertheless, such computer abilities have led to a redefining of, and a change in our understanding of intelligence [5]. What was once thought to be an intelligent act in humans, now comes directly into question when a machine clearly outperforms a human.

Technology has also been employed externally to improve on the humans' limited range of sensing the world around them. So technology can give a picture of what is going on in the infrared or ultraviolet spectra, even translating X-ray signals into visual images that human brains can understand.

Another factor is that human brains have evolved to think in at most, three dimensions, whereas computers are able to 'think' in n-dimensions. Space around us is, of course, not three dimensional, as categorised by humans, but can be perceived in as many dimensions as one wishes. Machines therefore have the ability of understanding the world in a more complex, multidimensional way when compared to humans. This is an extremely powerful advantage for machine intelligence.

Perhaps the biggest performance difference, in an intellectual sense, between humans and machines is that of communication. Each human brain operates on relatively complex electro-chemical signals, which are converted into mechanical signals, sound waves in speech or hand movements to operate a keyboard. In reality such mechanical signalling is a very slow, error prone means of communication. As a result, human languages are nothing more than finite coding systems that cannot hope to convey more than a small fraction of what we would really like to communicate with another including our thoughts, wishes, feelings and emotions. Problems occur due to the wide variety of different languages and the indirect relationships and cultures between them. In comparison, machine communication is tremendously powerful, not only because of its usually inherent parallel nature, as opposed to human serial communication.

Looking at these mental differences between humans and machines, it is clear that humans can benefit enormously by the use of external cooperation, as indeed we do now. However a direct link could offer so much more. For example, by linking human and machine brains together could it be possible for us in this Cyborg (part human, part machine) form to understand the world around us in twenty or thirty dimensions? Even four or five dimensions would be worth it. Could it be possible to tap the mathematical and memory capabilities of computers directly, thereby probably changing the operation of the human part of the Cyborg brain? What will the human brain make of extra sensory information being fed directly in? Perhaps most importantly of all, by linking the human brain directly with a computer, might it be possible to communicate directly between human and machine, and even person to person purely by electronic signals – something that could be regarded as thought communication?

All of these questions present an exciting new frontier for research linking humans and machines closer together. As a result, in the 1990's various scientists speculated on a future in which implant technology became a norm for all [6]. In one example Peter Cochrane, who was then Head of British Telecom's Research Laboratories wrote [7]; 'Just a small piece of silicon under the skin is all it would take to enjoy the freedom of no cards, passports or keys. Put your hand out to the car door, computer terminal, the food you wish to purchase and you would be dealt with efficiently. Think about it: total freedom; no more plastic'.

However, apart from heart pacemakers and the like to overcome a problem, no one had actually experimented with implants to provide extra abilities. Until that is, 24 August 1998 when, as reported in [8], a silicon chip transponder was surgically implanted in my upper left arm. With this in place, the door to my laboratory opened when I approached, the corridor light came on automatically and a voice box in the entrance foyer welcomed me with "Hello, Professor Warwick" when I entered the building.

But the identifying signals my 1998 implant transmitted were not affected by what was going on in my body and signals transmitted to the implant from the computer did not affect my body in any way. For that, we needed something more sophisticated. Hence, as soon as the 1998 tests were concluded, we immediately set to work on a new implant experiment.

2. Neural Implant Operation

On March 14, 2002, an array of one hundred silicon electrode needles was surgically implanted into the median nerve fibres of my left arm, at the Radcliffe Infirmary, Oxford, UK. Each one of the electrodes was 1.5 mm in length, the total array measuring 4 mm x 4 mm. With the entire median nerve fascicle estimated to have a maximum diameter of 4mm, this meant that each of the electrodes penetrated well into the fascicle.

During the two-hour operation, a first incision was made centrally over the median nerve for a length of just over 4 cm, directly up to the wrist. A second incision was then made, proximally to the first, 16 cm up the inside arm towards the elbow. This second incision was 2 cm in length. Following a tunnelling procedure to connect the two incisions together, a piece of open tubing was run between the incisions, creating a clear passage. The array, with its connecting wires, was then passed down the tubing from the incision nearest the elbow to that nearest the wrist.

Once the array had been successfully passed down the tubing, the tubing was removed from the wrist end, leaving the array in position over the exposed median nerve fascicle by the wrist. Wires from the array travelled up the inner arm, exiting at the second incision where they were attached to an electrical terminal pad. The array was pneumatically inserted into the radial side of the median nerve fascicle under microscopic control. Once the array was successfully in position, both incisions were closed.

3. Input/Output Signals

With the array acting as a direct electrical connection into the human nervous system, it was found to be eminently possible to transmit neural signals directly from the peripheral nervous system to a computer. These neural signals could be readily generated by simple finger movements. The signals were transmitted to a computer, either by a straightforward hard wire from the terminal pad via an interface unit, or though a radio transmitter attached to the pad.

It was, however, also possible to stimulate the nervous system, via the array, transmitting current signals from the computer to bring about sensations. In experiments to investigate appropriate current signals to be input, it was found that currents of less than 80 uA in magnitude had little perceivable effect at that value, though certain of the electrodes produced a recognisable effect, the associated applied voltage being 40 to 50 volts. The exact voltage applied depended on the input resistance being encountered on each particular electrode. Due to the variability of the human nervous system this resistance was though, not identically the same on a day-to-day basis.

Stimulation currents above 100 uA had little extra effect on nerve stimulation, indicating that a non-linear thresholding characteristic was being exerted by the nervous system in response to the current. The current was in fact being applied as a bi-phasic signal with 100 usec inter signal break periods. It could be said, in fact, that this signal waveform, which was the most successful tried, closely emulated the first harmonic of motor signals recorded.

The array allowed motor neural signals to be detected from the small collection of axons around each electrode. Because the majority of signals of interest occurred at frequencies of below 3.5 KHz, low pass filters were employed to ensure that higher frequency effects, including those due to noise, were either removed from the procedure or, at least, significantly reduced. In this way, it was relatively easy to generate useful motor neural signals simply by making controlled finger movements. In the cybernetic experiments carried out, these motor neural signals were transmitted directly to the computer, where they could be made use of to operate a variety of networked technological implements [9].

Whilst motor neural signals could be generated and employed from the first day of experimentation onwards, in the first stimulation tests, whilst wearing a blindfold, a mean correct identification rate of 70% was achieved. What this means is that without prior warning, on average, seven times out of ten I could successfully detect when a current stimulation had occurred and when it had not. Further details on this are given in [10]. These stimulation tests did not commence until six weeks after the implant operation, and it took approximately two weeks of continued testing to arrive at suitable current types to obtain this detection rate.

An important feature of obtaining suitable current signals, recognisable on the nervous system, was, effectively training of the brain to decipher the signals. In a sense, therefore it was a mutually convergent exercise with, over a period of weeks, more recognisable signals being inserted with, at the same time, the brain learning about the signals patterns and what they meant. This learning continued in the further weeks of the experiment.

Towards the end of the entire experiment, which concluded with the implant being extracted on 18th June 2002, over three months after the original implantation, a mean perception rate of stimulation of over 95% was being achieved. To all intents and purposes though, because of several factors apparent in the method of experimentation [10], realistically this figure should be seen, in a practical sense, to be as near to 100% as could be achieved.

Before discussing the cybernetic applications actually carried out with the implant in place, it is important to realise that the whole project was conducted in association with the National Spinal Injuries Centre at Stoke Mandeville Hospital, Aylesbury, UK. One aim of the project was therefore to assess the practicability of employing the same type of implant to help those with a spinal injury. The aim was not so much one of attempting to restore movement to otherwise motionless limbs, but rather to consider the possibilities of using motor neural signals to control technology and thus bring about a considerable lifestyle improvement.

The long term goal would therefore be, where necessary, to direct brain implants to allow an individual who is paralysed to control their local environment by neural signals – in popular terminology, to switch on lights or perhaps drive their car just by thinking about it. In this sense, our experiment was useful in assessing the present state of technology.

4. Application Studies

In order to demonstrate the sort of applications possible, thereby indicating the range of potential use for implant technology of this type, a variety of applications were performed.

The first implementation was to make use of the neural signals being transmitted to control an articulated hand. The aim of the hand, referred to as the SNAVE hand, is to mimic the operation of, in particular the control mechanisms inherent in, the human hand. Effectively, neural signals responsible for moving fingers in my own left hand were also used to operate the articulated hand.

Sensors in the fingertips of the hand allow for the grip shape to be adapted as well as the applied force being modified as necessary. Hence appropriate tension can be applied via the hand in order to avoid object slippage. In tests, whilst wearing a blindfold, sensory data from the fingertips was fed back down on to my nervous system. As more force was applied to an object, so the amount of neural stimulation was increased. At the same time, the hand's movements were being controlled from my own nervous system. Over a two week period of regular experimentation I learnt to judge, to very fine detail, within ±5%, a force just sufficient to grip an object.

As a follow on from the articulated hand investigation, on 20th May 2002 a team at Columbia University, New York City, teamed up to bring about an internet link. With myself in the Internet real-time labs in the Computer Science Department of Columbia University, the implant was put on-line onto the Internet. The articulated hand experiment was then repeated, although this time, signals from the neural implant were transmitted via the Internet to directly control the articulated hand back in the Cybernetics Labs at Reading University in the UK. As well as this, feedback information was transmitted from the hand's fingers in the UK to stimulate my nervous system in New York. A 100% success rate in signal recognition was achieved in this one off trial and the articulated hand was controlled adequately despite the delay in signal transmission due mainly to the distance involved.

Neural signals were also employed to control the directional movements of an electric wheelchair. For this purpose a sequential state machine provided a simple solution, the machine being halted, by neural signals, to select the desired travel direction – forward, backwards, left, right. Experiments were also carried out to selectively process signals from several of the implant electrodes over time in order to realise fine control.

Due to the chair mobility, a short-range digital radio link was brought about between the implant and the wheelchair driver control mechanism. The radio transmitter/receiver unit was worn as a gauntlet arrangement on my lower left arm. After about one hour of learning time, quite reasonable control of the wheelchair was achieved. Subsequently, considerable success was achieved in driving the wheelchair around a cluttered, external environment.

One further experiment was to investigate the possibility of extra sensory input to the human nervous system. To this end, ultrasonic sensors were positioned on a baseball cap. The output from these sensors was fed down on to the radio transmitter/receiver gauntlet to provide neural stimulation via the implant. When an object was in the vicinity of the sensors, the stimulation rate was high, whereas as the distance increased, the stimulation rate decreased. With no object present, no stimulation occurred.

Tests were carried out in a normal (untidy!) laboratory environment. Whilst wearing a blindfold, I was able to readily navigate around objects in the laboratory by means of, what turned out to be, a highly accurate ultrasonic sense of distance. Obviously, drawing universal conclusions from a one off experience would be wrong, however what can be reported is that my brain adapted very quickly, within minutes, to its new sensory input.

Importantly, the stimulation pulses being received were linked directly with the ultrasonic detection, in terms of an indication of how far away any objects were. The pulses were not witnessed as one of the normal five human senses. When an object was brought rapidly into my ultrasonic 'line of sight', a reactive, automatic recoil occurred to, what felt like, a dangerous situation.

The final experiment carried out involved my wife, Irena, who had two electrodes inserted in her median nerve through microneurography, in roughly the same location to my own implant.

By means of one of the electrodes in particular, strong motor neural signals could be obtained when she moved her fingers. The output from this electrode was linked directly to a computer and was connected such that my own nervous system was stimulated each time

Irena moved her fingers. The process was also linked up in the reverse direction, with Irena's nervous system being stimulated when I moved my fingers. So when Irena moved her fingers three times, I felt three pulses on my nervous system, and vice versa.

What we had brought about was a direct electrical connection between the nervous systems of two individuals. Through this connection, motor neural signals were transmitted from person to person to successfully achieve a simple radiotelegraphy signalling system.

It is apparent that with implants fitted not in the peripheral nervous system, but rather directly in the motor neural area of the brain, the same type of signalling between two individuals could be considered to be the first, albeit rudimentary, steps in thought communication.

5. Conclusions So Far

The practical implant study carried out gives rise to a host of implications [11]. Firstly, by positioning such arrays in the motor neural area in the brain, this should bring about a variety of technological control systems operated merely by the individual thinking about moving. In essence, just about any technical device that can be controlled should be operable in this way, domestic implements providing the obvious immediate application field.

For those people who are paralysed, implant technology should therefore open up a whole new world. Whilst we should not be overenthusiastic in claiming that it will all happen today or indeed tomorrow, at least we can say that a number of things appear to be technically quite possible. Directly from the results of our experiments, it should be possible for a paralysed person to switch on lights, make the coffee and even drive their, suitably modified, car.

In the tests carried out, a wheelchair was driven around under the control of my neural signals. The same should be possible for someone who is paralysed. Also an articulated hand was controlled from my nervous system. The same should be possible for someone who has had their hand amputated. Further, I benefited from an extra (ultrasonic) sense. The same should be possible for someone who is blind – not to repair their blindness in any way, but to allow them an alternative sense.

One part of the study was the investigation of infection and rejection as regards the interaction between my body and the implant. The run of wires up the inside of my arm was an attempt to reduce the effects of infection. In fact, no indication of infection was witnessed during the trial period, the two operation sites on my left arm being monitored closely over that time.

As for rejection, results were far more encouraging than could have been imagined. Firstly, mentally my brain had tuned in more and more to the signals used for stimulation. Secondly, when the extraction operation took place it was found that scar tissue had grown round the implant, pulling it tightly into the median nerve fibres. When the scar tissue was removed, it was discovered that the implant had neither lifted nor tilted from the nerve fibres – it was exactly where it had been positioned over three months earlier.

On the negative side, where the wires exited from my arm they were subject to quite severe mechanical bending stresses and this resulted in gradual breakage of the wires [12]. In fact by the end of the experiment only three wires (therefore three electrode connections) were still operative. Clearly the mechanical strength of the wires will need to be improved if long-term implants are to be considered. However, if a device were to be completely implanted, then perhaps this would not be a problem. A complete implant, of this type though, would need a light/compact power supply and aerial.

6. Implications for the Future

The programme of research presents quite an ethical dilemma. Very few people would argue against the use of implant technology, as long as it has been shown to be safe, to help those with a disability of some kind. However the use of the same technological base in order to upgrade humans raises some serious questions. Who gets an implant and who doesn't? Will it be left purely to commercial enterprises to push the technology on or is it something for which some key political decisions need to be made?

Our own research is now clearly focussed on motor neural brain implants as the next step. Many research questions arise though, in terms of number and positioning of implants. Also the extent and range of signals to be bi-directionally transmitted is of major concern. Of the tests to be carried out, thought communication ranks as something of a priority. However this will mean that more than one person will need to be implanted for scientific, rather than medical, purposes – which could be difficult from an ethical standpoint.

Giving humans extra abilities by technologically upgrading them (into Cyborgs!) [11] now appears to be becoming possible. Shouldn't humans be allowed to simply get on with it – as has (largely) been the case with previous technical improvements – and become superhuman? Humans are now in a position whereby we have the potential to evolve our own destiny. Perhaps issues affecting such a move are now as much social and ethical as they are technical.

References

[1] Chapin, J; Moxon, K, Markowitz, R and Nicolelis, M., "Real-time control of a robot arm using simultaneously recorded neurons in the motor cortex", Nature Neuroscience, Vol. 2, pp. 664–670, 1999.

[2] Talwar, S; Xu, S; Hawley, E; Weiss, S, Moxon, K and Chapin, J; 'Rat navigation guided by remote control', Nature, Vol. 417, pp. 37–38, May 2002.

[3] Nicolelis, M, "Actions from Thoughts", Nature, Vol. 409, pp. 403–407, 2001.

[4] Kennedy, P; Bakay, R; Moore, M, Adams, K and Goldwaithe, J; 'Direct control of a computer from the human central nervous system', IEEE Trans. On Rehabilitation Engineering, Vol. 8, No. 2, pp. 198–202, 2000.

[5] Warwick, K; 'QI: The Quest for Intelligence', Piatkus, 2001.

[6] Kurzweil, R: 'The Age of Spiritual Machines', Viking, New York, 1999.

[7] Cochrane, P, 'Tips for the Time Traveller', Orion Business Books, 1997.

[8] Bushko, R. (ed.), 'Future of Health Technology', IOS Press, 2000.

[9] Gasson, M; Hutt, B; Goodhew, I; Kyberd, P and Warwick, K: 'Bi-directional Human Machine Interface via Direct Neural Connection', Proc. IEEE International Workshop on Robot and Human Interactive Communication, Berlin, pp. 265–270, Sept. 2002.

[10] Warwick, K: "A Study in Cyborgs", Royal Society of Edinburgh 2003 Joint Lecture, ISBN 0 902198688, March 2003.

[11] Warwick, K., "I, Cyborg", Century, 2002.

[12] Warwick, K; Gasson, M; Hutt, B; Goodhew. I; Kyberd, P, Andrews, B; Teddy, P and Shad, A: 'The Application of implant Technology for Cybernetic Systems', Archives of Neurology, to appear, 2003.

Future of Intelligent and Extelligent Health Environment
R.G. Bushko (Ed.)
IOS Press, 2005

Future of Caring Machines

Timothy BICKMORE, Ph.D.[a] and Rosalind W. PICARD, Sc.D.[b]
[a]*Assistant Professor, College of Computer and Information Science,*
Northeastern University, Boston, MA, USA
[b]*Director, Affective Computing Research Group,*
MIT Media Laboratory, Cambridge, MA, USA

Abstract. Feeling cared for has profound effects on physiology, cognition and emotional state, and has significant health ramifications whether the source of this feeling is an intimate other, friend or health provider. Unfortunately, not everyone has access to social networks populated with caring individuals or has health providers who are patient, empathic and reliably available when emotional support is needed. Over the last decade, a range of computational artifacts and technologies have been developed that could help fill this unmet need in many peoples' lives. *Caring machines* are technologies that interact with an individual to accomplish a goal while also behaving in ways that give the individual the feeling of being cared for. This chapter presents evidence that these machines can begin to lead to significant health benefits, such as increased adherence to prescribed health behavior change and medication regimens.

1. Introduction

People cannot always get the support that they need. As families become more geographically dispersed and as the population ages, social isolation is becoming more and more prevalent. In addition, even those who are surrounded by people may not always get the comfort, caring and attention they need to thrive. These unmet emotional needs are not just frivolous desires whose neglect is inconsequential; a significant body of research now indicates that addressing an individual's needs for emotional care-taking is essential for maximizing their health and well-being.

Over the last decade, researchers in affective computing—that which relates to, arises from, or deliberately influences emotions [1]—and related disciplines have developed a number of technologies and performed a wide range of experiments that demonstrate that an individual's need for caring could be met (at least partially) by computational artifacts ranging from computer agents to wearable computers to robots.

In this chapter, we first review the literature on human-human and animal-human caring and their known effects on health. We then review the research that has been conducted over the last decade on technology development and experiments that serve to work towards the goal of building machines that people feel care about them. We close with some observations and visions about the possible futures of caring machines.

2. Human-Human Caring and Health Implications

Feeling cared for has profound effects on physiology, cognition and emotional state in humans. It plays an especially crucial role in the helping and medical professions. According to Levinson, et al., "A growing body of literature suggests that outcomes of care are optimal when physicians address patients' emotional and personal concerns in addition to their biomedical problems. Patient satisfaction, patient adherence, and biological outcomes can be improved with a patient-centered model of care that demonstrates respect and caring for patients" [2].

Social support is the name given to those behaviors that take place within the context of a personal relationship, and that serve to provide aid and assistance. This group of behaviors has been broken down into several subtypes of support including: emotional support (expressions of empathy, trust, esteem, reassurance of worth, affection, attachment, intimacy); instrumental support (material assistance); informational support (giving advice and information); appraisal support (information that is useful for self-evaluation); and social network support (e.g., providing introductions to other people) [3,4]. Of these, emotional support is the most strongly and consistently associated with health and well-being. For example, a number of studies have demonstrated that emotional support, provided in the context of intimate relationships, increases survival rates among people with severe cardiovascular conditions [5]. The effects of all kinds of social support are primarily a function of the *perception* of support by the one receiving it, rather than the perceptions, intentions or actual behavior of the person providing it [6]. For example, in studies in which both the provider and the recipient of social support were asked about the kinds of support provided in a relationship, the recipient's reports are always the most strongly correlated with the positive effects.

Studies have consistently found a relationship between social isolation and mortality, and this effect is most profound for those individuals who are the most isolated. One study found that older women who lived alone and did not have contact with family or friends had mortality levels three times greater than those who lived with others or had more frequent contact with family and friends [7].

Note that while social support can involve attempts at persuasion (e.g., via informational support), it is fundamentally different from other types of social influence in that it is always provided in a context of caring, trust and respect [4], and thus the technologies that may be involved in artificial caring need to be concerned with a much richer and deeper set of issues than those involved in argumentation or "captology" [8].

2.1. Caring by Health Professionals

There is also a known association between patients' perception of caring by health professionals and patient satisfaction, treatment regimen adherence and outcomes, across a wide range of health disciplines. The most significant empirical support of this phenomenon is in the field of psychotherapy, in which measures of "working alliance" –the trust and belief that the therapist and patient have in each other as team-members in achieving a desired outcome—show consistently high correlations with successful outcomes [9]. Even in physician-patient interactions, physician empathy for a patient plays a significant role in prescription compliance, and a physician's *lack* of empathy for a patient is the single most frequent source of complaints [10].

However, health professionals cannot provide an individual's primary source of social support. Professionals are rarely available to provide support over long periods of time, and the power differential in the provider-patient relationship may hamper empathic understanding [4]. Additionally, professionals are under significant demands to reduce costs and to see more patients in less time. Time spent with a machine costs significantly less than time with a health professional. As the time that patients interact with machines increases, it is prudent to consider how that interaction can be designed to contribute to helping the patient feel cared for.

2.2. Caring Behavior

There are several human communicative behaviors that are known to elicit the perception of feeling cared for by a person. Although providing any kind of social support can indicate caring, demonstrations of empathy and comforting behavior are perhaps the quintessential examples, and are widely cited in the helping literature as being key in achieving desired outcomes [11,12]. Other behaviors that can contribute to an impression of caring include social dialogue, self-disclosure, emphasizing commonalities, meta-relational communication (particularly emotional aspects) talking about the past and future together, continuity behaviors (appropriate greetings and farewells and talk about the time spent apart), and reference to mutual knowledge, as well as explicit messages of esteem (see [13] for a summary).

There are also nonverbal behaviors indicative of caring such as facial expressiveness (including displays of concern), head nodding, and tone and timing of speech. Nonverbal "immediacy" behaviors—including close conversational distance, direct body and facial orientation, forward lean, increased and direct gaze, frequent gesturing and postural openness—have been found to project liking for the other and engagement in the interaction, and to be indicative of caring [14].

3. Animal-Human Caring and Health Implications

Pets can also provide a sense of caring and emotional support, and have been found to be correlated with several kinds of beneficial health-related effects, although the specific mechanisms of these effects have not been determined [15]. Candidate mechanisms for the health-related benefits of pet ownership include: the opportunity for people to provide nurturance, since it can increase their self esteem; the ability of pets to provide network support through their role as social catalysts; and their ability to instill a perception of social support in their owners, given that they are always available and reliable, nonjudgmental, perceived as caring about and needing their owners, and can provide tactile comfort and recreational distraction from worries.

4. Progress Towards Caring Machines

Although the literature cited above describes the significant positive health effects of perceived caring by humans and pets, these sources of support also have many drawbacks associated with them. First, other people may not be consistently available or reliable to provide support when needed. Human helpers may react negatively if their help is rejected [4]. For older adults, the problem of physical and mental abuse by those who are otherwise supportive is also a real problem [16]. Finally, many individuals may simply not have a network of friends available, or may live in a location in which pets are not allowed. For all these reasons, computer agents that provide people with the perception of feeling cared for may be able to help fill this emotional void in the lives of many individuals.

Before a machine can provide effective emotional support or caring, it is first helpful for the machine to have some idea of what kind of emotions an individual is expressing: Is he upset? Is he pleased? In the following sections we first review the state of the art in sensing human emotional state, then move on to a review of technologies designed to intervene at the appropriate time.

4.1. Technologies for Sensing Human Emotional State

In order to respond in a caring way to people's feelings, it is important first to have a reasonable assessment of what they might be feeling. While there is no instrument that can directly read an individual's feelings, there are a variety of ways that people communicate their feelings to each other (often imperfectly), and these modes of communication are becoming increasingly accessible to machines. These ways range from dialogue and verbal expressions to non-verbal cues such as facial expressions, postural shifts, gestures, and more.

Machine conversational agents are computer characters designed to carry on a dialogue with a person, and this dialogue can help the machine to sense emotional information. While machines remain very limited in their ability to understand most of language, they can already engage successfully in quasi-scripted dialogues about feelings [17–19]. There are times when it is appropriate to overtly ask how somebody is doing, which can lead to disclosure of feelings, e.g.,

"How's it going?"
"Not so great."
"Oh dear. Sorry to hear. Anything I can do to help?"
"I don't know, I just feel terrible about ..."

Sometimes feelings are not communicated through *what* is said as much as *how* it is said, e.g. "Good Morning!" can be spoken with genuinely cheery enthusiasm or with annoyance, disdain, and other kinds of inflection that may very clearly contrast the words used. Dialogue systems have a chance to sense the words selected by a person and reason about the associated affect [20–22], and also have the opportunity to listen to para-linguistic aspects of speech for indications of a person's feelings [23,24].

Clearly if there is no dialogue, then speech won't work, and other modes of sensing will be needed. In many medical situations, it is natural to sense aspects of a person's physiology. Physiological information has been shown to carry information that can be used to classify an individual's affective state. Picard, et al., built a recognition system using four physiological signals, which learned patterns for an individual over time, and achieved 81% recognition accuracy classifying one of eight states (anger, joy, sadness, hatred, platonic love, romantic love, reverence, and neutral) that an individual was having [25]. (The person was seated, and deliberately focusing on having each of the eight emotions.)

Signals such as skin conductance and heart rate variability have also been shown to be indicators of stress in natural situations, e.g., driving in Boston [26], and recently it has been shown that an agent's empathetic responses can influence skin conductance in a way that is associated with decreased stress [27]. Stress and anxiety are increasingly being recognized as common in medical interactions and are also linked to a number of significant health problems; hence, the new ability of empathetic technologies to help reduce stress has many implications for health care.

Other forms of affect sensing technologies have been developed for specific environments. Physiological sensors have been put into computer mice [28] and sensors have been put into a chair to sense postural changes related to levels of high or low interest in young learners working with educational software on a computer [29]. There is also lots of research on automated recognition of facial expression and on head gestures to discern states such as "concentrating," "disagreement," "thinking," "unsure," and "interested," [30] all of which could also be helpful to a machine trying to appear more caring by adjusting its responses to those of the person with whom it is interacting. Stronger results can be obtained by combining multiple channels, e.g. face with voice [31] or face with chair, mouse and task [32]. Different kinds of sensing may be more or less natural in different kinds of envi-

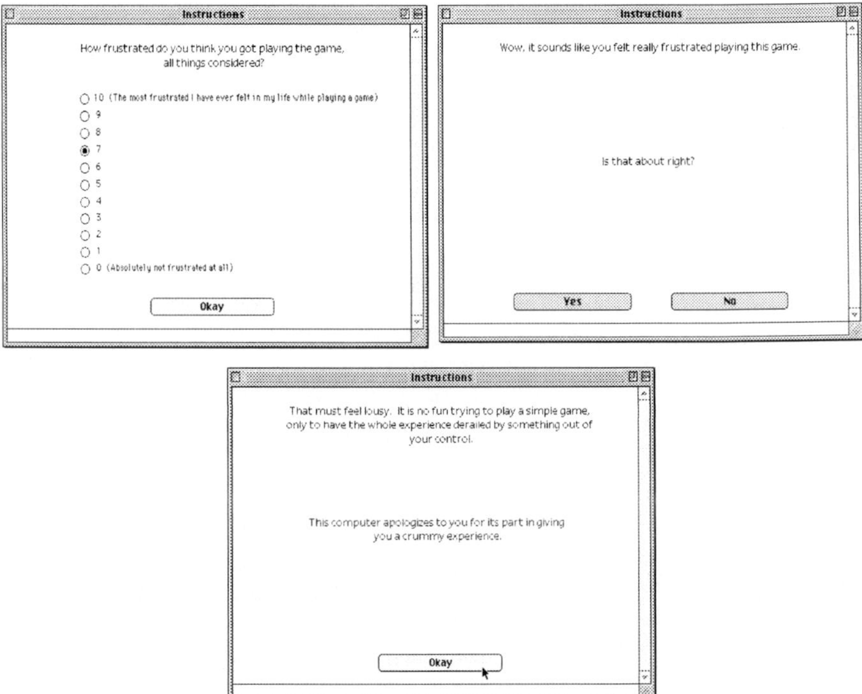

Figure 1. Klein et al. used simple dialogue boxes to convey the impression of active listening, empathy, and sympathy to frustrated computer users.

ronments, and confidence that the computer has properly recognized the person's affective state tends to increase with more than one mode of sensing.

4.2. Technologies for Influencing the Perception of Being Cared For

Once a computer agent has detected that a user is in need of caring, it may engage in some caring behaviors even without detecting the person's state, although knowing more about their state enhances chances of success. There are a wide range of comforting behaviors a computer could use to intervene (as outlined in Section 2.2), with the quintessential example being the expression of empathy. Here, we review some of the systems and studies in which a computer used empathy and other caring behaviors in its interaction with users. Additional examples include the work of Lisetti, et al. [33], Paiva, et al. [34], and Prendinger, et al. [27,35].

4.2.1. CASPER

One of the earliest empathic agents was the CASPER affect-management system developed by Klein et al. [17,36], which was demonstrated to provide relief to users experiencing frustration. The system presented a frustrated user with a series of menus (e.g., see three examples in Fig. 1) that prompted the user to describe his or her affective state, provided paraphrased feedback, allowed users to repair the computer's assessment and provided empathetic and sympathetic feedback. This agent was found to be significantly better than a venting-only agent (to which users could simply describe how they felt in an open-ended manner without feedback), or an agent that ignored their emotions completely, in relieving frustration, as measured by the length of time users were willing to continue working with a computer after a frustrating experience.

4.2.2. Computers as Social Actors

In their seminal series of studies and resulting book—*The Media Equation*—Cliff Nass and Byron Reeves at Stanford have demonstrated that when computers produce social cues that people respond in fundamentally social ways, even though this reaction is entirely unconscious [37]. In their book, they describe studies that demonstrated the following relational effects:

- Computers that use flattery, or which praise rather than criticize their users are better liked.
- Computers that praise other computers are better liked than computers that praise themselves, and computers that criticize other computers are liked less than computers that criticize themselves.
- Users prefer computers that match them in personality over those that do not (the "similarity attraction" principle).
- Users prefer computers that become more like them over time over those which maintain a consistent level of similarity, even when the resultant similarity is the same.
- Users who are "teamed" with a computer think better of the computer and cooperate more with it than those who are not teamed (the "in-group membership" effect, which can be achieved by simply signifying that the user and computer are part of a team).

Since the Media Equation was published, Reeves and Nass and their students have continued doing studies within this "Computers As Social Actors" paradigm. Morkes, Kernal and Nass demonstrated that computer agents that use humor are rated as more likable, competent and cooperative than those that do not [38]. Moon demonstrated that a computer that uses a strategy of reciprocal, deepening self-disclosure in its (text-based) conversation with the user will cause the user to rate it as more attractive, divulge more intimate information, and become more likely to buy a product from the computer [39].

In one of their most recent, and relevant, studies in this paradigm, Brave, Nass and Hutchinson compared the use of empathic facial displays and text messages by an embodied computer agent (using images of a person's face with different emotional displays) with self-oriented emotional displays and messages [40]. They found that the empathic agent was given more positive ratings, including likeability and trustworthiness, as well as greater perceived caring and felt support, compared to either an agent that used self-oriented displays and messages or an agent that performed no emotion-oriented behavior.

4.2.3. Mobile System for Sensing and Responding to Stress

Can machine empathy make a positive difference in people's acceptance of a highly interruptive device designed to collect information related to stress? Liu and Picard modified a handheld device (HP IPAQ) to receive signals wirelessly from a set of FitSense sensors for monitoring the heart, foot acceleration, and location context, and to associate this data with what users reported about their stress and how interruptible they were [19]. The device would interrupt people on average a dozen times a day, in order to query for their stress levels and acquire a better understanding of whether or not it was a good time to interrupt. Two versions of the system were built, one designed to be empathetic and one not, and both of which were friendly and polite, and engaged in brief text-only dialogues with the user, for example:

System: Morning, Jane! Do you have a minute?
Jane: Yes
System: You know the drill – feeling stressed?
Jane: It's there – but not the worst.
System: Wish it was better. Hope things start looking up.
System: Thanks so much for all your input.

The above dialogue differed in only one respect in the two conditions: In the empathetic condition all six of the above lines were exchanged. In the non-empathetic condition, the next to last line was omitted by the system. Thus, the empathetic condition took an extra second or two to respond to the user's feelings before thanking the user, while the non-empathetic condition only gave the last line, a polite thank you, in response to the user's statement of her feelings. The presence of an extra empathetic line happened in each interruption during all the days a user interacted with the empathetic system.

The empathetic system also used a slightly different algorithm to trigger when the interruptions would occur; however, this inadvertently led to the system interrupting people significantly more. Each subject was given each system to use for four days, in counterbalanced order. (Half the subjects used "A" then "B", without us indicating anything about any differences in the two systems, while the other half used "B" then "A".) After the eight days, users chose which one – A or B – that they wanted to use for the next four days. Seven out of ten chose the empathetic system over the control. When asked at the end of each of the first eight days, "about how many times does it seem like the system interrupted you today?" the users significantly underreported the number when using the empathetic system, and not when using the control. Also, at the end of the eight days, those in the group currently using the empathetic system reported a significantly higher desire to continue in the study. While the group of subjects was small, these findings support our intuition that introducing even a single line of empathetic response could have a measurable impact on people's perception of how interruptive a technology is, and on people's desire to keep using the technology.

4.2.4. FitTrack

Evidence that computers can instill a sense of caring comes from a recently completed study on the longitudinal effects of relationship-enhancing behaviors used by a computer agent (a "Relational Agent") on measures of user-computer relationship quality [18,41,42]. In this study the agent—named Laura—played the role of an exercise advisor designed to help subjects through a behavior change program, which was designed to increase their physical activity levels. The agent appeared as an embodied conversational agent [43], whose speech and nonverbal behavior (including hand gestures, eye gaze behavior, posture shifts, head nods, proximity and facial expressions) were controlled using the BEAT text-to-embodied speech engine [44] (see Fig. 1). Subjects conducted a 5 minute interaction with Laura daily on their home computers for one month, during which Laura provided feedback on their exercise behavior, helped them overcome obstacles to exercise, provided educational content related to exercise, and obtained and followed up on commitments to exercise.

A RELATIONAL version of the agent used all of the caring behaviors described above. For example, if a subject indicated they were not feeling well (and thus unable to exercise), Laura provide appropriate empathetic feedback while exhibiting a concerned facial expression (as in Fig. 1). A NON-RELATIONAL version of the agent delivered identical health content but had all caring and relational behaviors removed.

The principal outcome measure used in the study was the Working Alliance Inventory, a 36-item self-report questionnaire used in psychotherapy that measures the trust and belief that the therapist and patient have in each other as team-members in achieving a desired outcome [11]. The bond subscale of this instrument assesses the emotional bond between the helper and helpee and includes questions that specifically address the helpee's feeling cared for.

Thirty-three subjects completed the month of interactions with the RELATIONAL agent and twenty-seven subjects completed interactions with the NON-RELATIONAL agent. Subjects were recruited from the MIT campus, were mostly (69%) students and were 60% female (balanced across the two conditions).

Quantitative Results

In this chapter we only describe results that are particularly relevant to the notion of caring; for a full description see [13]. These results include the following items from the bond subscale of the Working Alliance Inventory, evaluated after four weeks of daily interaction. Subjects in the RELATIONAL condition indicated significantly greater agreement (on 7-point Likert scales) with the following items, compared with subjects in NON-RELATIONAL:

- "I feel that Laura cares about me in her own unique way, even when I do things that she does not approve of." t(60) = 2.39, p<.05.
- "I feel that Laura, in her own unique way, is genuinely concerned about my welfare." t(60) = 2.19, p<.05.
- "I feel that Laura, in her own unique way, likes me." t(60) = 2.56, p<.05.
- "Laura and I trust one another." t(60) = 2.05, p<.05.

When asked at the end of the month if they would like to continue working with Laura, subjects in the RELATIONAL condition also responded much more favorably than the NON-RELATIONAL group, t(57) = 2.43, p=.009. This measure is of particular importance since continuing with a treatment program is related to outcome, and desire to continue Treatment is likely to facilitate that result as well.

One behavioral measure related to caring was evaluated. In the closing session, subjects were given a choice of farewell greetings to say goodbye to the agent. Significantly more subjects in the RELATIONAL group (69%) chose the most sentimental farewell ("Take care Laura, I'll miss you." vs. "Bye.") than in the NON-RELATIONAL condition (35%), t(54) = 2.80, p=.004.

Qualitative Feedback

After the experiment we asked subjects about their experiences with Laura. When asked whether they liked the overall concept of conversing with and relating to an animated character, subjects reported strong opinions on both sides of the issue. Representative responses included:

- "It was a really, really great idea to have some kind of animated character because it makes you feel like you're actually talking to a person rather than having words on the computer screen."
- "Personally I detested Laura."
- "I like talking to Laura, especially those little conversations about school, weather, interests, etc. She's very caring. Toward the end, I found myself looking forward to these fresh chats that pop up every now and then. They make Laura so much more like a real person."

When asked "Do you feel that she really cared about you?", many subjects responded affirmatively but qualified their responses with comments such as:

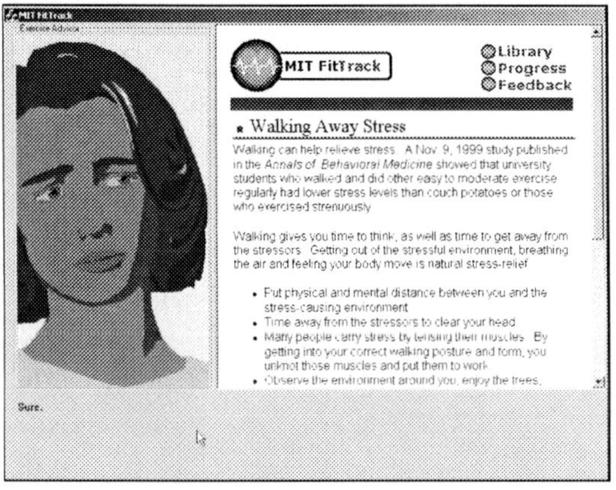

Figure 2. Exercise Advisor Agent.

- "Yes, as much as a computer can care."
- "Yea, I think there was an illusion there that she did."
- "As much as it mattered to ... I never forgot that it was a computer program, but you'll notice that I find myself calling her by feminine pronouns rather than calling her an 'it'. So, I definitely remembered that she was a computer program, but I did feel like it was a more personal interaction than that."

Other subjects responded with uncertainty about the concept of Laura "caring":

- "I find 'care' to be a funny term to use with a computer character. I felt like it was helpful to have positive reinforcement, even if it was from a computer character."
- "She's a computer character. I don't know if she cared about me. I don't know if she feels. She's a character and has a role, but I don't know if she has feelings. But, it worked for me and I'm happy."

Finally, there was a group of subjects who answered negatively, emphasizing Laura was a machine.

- "No, not really, because I plugged in a number and she had a script."
- "No. I felt like I was talking to a robot, to a machine."

These responses illustrate a range of user feedback about a system that might evoke feelings of caring – from liking to disliking, from acceptance of the effects to denial of any effects. While clearly the technology did not lead to strong reports of caring in everyone, nonetheless the effect was significant across the group when the caring behaviors were included.

4.2.5. FitTrack for Older Adults

Relational agents may provide an accessible user interface for much of the older adult population, and an especially effective channel for health communication and behavior change interventions. To test this hypothesis, a pilot study was recently conducted to evaluate the acceptance, usability and efficacy of a version of the FitTrack system used by patients from the Geriatric Ambulatory Practice (GAP) at Boston Medical Center, the primary safety net hospital in the Boston area [45,46].

Several modifications were made to the FitTrack system for older adults including: use of large fonts, a touch-screen interface, and modifications to the dialog content (see Fig. 2).

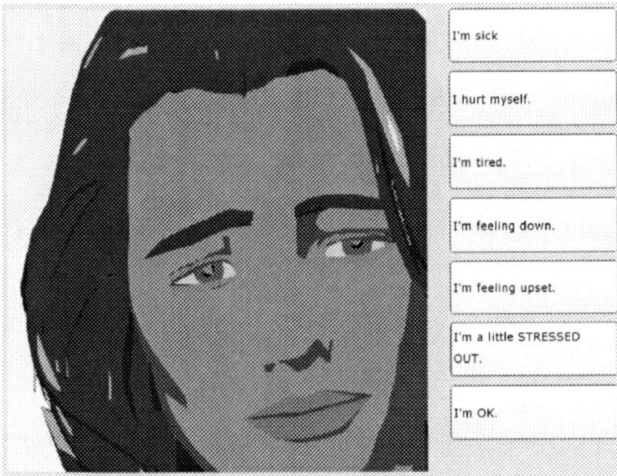

Figure 3. FitTrack for Older Adults.

A randomized trial compared subjects who interacted with the relational agent daily in their homes for two months (RELATIONAL) with a standard of care control group who were only given pedometers and print materials on the benefits of walking for exercise (CON-TROL). The subjects were twenty-two participants recruited into the study based on referrals from the GAP clinic. Participants ranged in age from 62 to 84, were 86% female, and 73% were African American. Seventeen (77%) were overweight or obese, and nineteen (86%) had low reading literacy [47]. Eight (36%) never used a computer before and six (27%) reported having used one only "a few times".

Comparisons between the RELATIONAL and CONTROL groups on daily recorded pedometer steps were based on generalized estimating equations (GEE) regression models for longitudinal data for increases in mean steps walked per week for each subject. The estimated slope (increase per week in mean weekly steps walked) for the CONTROL group was estimated as 83.9, while the slope for the RELATIONAL group was estimated as 411.1. The difference in slopes is significant ($p = 0.004$). The slope in the control group was not significantly different from 0 ($p = 0.295$), while the slope in the RELATIONAL group showed significant increase in steps over time ($p = 0.001$).

When asked if they liked Laura, RELATIONAL subjects scored this 6.3 on a scale of 1 (not at all) to 7 (very much), and scored their relationship with her a 5.6 on a scale of 1 (complete stranger) to 7 (close friend). When asked if they felt that Laura cared about them, they gave this an average score of 5.9 on a scale of 1 (not at all) to 7 (very much).

Post-experiment semi-structured interviews conducted with subjects in the RELA-TIONAL group indicated that most subjects liked the agent and felt that the feeling was reciprocal:

"By the way that she sound, she sound like she like me."

"I remember one weekend I went to Wareham... You know, I began to feel bad about Laura, stuck in that box."

4.2.6. Caring Robots

Several recent efforts in academia and industry have focused on creating robotic pets for older adults in order to achieve the same beneficial effects found in animal-assisted therapy, namely to decrease stress, anxiety and loneliness and improve mood, e.g. [48]. The "mental commit" robots take the form of cute stuffed animals such as a cat or a harp seal pup, and are designed to foster an attachment with users. One study compared the effects of these robots on older adults in a nursing home with the effects of an identical robot that had a much simpler behavioral repertoire, however no significant differences were found [49]. Although the robot was used in group sessions by the same individuals four days per week for three weeks, and has long-term memory and a reinforcement learning mechanism, it is not possible for it to model a relationship with any particular user given that it does not have the ability to discriminate between users. Another study compared the use of a Sony AIBO robotic dog with a stuffed toy dog and a "clothed" AIBO by a group of older adults with severe dementia. This study found that patients actually interacted more with the stuffed toy than either of the AIBOs, but the differences were not significant [50].

There is also an emerging commercial market for robotic dolls targeted at the older adult caretaking market, particularly in Japan. Bandai launched the Primopuel doll in 1999, which is designed to resemble a five-year-old boy who continually asks to be hugged and entertained. Dream Supply released the Snuggling Ifbot in 2004, intended to be a speech-based conversational partner for the elderly. Tomy recently announced the release of the Yumel doll, which also converses with older adults using speech, and assists users in maintaining healthy behaviors such as good sleep hygiene [51]. None of these systems have been reported on as being formally evaluated.

5. The Future

Our machines will undoubtedly continue to improve in their ability to calm, comfort and soothe us, to gain our trust and attachment, and—consequently—to help us in times of sickness and crisis. They may even surpass the ability of many humans to do so, given that they are always available and reliably consistent. In addition, since they can be a persistent part of our lives over many years or even decades, they can have perfect memories of our past history, personal needs, values and aspirations (in human relationships, long-standing intimates are the best source of social support [4]).

Caring machines can certainly make use of more sophisticated techniques in how they address our problems. For example, rather than just offering canned empathetic messages or messages indexed to degree of emotional upset (as in [17,18,40]), they can offer comforting messages that are indexed or formulated according to a much more fine-grained set of emotional criteria, such as: extent to which a user's feelings are explicitly acknowledged, elaborated and legitimized; extent to which the messages are centered on the user's emotions (vs. the computer's feelings or the causes of the upset); and whether the empathic messages also contain a cognitively-oriented explanation of the user's emotions or not [52]. These cognitive explanations can also help users re-examine the events that gave rise to their negative emotions in the first place so that they can better cope with the situation.

Of course making people emotionally dependent on their machines has many ethical implications. In addition to the possible malicious use of these machines for manipulation of their users (e.g., see [53]), computer crashes, repairs and upgrades—commonplace events in our current world of computers—suddenly become potentially traumatic events for their users.

Another ethical issue is that this kind of technology may serve to further socially isolate users from other people, even though the potential exists to use the technology to help bring people together. For example, in the FitTrack study involving older adults, one subject involved her friends in her discussions with Laura, and her friends would often ask her about her ongoing interactions with the character [46]:

> *"I brought my friends up here a couple of times to listen to her. My girlfriend she came upstairs with me and I show it. She say 'what's that?' and I say 'let me show you.' So I talk to her. So every time she talk to me she say 'Did you talk to Laura last night?.'"*

In addition, computer agents can serve in the capacity of match-makers, introducing people to others with similar interests, contacting friends when it thinks someone could use some human social support, and even pro-actively helping someone maintain their social network by reminding them to contact their friends periodically and helping them work through relational problems.

These caring agents will not only reside on our computers, but in our home robots, our mobile devices and in our health care facilities. Caring home health care robots could be used to help users through physical rehabilitation regimens or to bring them their medication, with the warmth and gentle coercion used by a skilled nurse who needs to motivate her patient to take care of themselves. Mobile devices, such as smart phones or PDAs, provide a platform in which caring health interventions can be delivered anytime, anywhere, such as smoking cessation messages at the instant a user gets a craving, or when someone is walking by the stairs on their way to the elevator. Finally, caring machines have obvious uses in our health care facilities, where patients are often ill informed about what is happening to them during hospital or emergency room visits or about proper self care when they return home. Caring agents could provide a persistent comforting presence throughout a hospital stay, answering questions, giving advice and preparing a patient emotionally for diagnoses, procedures, and home care.

References

[1] Picard R. Affective Computing Cambridge, MA: MIT Press; 1997.
[2] Levinson W, Gorawara-Bhat R, Lambs J. A Study of Patient Clues and Physician Responses in Primary Care and Surgical Settings. JAMA. 2000; 284(8):1021–1027.
[3] Berscheid E, Reis H. Attraction and Close Relationships. In: Gilbert D, Fiske S, Lindzey G, eds. The Handbook of Social Psychology. New York: McGraw-Hill; 1998:193–281.
[4] Glanz K, Lewis F, Rimer B. Health Behavior and Health Education: Theory, Research, and Practice San Francisco, CA: Jossey-Bass; 1997.
[5] Berkman L, Glass T. Social Integration, Social Networks, Social Support, and Health. In: Berkman L, Kawachi I, eds. Social Epidemiology. New York: Oxford Press; 2000.
[6] Wethington E, Kessler R. Perceived Support, Received Support, and Adjustment to Stressful Life Events. Journal of Health and Social Behavior. 1986; 27:78–89.
[7] LaVeist T, Sellers R, Brown K, Nickerson K. Extreme Social Isolation, Use of Community-Based Senior Support Services, and Mortality Among African American Women. American Journal of Community Psychology. 1997; 25:721–732.
[8] Fogg BJ. Captology: The Study of Computers as Persuasive Technologies. CHI 98; 1998:385.
[9] Horvath A, Symonds B. Relation Between Working Alliance and Outcome in Psychotherapy: A Meta-Analysis. Journal of Conseling Psychology. 1991; 38(2):139–149.
[10] Frankel R. Emotion and the Physician-Patient Relationship. Motivation and Emotion. 1995;19(3): 163–173.
[11] Horvath A, Greenberg L. Development and Validation of the Working Alliance Inventory. Journal of Counseling Psychology. 1989; 36(2):223–233.
[12] Squier R. A model of empathic understanding and adherence to treatment regimens in practitioner-patient relationships. Soc Sci Med. 1990; 30:325–39.
[13] Bickmore T. Relational Agents: Effecting Change through Human-Computer Relationships. MIT; 2003.
[14] Richmond V, McCroskey J. Immediacy. Nonverbal Behavior in Interpersonal Relations. Boston: Allyn & Bacon; 1995:195–217.
[15] Wilson C, Turner D. Companion Animals in Human Health SAGE Publications; 1997.
[16] Ryan E, Hummert M, Boich L. Communication predicaments of aging: patronizing behavior toward older adults. Journal of Language and Social Psychology. 1995; 14:144–66.
[17] Klein J, Moon Y, Picard R. This Computer Responds to User Frustration: Theory, Design, Results, and Implications. Interacting with Computers. 2002; 14:119–140.
[18] Bickmore T, Picard R. Establishing and Maintaining Long-Term Human-Computer Relationships. ACM Transactions on Computer Human Interaction. to appear.
[19] Liu K, Picard R. Embedded Empathy in Continuous, Interactive Health Assessment. CHI Workshop on HCI Challenges in Health Assessment. Portland, OR; 2005.

[20] Ma C, Osherenko A, Prendinger H, Ishizuka M. A Chat System Based on Emotion Estimation from Text and Embodied Conversational Messengers (Preliminary Report). 2005 IEEE Int'l Conf on Active Media Technology (AMT-05). Takamatsu, Kagawa, Japan; 2005: 546–548.

[21] Liu H, Lieberman H, Selker T. A Model of Textual Affect Sensing using Real-World Knowledge. 2003 Int'l Conf on Intelligent User Interfaces (IUI). Miami, FL: ACM; 2003: 125–132.

[22] Elliott C. The Affective Reasoner: A process model of emotions in a multi-agent system. Northwestern University; 1992.

[23] Fernandez R, Picard R. Classical and Novel Discriminant Features for Affect Recognition from Speech. Interspeech 2005 – Eurospeech – 9th European Conf on Speech Communication and Technology. Lisboa, Portugal; 2005.

[24] Douglas-Cowi E, Cowie R, Campbell N. Special Issue on Speech and Emotion. Speech Communication. 2003; 40(1–2).

[25] Picard RW, Vyzas E, Healey J. Toward Machine Emotional Intelligence: Analysis of Affective Physiological State. IEEE Transactions Pattern Analysis and Machine Intelligence. 2001; 23(10).

[26] Healey J, Picard R. Detecting Stress During Real-World Driving Tasks. IEEE Transactions on Intelligent Transportation Systems. to appear.

[27] Prendinger H, Mori J, Ishizuka M. Using Human Physiology to Evaluate Subtle Expressivity of a Virtual Quizmaster in a Mathematical Game. Int'l J of Human-Computer Studies. 2005; 62:231–245.

[28] Ark W, Dryer DC, Lu DJ. The Emotion Mouse. HCI International '99. Munich, Germany; 1999.

[29] Mota S, Picard R. Automated Posture Analysis for Detecting Learner's Interest Level. Workshop on Computer Vision and Pattern Recognition for Human-Computer Interaction, CVPR HCI; 2003.

[30] Kaliouby Re, Robinson P. Real-time Inference of Complex Mental States from Facial Expressions and Head Gestures. Real-Time Vision for HCI: Springer-Verlag; 2005:181–200.

[31] Huang TS, Chen LS, Tao H. Bimodal emotion recognition by man and machine. ATR Workshop on Virtual Communication Environments; 1998.

[32] Kapoor A, Ahn H, Picard R. Mixture of Gaussian Processes for Combining Multiple Modalities, in Proceedings of Multiple Classifier Systems. In: Oza NC, Polikar R, Kittler J, Roli F, eds. 6th Int'l Workshop on Multiple Classifier Systems. Seaside, CA; 2005:86–96.

[33] Lisetti C, Nasoz F, LeRouge C, Ozyer O, Alvarez K. Developing multimodal intelligent affective interfaces for tele-home health care. Int J Human-Computer Studies. 2003; 59(1–2):245–255.

[34] Paiva A, Dias J, Sobral D, Aylett R. Caring for agents and agents that care: Building empathic relations with synthetic agents. 3rd Int'l Joint Conference on Autonomous Agents and Multi Agent systems (AAMAS-04). New York; 2004.

[35] Prendinger H, Ishizuka M. The Empathic Companion: A Character-based Interface that Addresses User's Affective States. Int'l J of Applied Artificial Intelligence. 2005; 19(3–4):267–285.

[36] Klein JT. (MIT). Computer Response to User Frustration. 1999 February.

[37] Reeves B, Nass C. The Media Equation Cambridge: Cambridge University Press; 1996.

[38] Morkes J, Kernal H, Nass C. Humor in Task-Oriented Computer-Mediated Communication and Human-Computer Interaction. CHI 98; 1998:215–216.

[39] Moon Y. (Harvard Business School). Intimate self-disclosure exchanges: Using computers to build reciprocal relationships with consumers. 1998. Report No.: Working paper 99-059.

[40] Brave S, Nass C, Hutchinson K. Computers that care: investigating the effects of orientation of emotion exhibited by an embodied computer agent. Int J Human-Computer Studies. 2005; 62:161–178.

[41] Bickmore T, Picard R. Towards Caring Machines. CHI'04. Vienna; 2004.

[42] Bickmore T, Gruber A, Picard R. Establishing the computer-patient working alliance in automated health behavior change interventions. Patient Educ Couns. to apear.

[43] Cassell J, Sullivan J, Prevost S, Churchill E, eds. Embodied Conversational Agents. Cambridge, MA: The MIT Press; 2000.

[44] Cassell J, Vilhjálmsson H, Bickmore T. BEAT: The Behavior Expression Animation Toolkit. SIGGRAPH '01. Los Angeles, CA; 2001:477–486.

[45] Bickmore T, Caruso L, Clough-Gorr K. Acceptance and Usability of a Relational Agent Interface by Urban Older Adults. ACM SIGCHI Conference on Human Factors in Computing Systems (CHI); to appear.

[46] Bickmore T, Caruso L, Clough-Gorr K, Heeren T. "It's just like you talk to a friend" Relational Agents for Older Adults. Interacting With Computers. to appear.

[47] Lobach D, Hasselblad V, Wildemuth B. Evaluation of a Tool to Categorize Patients by Reading Literacy and Computer Skill to Facilitate the Computer-Administered Patient Interview. AMIA. Washington, DC; 2003:391–395.

[48] Banks M, Banks W. The effects of animal-assisted therapy on loneliness in an elderly population in long-term care facilities. J Geronol Med Sci. 2002; 57A:M428–M432.

[49] Wada K, Shibata T, Saito T, Tanie K. Effects of Robot Assisted Activity to Elderly People who Stay at a Health Service Facility for the Aged. Proceedings of the 2003 IEEE/RSJ Intl Conference of Intelligent Robots and Systems. Las Vegas, NV; 2003.
[50] Tamura T, Yonemitsu S, Itoh A, et al. Is an Entertainment Robot Useful in the Care of Elderly People with Severe Dementia? The Journals of Gerontology. 2004; 59A:83–85.
[51] AFP. As Japan goes grey, toymakers design dolls for the elderly. AFP Online. 2005. Feb 23.
[52] Burleson B. The Production of Comforting Messages: Social-Cognitive Foundations. J Lang and Social Psyc. 1985; 4(3&4):253–273.
[53] Picard R, Klein J. Computers that recognize and respond to user emotion: theoretical and practical implications. Interacting with Computers. 2002; 14:141–169.

Future of Intelligent and Extelligent Health Environment
R.G. Bushko (Ed.)
IOS Press, 2005

Cyber-Anthropology: A New Study on Human and Technological Co-Evolution

Alexander LIBIN, Ph.D. and Elena LIBIN, Ph.D.
Cyber-Anthropology Research, Inc., Georgetown University, Washington, D.C., USA

Abstract. For the first time cyber-anthropology is defined as a concept and a new field of study aimed at the analysis of person's reciprocal relations with the computer-generated (CG) world evolved as a result of technological progress. In the cyber-era, simulated reality has come to the point of becoming a force that has the potential to transform the human race. Digital beings such as virtual and embodied agents, although not a part of the natural human habitat, have become necessary elements of people's surroundings and life conditions. As a theoretical construct, Cyber-anthropology is concerned with the merger of natural and artificial worlds mediated by the human imagination, as well as compatibility between people and digital life they have created. As an empirical study, Cyber-anthropology deals with the psychophysiology and psychophysics, semantic and semiotics of human engagement with computer-generated reality that is viewed as a Complex Interactive System. Personal competence as a crucial element of any cyber-system underlines the importance of psychological culture in artificial world exploration. A newly developed concept of Psychological Culture is viewed as an essential part of Cyber-anthropology while concentrating on the following core issues: (1) ethical questions, such as whether or not technological tools can be employed to solve human problems; (2) moral consequences of bringing cutting edge technology into our every day life; (3) studies of individual differences regarding psychological competence of technology users through effective vs. ineffective, independent vs. addictive, and active vs. passive dichotomies. Psychological Culture is defined as the study of a person's competence associated with the use of modern technology and individual acceptability of technological innovations. Several crucial dilemmas arise when a human being is engaged in a simulated environment, and artificial agents inhabit a human world. The ultimate goal of Psychological Culture is to provide people with the knowledge necessary for adequate recognition of scientific innovations to overcome obstacles in the process of implementing technology to enhance human well being.

1. Computer-Generated Reality: A Personal Touch

Since ancient times people employed their imaginations to model fictitious realities filled with bizarre creatures and strange life forms capable of acting beyond human possibilities. When all the other necessary survival tools were exhausted, people used the power of their minds to gain the strength of the spirit when fighting unknown diseases or trying to understand unpredictable chains of events. Sometimes, the thin line between the real and imaginary worlds would became blurry or even disappear. The degree of self-immersion into one's own fantasy combined with people's ability to keep up with their actual life requirements would result either in total mal-adaptation or in the re-construction of the existing realities. Modern technological tools have enriched human abilities not only in exploration, but in altering our inner and outer worlds. With the development of digital vehicles for information technologies, we entered a realm never experienced before by the human mind or senses. How do these new experiences fit into the existing methodology of human studies? What are the conceptual frames for analyzing and interpreting a person – cyber-world interaction? Is it possible to predict the outcome of those interactions? Below are defined some primary coordinates of the emerging field of Cyber-anthropology – a theoretical and practical study of human-centered, digitally-based technological systems, their structure, development, and functioning.

1.1. On the Crossroad of Anthropology and Cybernetics

A clashing charisma of anthropological studies attracted materialists and idealists, empiricists and methodologists, naturalists and humanitarians. The term 'anthropology' (from Greeks 'anthro-' – a man, and 'logos' – a study) was coined by Aristotle more than 2000 years ago [1], and the new discipline of anthropology was formulated by Kant in 18th century [2] acknowledged the beginning of a science that focused on studying physical, psychological, and cultural trends in human development. The aims of anthropology include the whole range of analyses from cultural artifacts (i.e., archeological method) and diversity of customs and beliefs (i.e., ethnographical method) to the study of human kind's similarity to and divergence from the animal kingdom (i.e., methods of physical anthropology and sociobiology). The body of knowledge about human life phenomenology was greatly expanded by the explorations of philosophical, structural, psychological and semiotic anthropology (see Table 1). However, regardless of the scientific paradigm underlying the investigation of a particular aspect of human – world interactions, anthropological analysis strived to search for the answers to the two inter-related questions posed by our very existence: *How do human beings transcend themselves in their own experience?*, and: *How do people actually behave?* [3].

Over the last twenty centuries, the systematic study of *Homo sapiens*, specifically their physical, psychological, and socio-cultural functioning, went through numerous transformations. The recent one is associated with the rise of highly technological systems based upon electronic "brains" and digitally originated behaviors. In such hybrids, a person appears as a human agent who performs a peripheral or – sometimes – a central role in the complex system functioning. A concentrated view on the essence of relationships between artificial and living systems was formulated by Norbert Wiener in 1948 in a concept named cybernetics (from Greek *kybernet*(es) or steer(-s) man) [4]. Cybernetics is viewed as a science of control processes in organic, and technological, mechanical and electronic systems. Cybernetic principles are employed by psychology for exploring the phenomena of artificial intelligence and emotion-like behaviors, by social sciences for studying effective management, and by engineering for analyzing the optimizing possibilities of technology-based processes.

Both worlds – human and artificial – came to existence as a result of evolution: socio–biological or technological respectively. The development of two independent subjects of study – anthropological and technological – brought to life a new field of Cyber-anthropology. Its dual nature is an adequate systematic method for studying this hybrid phenomenon – the cyber world.

1.2. Cyber-Anthropology: Human World Through the Prism of Technology

The definition of the new phenomenon is unavoidably multi-semantic, for it has to account for the methodology and the epistemology of the variety of analyzed experiences, as well as their theoretical and practical implications. Bearing this in mind, we would like to present a unified framework that combines various meanings – or, rather, dimensions for the analysis – of the emerging field named Cyber-anthropology (see Table 1):

Table 1. Definitive classification of Cyber-anthropology.

Anthropological models of man	Cyber-anthropology elements		
	Focus of the computer-mediated analysis	**Subject of Cyber-anthropology study**	**Related cyber-phenomena**
Physical anthropology/ Cognitive anthropology	Reconstruction of human beings via virtual representations	Archeological and evolutionary aspects of human physical representations through the historical and geographic prospective	Digital reconstruction of human's predecessors, their behavior, and associated artifacts
Ethnographical anthropology/ Social anthropology	Analysis of computer-mediated social interactions	Social manifestation of interactions between humans and virtual agents	Virtual heritage and Internet culture
Philosophical anthropology	Methodological analysis of computer-generated phenomena such as presence and immersion	Reflection on human existence into digital world	Sense of immersion and presence produced by person's engagement in virtual reality or virtual communications
Structural anthropology/ Semiotic anthropology	Structural analysis of semantic and semiotic of digital artifacts	Functioning of digital symbols	Imaginary, virtual, and embodied personages; digital folklore; myths of computer era
Psychological anthropology	Study of compatibility between human and technology	Psycho-physiological, psychological, and social effects produced by human – computer interactions	Digital self and virtual identity; cyborg-dilemma; psychological aspects of people-robot co-existence

Cyber-anthropology for the first time is defined as a concept and a new field of study aimed at the analysis of human reciprocal relations with the computer-generated (CG) world which have evolved as a result of technological progress. In the cyber-era, simulated reality has come to the point of becoming a force that has the potential to transform the human race. Digital beings such as virtual and embodied agents, although not a part of the natural human habitat, have become necessary elements of people's surroundings and life conditions. As a theoretical construct, Cyber-anthropology is concerned with the merger of natural and artificial worlds mediated by human imagination, as well as the compatibility between people and the virtual and embodied forms of digital life they have created. As an empirical study, Cyber-anthropology deals with the psychophysiology and psychophysics, semantic and semiotics of human engagement with computer-generated reality viewed as a Complex Interactive System [5].

2. Cyber-Anthropology as a Science of Differentiation Between Living and Artificial Complex Interactive Systems

The importance of the notion that speaks to distinctions in origin, structure and ultimate goals of living and non-living, inanimate, artificial systems has been emphasized by many authors. The founder of differential psychology and inventor of the IQ (Intelligence Quotient) hypothesis, William Stern, pointed out that the biggest methodological mistake is to apply mechanistic interpretation to the analysis of '*a person*', which transforms it into '*a thing*' by eliminating a certain psychological component from the epistemological and phenomenological analysis [6,7]. A differing criteria, based upon the '*closed vs. open*' dichotomy, was offered by von Bertalanffy, a creator of the modern systematic approach, to distinguish between *non-living, closed* and *living, open complex systems* [8].

A study of the principles of mental representation revealed the fundamental role of tactile-kinesthetic gestalts in forming a hierarchical structure not only of sensory-motor, but emotional and cognitive mental phenomena [9]. Only the neuronal core of an open living system is able to produce tactile-kinesthetic sensation unavailable in the artificial systems. The latter is based exclusively upon information exchange in the form of electric impulses, which lie at the foundation of electronic-originated phenomenology. No matter how complex the system is and how high the level of the system's internal or external interactivity is, the ability of living beings to transform non-transitive physical properties of an object into the internal sensation through the tactile-kinesthetic mechanism [9], remains a major criteria that differentiates between natural and artificial phenomena, mental and virtual representations, real and unreal experiences.

It is notable that a concept of complexity brings two vitally significant components into the cyber-anthropological approach – the non-linear nature of examining phenomena and its interactive nature. Perhaps because interactivity is a main characteristic of the brain [10], mental functioning [9] and human development in general [11], an interactive nature of cyber-applications makes them natural – like part of our physical and social environment. On the other hand, having human personality as a main element in person–cyber-world interactions emphasizes the key role of psychological knowledge in understanding the character of cyber-anthropological models. In 1930, Vygotsky rightfully suggested that a study of psychological systems focuses rather on the analyses of relations between different functions and modifications of these relations over time, than on changes within each function and their structure [12].

Differentiation between living and artificial systems, based upon open–closed dichotomy and tactile-kinesthetic criteria, interactive complexity, and structural analysis of functional frames, outlines the theoretical part of Cyber-anthropological approach.

3. Practical Applications of Cyber-Anthropology

The artifacts produced by digital technologies form the subject for experimental and applied Cyber-anthropology research. Primary classification of computer-generated phenomena sheds some light on the practical agenda of Cyber-anthropology, which includes an examination of:

A. *Cyber-space*, including: 1) computer-mediated communication such as Internet, Email, Chat groups, Virtual communities, 2) World Wide Web as a mediated form of immediate social contacts, 3) cyber-culture

B. *Virtual environments* as part of 1) VR-based application (i.e., database representations, cyber-therapy products), 2) video games, and 3) virtual projection of digital structures

C. *Digital representation* or reconstruction of real experiences associated with 1) living beings such as humans – ancient in case of traditional physical anthropology and archeology, or modern in case of virtual medicine, and 2) material objects (i.e., virtual heritage or modern architecture)

D. *Human-computer interactions* as constellation of psychological and ergonomic factors including multi-modal interfaces

E. *Embodied agents* in the form of interactive robotic creatures with artificial intelligence and sensory feedback, e.g., lifelike robots imitating living beings, humanoids, etc.

The first three sub-groups (A-C) are organized in a class of virtual phenomena, the fourth group is structured as a transitional class combining both virtual and embodied elements, and, finally, the last group (E) presents a newly emerged class of embodied agents – a materialized form of digital activity. Cyber-anthropological studies of person – robot interactions are carryied out in two modes recognized as *Robotic Psychology* and *Robotherapy*. Robotic psychology focuses on the compatibility between humans and robots [13], while Robotherapy concentrates on using interactive robots as therapeutic agents for people with psychological problems or limited physical, cognitive, or emotional resources [14,15].

4. First Research Priorities from the Cyber-Anthropologist's Point of View

Although traditional approach has proved the effectiveness of the formula 'All's well that ends well', a more important rule at the beginning of new ventures (ought to sound like) sound like: "It's better to start well". Presented below is a brief schema for the Cyber-anthropology research necessary to establish a systematic techno-knowledge [16] about the field:

- Emotional experiences triggered by both virtual and embodied digital interactions;
- Criteria of differentiation between real and imaginary worlds;
- Symbolic meaning of computer-mediated interactions and digitally-generated experiences;
- Stereotypes and myths about the origins and functioning of cyber-reality;
- Psychological and psycho-physiological effects produced by person interactions with virtual and embodied agents;
- The nature of presence and immersion;
- Classification of cyber-phenomena based on tactile-kinesthetic and visio-geometrical gestalts and related studies on multi-modal interfaces.

Finally, the concept of Psychological Culture deserves a special attention in Cyber-anthropology study program.

5. Psychological Culture as a Subject for Cyber-Anthropology Studies

In the technological age, Psychological Culture plays an essential role in balancing real and artificial worlds' co-existence through mediated interactions. Personal competence underlines the importance of psychological culture in artificial world exploration as a crucial element of any cyber-system. From this point of view, Psychological Culture is defined as the study of a person's competence associated with the use of modern technology and individual acceptability of technological innovations. Special consideration is given to the study of individual differences in people's interactions with the artificial world. The personality-oriented focus of Psychological Culture makes it an integral part of Cyber-anthropology. One of the fundamental standpoints of Cyber-anthropology is that our co-existence with the artificial world, though highly complex, complies with physiological, psychological and cultural regularities of the individual and social life. Psychological Culture is based upon a humanistic approach and concentrates on investigating the following Cyber-anthropology related issues:

- Exploring advantages and disadvantages of human-cyberworld co-existence;
- Understanding the psychological specifics of interactions between persons and their artificial partner (i.e., virtual or embodied agent) on all levels: sensory-motor, emotional, cognitive, behavioral and social;

- Studying how the rich diversity of our personalities justifies a broad variety of environments and agents;
- Searching for possible solutions of moral dilemmas stemming from human- technology interactions;
- Providing people with knowledge required for the further virtual space expansion and effective person–artificial agent collaboration.

First of all, Psychological Culture concentrates on ethical questions such as whether or not technological tools can be employed to solve human problems. The next important issue relates to the study of the moral consequences of bringing cutting edge technology into our every day life. The third core question involves a study of individual differences with relation to psychological competence of technology users through effective vs. ineffective, independent vs. addictive, active vs. passive dichotomies.

Among the main topics that catch the attention of psychological culture researchers are such questions as *'Why does one person maintain a lifestyle independent from modern technologies while others develop technology (TV, computer, internet etc.) addictions?'*, *'What are the psychological parameters that can predict effective or ineffective technology usage?'*, and *'How technology can help people cope with their problems without putting an extra burden on them?'*

In sum, Psychological Culture studies the extensive range of psychological aspects of technology–mediated communication that arise on the merge of artificial and human worlds.

6. Technology–Mediated Solutions for Human Problems

In recent decades, the merger of artificial and human worlds has shown its promising results. Many researchers, engineers, and practitioners have already proven the productivity of technological applications in such areas as health, education, therapy and entertainment. In particular, exploration of virtual reality advantages known as 'immersion' and 'sense of presence' promoted a creation of original VR-based methods of psychological therapy. A new approach named Cybertherapy [17] showed effectiveness of VR-applications employed for treating psychological disorders including phobias (i.e., fear of flying, agoraphobia, etc.), social anxiety, different kinds of addiction (i.e., gambling, tobacco addiction), and cognitive and emotional deficits (i.e., autism, attention deficit hyperactivity disorder, sensory disintegration, etc.). Computer-generated reality has proven to be a useful therapeutic tool for a wide variety of populations such as children and the elderly, persons with physical and mental disabilities, and people who live both in home environment and clinical settings.

Success of early VR-based therapeutic interventions has inspired designers to further investigate the potential of artificial tools to provide real-life benefits. This is a vivid example of mutually advantageous collaboration between technology and psychology.

Another promising technological application concerns the development of embodied digital agents or interactive robots. The contemporary world of robotics is inhabited by a broad variety of artificial creatures designed for the purpose of helping people with special needs to overcome their limitations and enrich their quality of life. Nowadays, robotic creatures are used as mediators in the treatment of mood disorders, loneliness and depression, and as rehabilitation aids. The concept of an artificial partner [5] places person-robot interactions into a psychological, rather than a technological, context. Beneficial features of robots as human companions lie at the foundation of a new field of study named Robotic psychology and Robotherapy [13,14]. Even so, interactive robots serve as therapeutic agents or stimulating companions, the effectiveness of people's communication with their artificial partners depends on their compatibility. Therefore, the robot's design should take into an account a whole range of both psychological and ergonomic parameters. This means performing a comprehensive analysis of human differences that underlie preferences in communication mode or intensity of interactions, degree of emotional or tactile stimulation, and the specifics of personal needs that are essential for maintaining effective person–robot compatibility.

Obviously, the broad diversity of people's personalities justifies the creation of a wide variety of virtual and embodied agents. Since a person is the central part of technology-mediated communication, human factors define the adequacy and effectiveness of the process' organization *per se*. An outcome of computer-mediated interactions depends on two inter-related issues:

- whether or not the person's individuality matches the specifics of artificial environment or agent;
- the level of the person's psychological culture based upon an understanding of the role and place technology takes in human life.

7. Moral Dilemmas of Human Engagement with the Artificial World

Without doubt, exciting virtual reality (VR) and robotics' applications have enriched science and engineering, industry and public service, medicine and entertainment, psychology and psychiatry, education and therapy. Technological agents positively influence the quality of human life by bringing accessibility and comfort, inspiration and enjoyment. Computerized tools have greatly expanded the human capability to visualize desires, materialize images, and observe the hidden processes. However, several crucial dilemmas arise when a human being is engaged in the simulated environment, and artificial agents inhabit the human world.

7.1. Virtual Presence vs. Reality Absence

Cyber-phenomenon known as 'presence' is a subjective sense of being in a virtual environment. Sheridan defines presence as 'sensory information generated only by and within a computer... a feeling of being present in an environment other than the one that person is actually in' [18]. Visual, auditory and haptic sensations produced by virtual reality applications are a part of an artificially simulated environment, otherwise known as artificially simulated illusions, which allow persons to experience 'presence'. Artificially triggered senses of presence may create positive, though illusory, experiences (i.e., VR-based treatment of phobias), or create false experiences resulting in a new chain of real problems (i.e., MUD-addiction based on false identity). One of the main psychological problems and moral dilemmas associated with the phenomena of presence stems from the person's inability to distinguish between real and artificial words. Individual inability to understand that those two worlds are not identical, but different, creates a barrier for implementing the achievements of engineering science. Psychological culture aims at studying the nature of simulated illusions and elaborating criteria for experiencing the sense of presence without side effects.

7.2. Coping with Difficulties vs. Escaping from Life

Technological applications provide people with new tools for coping with life's difficulties.

The level of individual psychological culture or psychological competence depends on understanding the meaning of technological progress for one's own life. If used appropriately, artificial reality expands human possibilities and enhances quality of life. However, there is much evidence of using technological innovations as an excuse to escape from real life problems into an illusory world. Psychological Culture is aimed at studying the criteria of differentiation between technology–mediated coping and defensive strategies. Coping strategies are defined as cognitive, emotional, and behavioral efforts *directed toward resolving an experiencing difficulty*. Defensive strategies are cognitive, emotional and behavioral efforts *directed away from actual problem solving* [19].

7.3. Assistance vs. Substitute

The next main task of Psychological Culture is to bring awareness to an individual as well as social consciousness about the value of both technology–mediated assistance and human support. Neither artificial reality nor any of its superlative products may serve as a replacement for genuine human relationships. Lack of psychological competence necessary for the adequate use of technical innovations in our daily life leads to various side effects, such as computer dependence, mixed identities resulting from rejection of real self in favor to the virtual persona, replacing human communications with electronic message exchanges and interpersonal relationships with person–machine interactions.

In particular, the moral dilemma of 'assistance vs. substitute' stressed in the use of robotic creatures for therapeutic purposes. The most important concern many researchers and practitioners pose is that robots would become a substitute for human caregivers [20,21]. This is true for any kind of robotic assistance. For instance, the use of robotic pets poses a question: '*Are robotic pets designed with the intention of replacing our favorite cats and dogs?*' This dilemma requires special attention from psychological culture research. When a robotic creature is employed in therapeutic practice, it is necessary for a therapist to keep in mind that any state-of-the-art robot is only a technological tool. The use of technological innovations establishes special requirements for psychological culture of the therapist or professional caregiver. It is especially important to not delegate a therapist's function to a robot. Humanistic robotherapy considers innovative technological tools as an additional resource essential to human care, but not the other way around. Robotherapy cannot be interpreted as an excuse for a therapist to avoid responsibility or deprive caretakers from human assistance. Effective technology–mediated health intervention of any kind is based upon conscious preference of technological means viewed as a way to improve human assistance while providing compassionate professional treatment [22].

Thus, a concept of Psychological Culture based upon an idea that human engagement with an artificial world is not an escape from reality and an excuse to avoid life's challenges, but an opportunity to expand coping resources.

8. Conclusion

Cyber-anthropology can be defined as a study of how humans are influenced by the artificial world produced by the technological evolution. In a broad sense, Cyber-anthropology is the science of investigating physiological, psychological, and socio-cultural phenomena that occur as a result of interactions between human mind–body systems and artificial computer–generated reality.

To gain benefits from cyberspace exploration, as well as from interactions with virtual and embodied agents, one needs to employ a systematic analysis of psychophysiology and psychophysics, semantic and semiotics of human–artificial world co–existence. Cyber-anthropology, while studying a complexity of person–machine interactions, employs principles of Psychological Culture. The ultimate goal of the new approach is to provide people with the knowledge necessary for adequate recognition of scientific innovations to overcome obstacles in the process of implementing technology to enhance human well–being.

Acknowledgments

Authors would like to thank the Faculty at the Department of Psychology at the Georgetown University, and especially our dearest friend and colleague Professor James T. Lamiell, and Professor Lee Ross at the Department of Psychology at Stanford University for their continuing support of our projects and for their enthusiasm so necessary at the beginning of any new venture.

References

[1] Encyclopedia of Philosophy, volume 1, Nauka, Moscow, 1960, p. 79 (in Russian).

[2] E. Kant, Anthropology from a Pragmatic Point of View. Leipzig, 1797/1926 (in German).

[3] E. Kant, Critique of Pure Reason. St.Martin's Press, New York, 1781/1965.

[4] N. Wiener, Cybernetics, Wiley, New York, 1948.

[5] A, Libin, Virtual Reality as a Complex Interactive System: A multidimensional model of person-artificial partner co-relations. In: H. Thwaites, & L. Addison (eds.), *Proceedings of the Seventh International Conference on Virtual Systems and Multimedia*. IEEE Computer Society, Los Alamitos, CA, 2001, pp. 652–657.

[6] W. Stern, Person und Sache. System des Kritischen Personalismus. Leipzig, 1923 (in German).

[7] J. Lamiell, Critical Personalism, Sage, San Francisco, 2003.

[8] von Bertalanffy, Robots, Men and Minds. Psychology in a modern world. George Braziller, New York, 1967.

[9] L. Vekker, and A. Libin, The Nature of Mind: Principles of Mental Representation, unpublished manuscript. Monographs of the Complex Interactive Systems Research Inc., 2002.

[10] K. Pribram, Languages of the Brain, New York, 1971.

[11] M. Bornstein, and J. Bruner (eds.), Interaction in Human Development. Lawrence Erlbaum Associates, Publisher, Hillsdale, New Jersey, 1989.

[12] L. Vygotsky, On Psychological Systems. In: Selected work, volume 1, Pedagogic, Moscow, 1989, pp. 109–131 (in Russian).

[13] A. Libin and E. Libin, Robotic Psychology. In: Encyclopedia of Applied Psychology, Academic Press, San Francisco (in print; expected in 2004).

[14] E. Libin and A. Libin, Robotherapy. In: Encyclopedia of Applied Psychology, Academic Press, San Francisco (in print; expected in 2004).

[15] E. Libin and A. Libin, A New Tool for Robotic Psychology and Robtherapy Studies, Cyber-Psychology and Behavior, volume 6, 4, Media Institute, San Francisco, 2003, pp. 124–131.

[16] E. Schraube, The Politics of TechnoKnowledge: An Experimental Moment in Psychology. In: N. Stephenson, R. Jorna, L. Radtke and H. Stam (eds.), Theoretical Issues in Psychology. Captus University Publication, Toronto, 2003.

[17] Wiederhold, B. & Wiederhold, K. (1998). A Review of Virtual Reality as Psychotherapeutic Tool, CyberPsychology & Behavior: The impact of the Internet, Multimedia and Virtual reality on Behavior and Society, 1(1), 45–52.

[18] Sheridan, T. (2002). Defining our terms. *Presence* 1(2):272–274.

[19] Libin, E. (2003). Individual differences in coping-defense strategies related to solving life difficulties. Ph.D.Thesis, Institute of Psychology at the Russian Academy of Education (in Russian).

[20] Libin, A., Libin, E., Ojika, T., Nishimoto, Y., Takeuchi, T., Matsuda, Y., Takahashi, Y. (2002). On Person – Robot Interactions: Cat NeCoRo Communicating In Two Cultures *(Phase 1. USA – Japanese study)*. Proceedings of the 8th International Conference on Virtual Systems and Multimedia, Creative Digital Culture, VSMM Society, Seoul, pp. 899–905.

[21] Libin, A., Cohen-Mansfield, J. (2004). Therapeutic robocat for nursing home residents with dementia: Preliminary inquiry, pp. 111–117. American Journal of Alzheimer's Disease and Other Dementias, 19 (2).
[22] Libin, A., Libin, E. (2004). Person – Robot Interactions From the Robopsychologists Point of View: The Robotic Psychology and Robotherapy Approach. In: Person – Robot Interactions for Psychological Enrichment, IEEE Special Issue (expected in 2004).

Hi-Tech Cure and Care Era – Examples: Future of Cancer and Addiction Control

Future of Intelligent and Extelligent Health Environment
R.G. Bushko (Ed.)
IOS Press, 2005

Harnessing the Power of an Intelligent Health Environment in Cancer Control

Bradford W. HESSE, Ph.D.
Acting Chief, Health Communication and Informatics Research Branch,
National Cancer Institute, Rockville, MD, US

Abstract. In 1971, when Congress declared "war on cancer," the public's perception was driven by an image of a single cure for a single disease. What researchers have learned since that time is that cancer is a formidable enemy made up of more than 100 different disease etiologies. The war on cancer became a war of the 21st century; a war to be fought on multiple fronts against a diffuse enemy and for which prevention was the most judicious path to victory. To fight this new war on cancer, the National Cancer Institute must seek to harness the power of health informatics to create a supportive environment for transforming science, delivering safe and patient-centric health care, and creating an environment of personal empowerment in public health. Three different types of health informatics applications are implicated: (a) applications in bioinformatics, which are intended to revitalize the engine of scientific discovery; (b) applications in medical informatics, which will create a safer and more effective environment for delivery; and (c) applications in consumer informatics, which will enable individuals to advance the charge of their own ongoing health care over the course of their lives. To keep these applications on track, health care administrators must take a sociotechnical approach to implementation. The new systems must be built into the health care environment in such a way that they support human capacities, provide failsafe backups in the face of cognitive and physical limitations, and support continuous quality improvement.

1. Introduction

In July 2001 the Institute of Medicine released "Crossing the Quality Chasm," its landmark prescription for health care in the 21st Century. The major theme of the report was far reaching: "Health care today is characterized by more to know, more to manage, more to watch, more to do, and more people involved in doing it than at any time in the nation's history." No one individual can expect to grasp the complexity of modern medical science, nor can any one individual stay abreast of the tsunami of data and findings that comprise effective health care over the life span of a typical patient [1].

Changes must be made, authors of the report argued, to the very system in which health care occurs to deal with the sheer volume of mounting medical information, and to ensure that the right information is brought to bear at the right time on every health decision made throughout an individual's lifespan. The only way this is going to happen is through advances in information technology. At the very least, the health care system has to be redesigned to make the same essential use of information technology—through computerized records management, electronic data interchange, and safety systems—that are already standard in other industries [2]. More critically, to win the health battles of the 21st century, the system will need to make substantive leaps forward. It must grow to accommodate the terabytes of data associated with analyses from the microcellular level of the human genome, while scaling up to accommodate the petrabytes of data needed to array medical data across individuals equitably and safely throughout the population. In short, the information-rich environment of health care must be supportive of health and wellness in the 21st century.

This chapter illustrates how the role of an intelligent health environment will be crucial for sustaining victory on one of the more significant health battles of the 21st century, the fight against cancer. It begins by explaining how the fight against cancer is conceptualized by researchers and practitioners at the National Cancer Institute (NCI), the institution that is tasked by thc US Federal Government to lead research efforts against the disease. It then explains how the development of a coordinated health informatics infrastructure will be a necessary, enabling step for transforming the research enterprise, improving practice, and enabling personal health decision-making.

2. Understanding the "War on Cancer"

In 1971, with the passage of the Cancer Act, the U.S. Congress declared "war on cancer." [3] Using a popular metaphor that resonated with a population only two and half decades removed from World War II, the battle cry galvanized the nation's resolve in combating a pernicious, biological foe. New resources poured into the NCI, while an army of scientists worldwide stepped up efforts to find an otherwise elusive cure.

The scientific progress made since that time has been astounding, but what the biomedical community learned was just how formidable and sophisticated the enemy was. What we now know to be cancer is really a family of 100 + diseases, each with parallel yet distinct etiological paths, and a lethal tendency to spawn new malignancies through an insidious process of metastasis. Rather than resemble the "Great War" against a single enemy, the war on cancer looks more like the 21st century "war on terror" – a protracted battle that requires a high level of intelligence and monitoring to avert threat altogether or detect and eliminate threat early before damage becomes widespread.

2.1. The Disease Process

To understand the opportunities for intervention in the new war against cancer, it is important to understand the common course of the disease. The common pathology of cancer is illustrated in Fig. 1. In essence, cancer occurs when the process of normal cell division goes awry, leading to uncontrolled and unchecked cellular growth. Cell division occurs throughout the life span, with predictable intracellular processes in place to transcribe genetic code into new growth throughout the body [4]. With such a great number of cell divisions occurring over the life span it is natural that some errors will occur in the process. Certain influences from the environment – say tobacco smoke or radiation – can exert a mutative pressure on groups of cells that can subvert normal regulatory processes. When this happens, anomalous cell growth will continue unabated forming neoplasms, or tumors. For some people, the genetic blueprint guiding cell division may itself contain inherited anomalies that can make these individuals more susceptible to disruptions in the growth process than others. For these people, the combination of genetic predisposition and exposure to toxic influences in the environment can prove to be lethal [5–7].

Usually, biologic safeguards are in place to identify offending cells and remove them before systemic damage occurs. If that does not happen, the growth process can result in new or extraneous tissue. If the extraneous tissue, or tumor, remains localized and does not invade surrounding tissue it is considered benign; if the new tissue continues to expand into

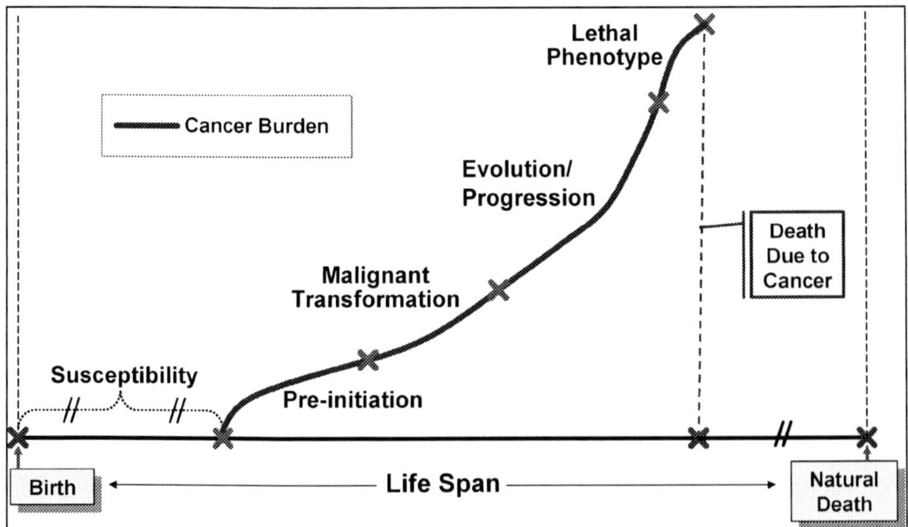

Figure 1. The disease process underlying most cancers.

surrounding areas it is considered malignant. Malignant tumors will often stimulate the growth of new blood vessels that bring nutrients and oxygen into the growing tumor, a process referred to as angiogenesis [8]. The growth of new capillaries and blood vessels can create a conduit by which cancerous cells may break off from the original site and metastasize into other sites within the body. It is this process that makes cancer so deadly. Locally constrained growths can often be tolerated with only mildly debilitative effects or can be excised completely through carefully targeted surgery. Metastatic disease poses a more systemic threat by spreading the malignancy to other sites in the body. When a cancer reaches a stage of uncontrolled growth and diffusion, it usually becomes lethal [9].

2.2. Windows of Opportunity for Intervention

Understanding the pathology of malignant neoplasms provides an enlightened view of where the windows of opportunity are for controlling the disease as illustrated in Fig. 2. For example, identifying the agents and genetic predispositions that make an organism susceptible to premalignant growth can make it possible to avert or delay development of the disease entirely [10]. Public health efforts can then be focused on promoting healthy behaviors and shielding individuals from the mutative effects of carcinogens in the environment.

Perhaps the most striking example of success in the prevention arena is the ongoing public health effort to limit the public's risk from exposure to tobacco. In 1964, the U.S. Surgeon General released a report documenting the link between cigarette smoke and a number of debilitating and fatal diseases, including lung cancer [11]. Following the release of the report, public health officials began a long but unrelenting campaign to inform the public of the risks inherent in smoking cigarettes, and in combating the persuasive messages of the tobacco industry, especially when aimed at minors. The public health success from exploiting that window of opportunity has been astounding. In 1964, roughly 45% of the population reported to be smokers. By 1995 that number had dropped in half to 25% of the U.S. population. It has been estimated that changes to smoking behaviors since 1986 have resulted in the prevention of nearly 2.1 million smoking-related diseases [12].

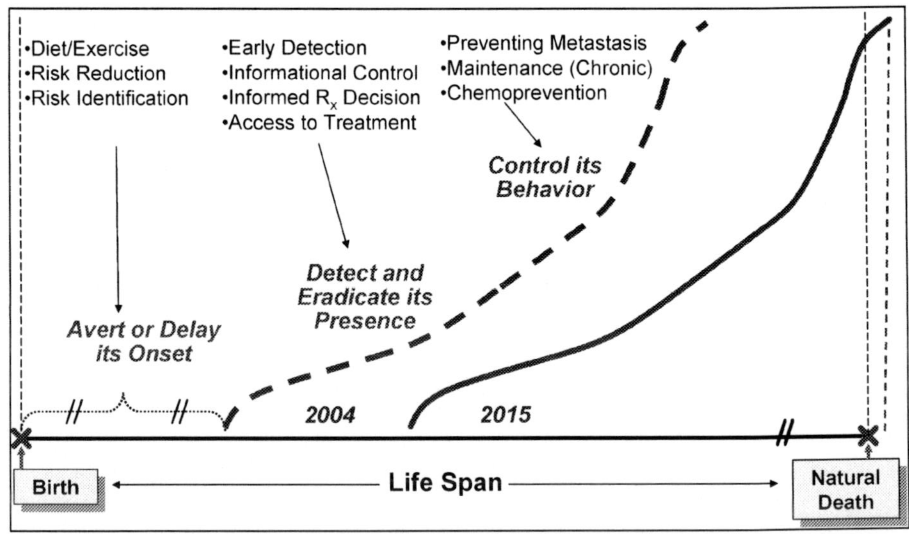

Figure 2. Windows of opportunity in the war against cancer.

The elimination of tobacco smoke as an active carcinogen for millions of people in the U.S. led to the first significant reduction in age-adjusted deaths due to cancer in the 20th century. Although the window of opportunity remains open — lung cancer accounts for the majority of deaths from the disease in men and women — the tide has begun to turn.

Similar opportunities for prevention exist in other areas. Epidemiologic data suggest that obesity and poor diet are predisposing risk factors for cancers of the GI track, that excessive drinking can be a predisposing factor for liver cancer, that radiation can catalyze risk in almost any body site exposed, and that overexposure to the sun can accelerate risk for melanoma [13]. The implication is that there is ample opportunity for controlling cancer in the population through a broader use of current knowledge and existing prevention strategies. Some estimates suggest that up to 50–75% of cancer deaths can be eliminated through behavioral interventions alone [14,15]. The preeminent role of effective health communication strategies in reducing personal and public burden from these cancers cannot be overstated.

The next most significant window of opportunity comes in identifying cancerous cells early in their life cycles, before they have evolved to a stage of aggressive growth and metastasis. Cancerous cells that are detected early enough can be removed entirely, often through relatively minor surgical procedures, thus eradicating the presence of the disease in the body altogether. From a public health perspective, the wide scale adoption of cervical cancer screening has been credited with dramatically reducing mortality from cervical cancer. Similar reductions in mortality are being achieved through early detection of breast, prostate, and colorectal cancers [16,17]. One of the more significant areas of research through the NCI is in the area of proteomics, and in identifying the telltale proteins and other markers that signal the formation of early-stage cancer cells.

Given the promise of early detection as a second line of defense, it is tempting to formulate a policy that would advocate for broad spectrum screening procedures routinely for the majority of the population. It does not take long, however, to figure out that the expense of such an approach, not to mention the undue disruptions from false positives for those not at risk, would be prohibitive. This is where completion of the Human Genome project holds such promise. Advances in genomics, tracing the relationship between chromosomal abnormalities and increased risk for the disease, hold the promise of reducing the cost by targeting screening efforts on an individual basis to those areas in which elevated risk has been detected.

If it is the case that the cancer does go beyond early stages of growth without detection, the next line of defense is to control the tumor's behavior. If the aggressive nature of the malignant cells can be tamed — that is, growth can be checked and metastasis curbed — then it should be possible to reduce cancer to the status of a chronic, but imminently survivable condition. One promising area of investigation is in studying therapeutic agents that inhibit the process of angiogenesis, essentially preventing the growth of existing tumors by preventing the spread of new vasculature. A number of antiangiogenic and antivascular therapies have shown great promise in preclinical experimentation. Though these therapies have met with mixed success in clinical trials, there is hope that the process can be perfected to the point of curbing the growth of existing tumors in patients who have been diagnosed with inoperable cancers. The strategy would turn cancer from automatic killer, to a controlled chronic condition [8,10].

3. The Role of Health Communication and Informatics

If so many cancers are avoidable through primary and secondary prevention strategies, and the mapping of the human genome is unlocking the secrets of more effective screening tests, then why has cancer eclipsed heart disease as a number 1 killer of Americans aged 85 years and younger? One of the answers may be that our ability to generate data may have outstripped our ability to utilize and integrate new knowledge. Journalist David Schenk referred to this as *"Data Smog,"* a condition that exists when too much raw data precipitates "paralysis by analysis" among scientists, and too many news stories describing the latest "scientific finding" leave consumers bewildered and bedraggled [19].

The notion that members of the public might be getting overloaded with too much raw data, without a clear organizing sense of what the relevance of the information would be in their own lives was borne out by answers to the NCI's Health Information National Trends Survey (HINTS) in 2003. HINTS is a biennial, random digit dial telephone survey designed to assess adults' usage of different communication media and their resulting knowledge, attitudes, and behaviors relevant to cancer control [20]. In the 2003 administration, respondents were asked on a one to five scale how much they agreed with the statement that "there are so many different recommendations it is hard to know what to do to prevent cancer." Almost 75% of the sample indicated they "strongly agreed" or "agreed" with the statement that there were too many recommendations to know what to do [21].

If the public is perplexed about what to do to prevent cancer, the situation may not be much better for health care practitioners or biomedical scientists. Practitioners are expected to keep up with the deluge of new technologies, pharmaceuticals, procedures, treatments, and regulatory requirements while integrating them into the crowded workflow of a patient-centered medical practice. Just keeping up with information on patients — their histories, medical status, check-ups, and preferences — in a system with antiquated records keeping practices is daunting enough [22]. Keeping up on best practice in a system that is exploding with new results daily is untenable without some assistance in integration or synthesis.

On the science side, biomedical researchers are expected to keep up on the latest results of research conducted at other institutions within the "invisible college" of their specialty, while monitoring at least some of the half million new medical articles added to the NLM database yearly. At the same time, basic scientists are being urged to integrate their findings with those of other disciplines in order to solve bigger problems. Integration and application will be essential if cancer researchers wish to move innovation into practice and to have an impact on the national cancer burden. All scientists, but especially those in the biomedical fields, will have to stay abreast of new technologies and data collection techniques. Often this means revisiting the methodological assumptions underlying the new techniques, and looking for new analytic processes to use in keeping up with a broader and more instantaneous data stream. Basic and applied scientists alike will need to stay abreast of the assumptions and technical implications associated with embedding these new techniques into their own discovery engines.

In each of these instances, the data and the innovations are coming. What is needed is a way of harnessing the power of intelligence embedded within these environments in manageable, safe, and effective ways. The solution lies in offering returns [23] back to the biomedical enterprise by harnessing the power of discovery through enhanced capacity for delivery. The solution lies in harnessing the power of health-related informatics.

3.1. Health Informatics

The French term "informatique" was coined in the early 1960's to describe an emerging technology that would allow scientists to communicate data via computer networks. Heavy investment in the 1960's and 1970's in the United States led to the development of a robust network protocol (Transmission Control Protocol – Internet Protocol) that would build on the informatics concept by enabling defense researchers and contractors to communicate data with each other over widely distributed and broadly interconnected computer networks. Further investments in the U.S. during the 1980's and 1990's enabled the National Science Foundation to extend the benefits of informatics infrastructures to basic science researchers and to educators. That period culminated in the development of the NSF high speed backbone, a public infrastructure designed to enable high speed transmission of data and messages across the US and to selected laboratories internationally. Further pressure on the US Congress led to the formation of plans to enable a broad informatics infrastructure for public use, which led to a privatization of a national informatics infrastructure (NII) and an acceptance of TCP-IP as the standard for inter-network connectivity. On November 15, 2001 the U.S. Department of Health and Human Services (DHHS) published a report by the National Committee on Vital and Health Statistics calling for the development of a National Health Information Infrastructure, or NHII [26]. On May 11, 2005, DHHS Secretary Mike Leavitt was quoted as saying that "information technology is a *pivotal* part of transforming our health care system." [27]

In the fight against cancer, this maturity of interests in informatics development will play out across three distinct, albeit interconnected, domains [24,25]. The first of these is a raise of investment in *bioinformatics*, or the use of advanced computing techniques and wide area connectivity to support basic biomedical research in studying the cause, diagnosis, and treatment of cancer. The second is the promulgation of *medical informatics*; a term that was originally coined in the late 1970's to describe the application of computer technologies to the delivery of medicine. The third is the relatively recent uptake of *consumer informatics*, a broad term used to describe the application of computer delivery systems – especially over the World Wide Web – to individual patients and their caretakers. Each of these aspects of the overall field of health informatics will be described below.

3.2. Bioinformatics and the War on Cancer

The challenge of deriving insights from a rapidly expanding information space is no more apparent than in the conduct of cancer-related research. Biomedical oncology is by its nature a data-intensive science, with vast data repositories and tissue banks emerging as a national asset to be shared among those researchers who are in the front lines of the war against cancer. The breadth of this data structure is aptly illustrated by the completion of the Human Genome Project, which effectively made data on up to three billion base pairs within the human genetic blueprint available to cancer researchers. Up until now, the tools for storing and analyzing data in these massive data repositories have been largely isolated within individual laboratories and clinics. To expand access to the data, and to save time and expense from reinventing the same computer resources across laboratories, the NCI has invested in a common informatics infrastructure among its funded comprehensive cancer center institutions. Termed caBIG (for the cancer *Bio-Informatics Grid*), this ambitious bioinformatics infrastructure will serve as a common data platform through which participating labs may share protocols, metadata (i.e., data about data), contacts, computer applications, vocabularies, repository data, and instruments [28].

Underlying the creation of a national bioinformatics grid is the vision of creating a national "collaboratory" among NCI-funded researchers. As envisioned by the National Science Foundation, a national collaboratory is an online meeting place that can be used (a) to support collaboration among similarly situated researchers (i.e., a "collaborat-ory") and (b) to provide community access to scarce and expensive laboratory resources (i.e., a "co-laboratory). [29,30] One of the fundamental justifications for creating a national collaboratory is to accelerate the discovery process and to facilitate the creation of new knowledge. For that purpose, the NCI has developed a "knowledge stack" through which data can be combined to generate new informational components, and the components can be combined to generate new types of cancer knowledge. This knowledge translation tool, known as the Common Ontologic Reference Environment, or caCORE, can be accessed openly through the NCI Web site (http://ncicb.nci.nih.gov/core).

The knowledge stack is itself made up of three interacting layers. At its foundation is an enterprise-wide vocabulary system referred to as EVS (Enterprise Vocabulary Services). Through the EVS researchers are able to code metadata (i.e., information about data) following guidelines for common terms and ontologies. NCI maintains its own medical thesaurus and cross-maps vocabulary in the thesaurus with widely accepted medical vocabularies such as MEDRA, SNOMED, ICD, and the National Library of Medicine's gene ontology and histopathology nomenclatures. The middle layer is composed of common data elements, built to store and redistribute data elements in accordance with ISO 11179 international standards. The top layer is made up of objects, built with open source programming tools, that capture by design the protocols and procedural knowledge within clinical oncology.

More broadly, the vision behind creating a layered knowledge-representation scheme, and developing a shared information grid of cancer research resources, should enable a brand new era of *in silico* research within the cancer research community [28]. *In silico* research represents a dramatic evolution to the environment in which cancer research will be conducted over the next century. Using resources made available through the bioinformatics grid, cancer researchers can push the envelope in the epidemiologic and genetic sciences to relate cancer incidence and mortality to very specific profiles of genetic risk in the population. Biomedical scientists skilled in the development of genetic assays can then build tests that would be distinctly predictive of risk for any one individual's distinct profile of genetic information. As embodied in recent speeches by the NCI director, scientists at the NCI envision a day when genetic tests will become so precise that health care providers will be able to sit down with patients and present an individually tailored behavioral prescription for managing their health risks, or prescribe a uniquely protective cocktail of preventive medications that will avert the risk of cancer altogether.

In an allied field, the field of proteomics, scientists are already accumulating data on the ways in which DNA interacts with the microcellular environment to produce proteins. Unlike the genome, which is relatively stable over time, the creation and behavior of proteins is highly dynamic. Subtle changes in the chemical makeup of a cell can lead to the transcription of an entirely new set of proteins; changes in the behavior of a single cell can lead to alterations in the intercellular environment and can signal changes within other cells. Bioinformaticians in the field of proteomics are striving to create a data infrastructure that will be comprehensive enough and fluid enough to track intercellular and intracellular changes over time. Linking proteomic data to data on microcellular growth processes will lead to new insights into how neoplasms are formed and how metastasis occurs. *In silico* research in the field will enable the development of ever-more precise screening mechanisms, and increasingly more effective treatment modalities.

Another goal of these connective technologies is to enable a new era of science in which researchers and clinicians, from different parts of the country and from wholly different disciplines, can combine forces. Thus, the technologies must be able to support an era of large-scale "team science." [31] One of the most striking examples of a tool designed to enable interdisciplinary research is the Cancer Molecular Assessment Project, or caMAP (http://cmap.nci.nih.gov). The primary goal of the caMAP project is to facilitate the identification of molecular targets for cancer treatment. To do this, genomic data are brought onto the network from UC Santa Cruz and the Cancer Genome Anatomy Project at the NCI. Those data are combined with information on molecular pathways obtained from BioCarta, a functional classification of genes as obtained from the Gene Ontology Consortium, and information on gene expression from the NCI's Developmental Therapeutics Program's cDNA microarray evaluation of the NCI 60 cell lines used for drug screening. Connections to molecularly targeted therapeutic agent information are made through the NCI's Cancer Therapy Evaluation Program, as is information on preclinical trial efficacy information from the Developmental Therapeutics Program, and information on formally announced clinical trials from the NCI's Office of Communication.

3.3. Medical Informatics and the War on Cancer

The next logical link in the chain is to bring the evidence garnered from biomedical science into the health care delivery system in timely, safe, and effective ways; that is, to expedite the "bench to bedside" delivery process. The task is more daunting than it first might appear. Work by the U.S. Agency for Healthcare Research and Quality (AHRQ) revealed that – given current systemic pressures – it takes anywhere from one to two decades to move new medical knowledge from research laboratories into medical practice within the U.S. [32] The task of effective dissemination is made even more difficult by the sheer expansion of the evidence base from which to draw in Medicine. In 2003 the National Library of Medicine estimated that it was adding somewhere in the neighborhood of 10,000 articles to its bibliographic databases per week [33]. Some observers have estimated that to maintain current knowledge a general internist would need to read 20 articles a day, 365 days a year; a task that is clearly impossible.

Unquestionably, information technology must play a crucial role in bringing the right information, into the right relationship, at the right time to take full advantage of windows of opportunity in cancer care. There are generally four types of computer applications that have been developed over the past two decades that can facilitate the discovery to delivery process. They include: (a) interoperable and interconnected records management systems, (b) bibliographic search and retrieval systems, (c) decision support systems, and (d) biomedical imaging systems.

With respect to *records management systems*, most hospitals have been maintaining administrative and cost records in electronic formats for years. These systems have been effective in helping administrators monitor costs, order supplies, seek reimbursement, and facilitate logistics. The goal of creating a truly interoperable and interconnected electronic medical record system has been more elusive. In his state of the union address to congress and the American people, the president of the United States announced on January 20, 2004 that developing an electronic medical record system would be a priority of his administration. "By computerizing health records," the president announced, "we can avoid dangerous medical mistakes, reduce costs, and improve care." [34] On April 26, 2005 the administration followed up on that promise by creating a subcabinet position to head up the nation's Health IT efforts, and by promising to make electronic health records a reality for at least half of the nation's health care providers within ten years' time.

In cancer care, the promise of developing portable electronic health record systems will enable new opportunities for intervention across the entire cancer care continuum. As advances are made in genetic testing, it is easy to envision a system that would create a tailored health management plan to follow a patient over the course of his or her lifetime. "Reminder systems," systems that promote action based on choice points implied by data in the medical record system, can be built to keep patients current with their suggested screening tests, and to promote healthy living. Cancer patients are especially at risk as they transition from one health care setting to another, and as they transfer care from general practitioners to medical oncologists. An interconnected medical record system, if executed correctly, will do a better job at supporting these transitions.

Regarding the utility of *bibliographic databases* in oncology, there is no doubt that advances made by the National Library of Medicine have played a pivotal role in giving physicians throughout and world unparalleled access to the medical literature. Future efforts will necessarily focus on creating newer and more efficient searching algorithms to help oncologists bring the best evidence to bear on every decision they make, regardless of how rare the cancer is they are treating or how removed their practices are from well-funded medical libraries. In a recent award from the Small Business Innovation Research Grant program, the NCI supported the development of an intelligent search tool that would allow patients to obtain search results from any large information space following preset criteria for quality and credibility. Access to bibliographic databases, organized using the same cancer-related vocabularies and ontologies as in the cancer bioinformatics grid, will allow researchers to distill the medical literature into usable knowledge products by conducting efficient meta-analyses. Online informatics tools, such as the Cancer Control Planet for public health administrators (http://cancercontrolplanet.cancer.gov/) will give decision-makers vetted access to evidence-based programs as contained within the medical and public health literature.

Decision support systems (DSS), often thought to be the core of an intelligent health care environment, hold important promise for the future but must be informed by lessons learned from the past. In the early days of medical informatics research, clinical informatics labs around the country began experimenting with the use of artificial intelligence to coordinate the burgeoning knowledge base of medicine into improved standards of care. The MYCIN project at Stanford University Medical Center, to use an often-cited example, was one of the first medically based expert systems to demonstrate how a rule-based production system could support diagnostic decisions for certain blood infections. Other noteworthy examples included the Quick Medical Reference (QMR) diagnostic system developed by Randy Miller at the University of Pittsburgh and the Iliad and Socrates systems developed by Homer Warner at the University of Utah [35,36].

What the early history of these AI systems taught health care designers was that physicians and patients were not trusting of a "black box" approach to computer support for decision-making. Neither patient nor provider would be willing to relinquish personal control over decision-making if the rules by which a system's inference engine reached a conclusion were not transparent. These early experiments in AI also provided lessons on the importance of workflow. Many of these systems required tedious interactions to input a patient's data. There was simply never enough time to enter the data, interact with the computer to orchestrate a response, and evaluate the merits of the decision; all while maintaining attentive interactions with the patient and responding to hospital administrators' demands for cost-effective throughput.

One of the fundamental mistakes underlying the assumptions of these early systems was that designers had hoped it would be possible to "automate" complex cognitive tasks. The assumption made sense from the perspective of an early industrial paradigm, wherein automation could often be implemented a cost-savings mechanism to replace human capital. In her book *"In the Age of the Smart Machine,"* social psychologist Shoshana Zuboff cautioned that assumptions of the industrial paradigm did not always translate to the ways in which organizations depended on computers in the information age. In the new era of work, computers will not be able to replace higher levels of thinking and judgment. To the contrary, computers can perform some of the tedious tasks associated with information management, but their true contribution will be in providing human decision-makers with better quality information so that they can make better decisions. To use Zuboff's terms, computers will not "automate;" they will "informate." [38]

In this respect, a review of decision support systems suggests that the best use of these technologies has not been to supplant clinical judgment, but to augment it. Reminder systems, in which the computer keeps track of scheduled appoints or treatments, have been especially effective in preserving the integrity of a healing relationship between health care providers and patients. Error checking systems, such as pharmaceutical look ups that check for potentially dangerous drug interactions, have also been useful in serving as supports to clinical decision making [39,40].

Breakthroughs in the future of clinical decision systems, then, will be focused on the work that must be done to create a better interface for higher quality information about patients, treatment options, and projected outcomes. Some of the more promising work in the area has to do with *biomedical imaging*, especially in using computer technology to aid in the construction and display of high fidelity images of tumors. The NCI's Cancer Imaging Program (http://imaging.cancer.gov/) is currently supporting breakthrough research in the areas of X-ray imaging, computer tomography scanning, nuclear imaging, and magnetic resonance imaging. Recent coverage in the national press highlighted the promise of the "virtual colonoscopy," a technique proposed that would remove the discomfort associated with physical procedures. The virtual imaging techniques use computerized construction tools to assemble 2D and 3D images from X-rays of organ systems and tumors. Advances in real time decision support systems will create a more intelligent and supportive clinical environment, with applications ranging from providing more precise and early diagnostic procedures to guiding the course of delicate operative procedures.

3.4. Consumer Informatics and the War on Cancer

Data from the 2003 administration of the Health Information National Trends Survey revealed a provocative pattern in the way in which the public consumes information about cancer. In a question asking respondents where they would likely go first if they needed to get information about cancer in an imagined scenario, an estimated 49.5% (95% CI, 48.1–50.8) of Americans indicated that they would likely go to their personal health care provider with the Internet as a close second choice. Indeed, physicians were the most trusted source of health information from among a number of sources named in the survey. When asked where they had actually gone to look for cancer information, though, 48.6% (95% CI, 46.1–51.0) of those who had looked for cancer information in the past said that they went to the Internet first. The pattern reversed [21].

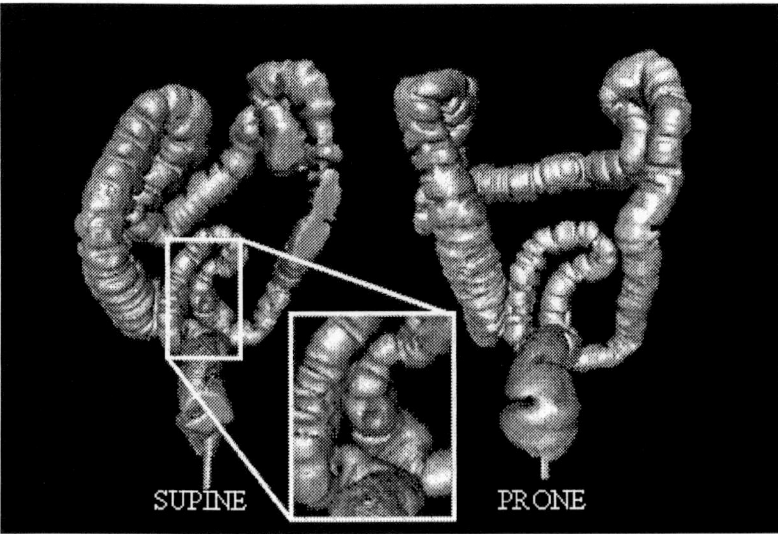

Figure 3. Example of a "virtual colonoscopy," an image constructed by computer from multiple X-rays.

These data are consistent with online health information trends reported from other surveys. In tracking the number of Americans going online, the U.S. Census Bureau noted a gradual incline from 22.2% in 1997 to 42% in 2000 and 51% in 2001. By 2003, the HINTS data placed the number of Americans online at 63.0% (95% CI, 61.7–64.3). Of those who report being online, 63.7% (95% CI, 61.7–65.8) reported having looked for medical information for themselves or for others sometime in the previous 12 months. Regarding what kind of health information people search for online, Rice reported that "cancer" was the third most popular health-related search term on the Web after "depression" (#1) and "allergies" (#2) [42]. These statistics drive home the importance of meeting information seekers' needs through multiple communication channels. The science of meeting the public's health information needs as enabled by advanced applications in health IT has been dubbed "Consumer Informatics" by some [43].

To support information seeking in complex environments [46,47], the NCI has been aggressive in its pursuit of evidence-based guidelines for interface development and has set up a fully equipped usability laboratory to conduct research and evaluation. During the initial phase of the lab, the NCI was instrumental in assembling an evidence base for the design of health related Web sites (www.usability.gov). In more recent years, the NCI has transitioned its efforts to conduct essential human factors research into new and more effective interfaces to the capabilities enabled by developments in bioinformatics and medical informatics.

For example, as the precision of individualized genetics profiles are made available to patients, more effective information designs will be needed to support decision making across levels of health literacy and innumeracy [48,49]. Research efforts are underway in collaboration with the institute's Centers of Excellence in Cancer Communication Research (http://dccps.nci.nih.gov/hcirb/ceccr) to understand the informational components of genetic risk portrayal needed for effective decision making.

A shift enabled by the diffusion of electronic medical records will be the development of online access tools allowing patients to monitor their own electronic medical information through the Web. These *Personal Health Records*, as they have been called, hold the promise of empowering a greater sense of self-advocacy among patients. Those who use a personal health record system will not only be better informed consumers, but should also become more vigilant in monitoring their own health conditions and can become more proactive in regulating their own health behaviors. Reminder systems embedded within the personal health record can prompt patients to see their physicians for routine screening tests or can provide instructions for behavior when laboratory values exceed safe ranges. In essence, the patient can become part of the medical team, monitoring his or her own health in more informed ways. Greater support for self-care, both for individuals and their caregivers, will be a necessity as the baby boom generation ages, and the population exhibits an increase in the prevalence of chronic disease [50,51].

An increase in sophistication within online media is only one facet of a fully supportive and healthy environment. Other media – newspapers, magazines, television, radio, brochures – will persist as new communication channels come online. In general, the new mix of media will appear more fragmented and specialized than the early days of mass communication. The new mix will also be more interactive than the preceding information environment and will be fueled by an underlying convergence of technologies. In the early days of the Internet health communicators thought of the World Wide Web as a final destination for health information seekers. The emphasis was creating content to be browsed onscreen in HTML. New evidence suggests that many health information Web surfers may actually be searching for someone else [21,52]. Using the Web as a delivery mechanism, rather than a destination, could mean providing Web surfers with downloadable, printer-friendly brochures that could easily be circulated to others. By supporting converging technologies, health information Web designers could extend their public health reach beyond the Digital Divide.

To understand how consumer health informatics can be used to empower individuals, it is instructive to review a psychological perspective on disease-oriented sense making. A theoretical framework that holds considerable promise in predicting the behavior of cancer information seekers within complex information environments is Howard Leventhal's self-regulation framework [44]. Leventhal's framework is built on the observation that much of human cognition and behavior can be characterized as being inherently purposeful. Humans, like other complex, self-organizing systems interact with their environment in ways that are intended to remove obstacles and pursue goals. As adaptive systems, humans inherently follow a cybernetic model of system regulation; that is, they *test, operate, test again,* and then *exit* (referred to as the TOTE model of adaptive behavior).

When confronted with the prospect of a disease, individuals go through a predictable sequence of questioning to determine the nature of the disease and their own course of action. Leventhal referred to the heuristic process that people use as a *Common Sense Model* of disease. From his observations, there are basically five questions that drive most people's information searching activities when the common sense model is activated. The questions, especially as they relate to cancer, are as follows:

- *Identity.* What is the disease, how do I interpret symptoms? Lay persons, like diagnosticians, work backwards from the presence of a symptom to a label for the illness condition. Since early detection is an important window of opportunity in cancer treatment, it is imperative that people obtain early support in interpreting the implications of an anomalous symptom, say a lump in the breast or blood in the stool. Online information systems should help users distinguish between normal conditions and conditions that truly are suspicious. Call centers, such as the NCI's 1-880-4CANCER, should be prepped and ready to support callers in determining what the next steps should be in confirming or dismissing a suspicious presentation.
- *Timeline.* What is the course of the disease? Cancers vary in their course. Some cancers are slow growing and amenable to control, while others are highly aggressive and are best treated through excision. Understanding the expected course of a

particular cancer will be an important part of the treatment decision. From a public health perspective, it is equally important for the public at large to understand that it is possible to live long and enjoyable lives with cancer as a controlled but chronic condition. The Lance Armstrong Foundation, an indispensable partner to the NCI, has helped change public perceptions life with cancer through its "live strong" campaign.

- *Consequences.* What are the consequences of the disease? Cancer is no longer the death sentence it used to be, and as progress continues in the war on cancer more and more people will hear the words "you have cancer" but come to understand they can live long and healthy lives in spite of the disease. For many, though, the word "cancer" evokes strongly negative images; images that may often dissuade people from going into their physicians for regular screening [45]. One of the goals of health communication will be to orient consumers to the consequences of their behavior and convey the notion that *not going in* for screening will have far worse consequences than *going in*.

- *Cause.* What caused the disease? Public messages about what leads to cancer are not always clear, but for a few causes the link is unambiguous. The link between smoking and lung cancer, for example, is inarguable at this point. Helping the public understand the nature of these causal links as the evidence becomes available will enable people to take corrective action early, before it is too late.

- *Control.* What can I do to control its consequences? From a "windows of opportunity" perspective, there is quite a bit that people can do to minimize the lethality of the disease. The first step lies in prevention: eating right, exercising, not smoking, and taking precautionary measures when working with toxic substances. The second lies in early detection: staying current with recommended screening tests, monitoring for lumps or skin abnormalities. If suspicion does arise, there will be plenty an individual can do to advocate for early treatment and to stay unswervingly compliant with treatment protocols.

4. Keeping the System on Track

In the wake of the "Dot Com" implosion of the late 1990's, successful entrepreneurs learned that no amount of new technology will replace a solid business plan for keeping an organization on track and productive. A recurring theme throughout this chapter is that the future of cancer control technologies must be guided by a perspective that is sociotechnical in nature [53]. Informaticians must recognize that health care environments are made up of people, tools, and conversations. Redesign efforts must keep the optimal balance between these three components firmly in mind if the efforts are to be successful; new technologies must be compatible with user attributes and they must be supportive of work flow and communication needs [54].

4.1. Create a Supportive Work Environment

The first point to consider when implementing a new technology is to understand thoroughly the work environment into which the technology will be integrated. Recent evidence suggests that many Health IT projects fail when deployed in real world settings. These are settings filled with conflicting work demands, time constraints, and attention-demanding medical emergencies [55–57]. These are also settings into which foisting a hard-to-use or error-prone computer system would wreak havoc. As the technology of medical science becomes more complex, the degree of risk associated with using the technology increases. So too, the need rises to ensure that the technologies are embedded within the environment of medical care in a seamless, effective, and safe way.

This exhortation was a core theme in the Institute of Medicine's companion reports to the medical community: *To Err is Human* and *Crossing the Quality Chasm* [58]. In *To Err is Human*, the IOM cautioned that the health care system is experiencing an epidemic of imminently preventable but, nonetheless, dangerous medical errors. The reports estimated that as many as 44,000 to 98,000 people die each year in the U.S. from preventable medical errors. That rate exceeds the number of people who die annually from breast cancer, AIDS, or automobile accidents. An explicit theme of the book was that these errors do not represent failures of individuals, but failures of the health care system; in fact, that mythos is what is preventing the system from repairing itself. Rather, the errors must be addressed from a systemic and a human factors perspective.

In *Bridging the Quality Chasm*, the IOM offered a prescription for solving the problem of unsafe medical systems nationally [1]. Authors of the book expanded on the theme that repairs must be made to the health care environment as a system, and looked to other high risk industries, most notably the airline industry, for clues on how to address the problem. What the authors noted is that human capacities – attention, memory, and physical strength – have predictable strengths and weaknesses. Environments that violate those capacities will put excessive strain on the human elements within the system thus causing the system to break down in predictable ways. Human factors engineers, who understand the strengths and capacities of the human element, must work together closely with health care administrators and systems engineers to create wholly new systems of performance.

In working with human capacities, rather than against them, systems engineers must focus on building the back-ups and failsafe procedures into their technologies that allow humans to operate within natural tolerances for cognitive capacity and physical limitations. Because variances are natural, the system must also be self-correcting. It should be infused with data monitoring systems that can inform continuous quality improvement, and it should make careful use of intelligent agents to inform – not take away from – human judgment and decision-making.

4.2. Provide "Deep Support" for Users

Another area in which systems engineers and health care administrators will need to focus is in providing levels of support that go beyond single transactions. Zuboff and Maxmin refer to the concept as providing "deep support," and have noted that it is this attribute that differentiates winners from losers in the new economy [59]. The point of focus in providing deep support is to emphasize the development of an ongoing trust-filled relationship between the service providers (in this case, the health care system) and their customers (the patients). In the Web economy, developers have often made the shortsighted mistake of trying to extract business value from each and every transaction. Thus, they have experimented with foisting "pop up ads" into the user's attention, often while the customers were trying to complete some other task; or they fail in providing any other level of support (say through a 1–800 number) beyond what pittance of forethought had been placed on the Web page.

Where program planners are failing is in moving beyond the myopic view of the single transaction to the more extended long-term view of the ongoing relationship. When a goal-directed visitor comes to a Web site looking for important health information, the last thing they want is to be bombarded with a barrage of targeted advertisements or to pick up on a health message that is incomplete, disconnected, or filled with uninterpretable words. Similarly, when someone is given a life-altering diagnosis of cancer within the comfort of a caring physician's office, but is not given an indication of where to go next or what to do, they can become paralyzed. Because they may be missing an opportunity for intervention during a time-urgent period, paralysis can be fatal.

Where informatics systems need to go next is to link all aspects of a patient's information environment together to form an unbroken cradle of "deep support" over time. The Institute of Medicine referred to this goal as creating a "healing relationship" with the health care system, in which some aspect of a coordinated care environment can be made available in patient-centric ways 24 hours a day, 7 days a week. If a person is feeling pain but it is infeasible to contact her physician, then she should be able to contact an advice nurse who would have immediate, electronic access to the patient's health record and would be able to offer sound, evidence-based advice. If a patient calls an interactive voice response (IVR) telephone system in order to request a prescription refill, then failsafe subsystems must guarantee that the necessary communication occurs between the IVR system, the physician's office, the pharmacist, and the mail room to guarantee delivery of the prescription within the expected time frame. If a new prescription is being ordered, then error-checking routines should be in place to guard against deleterious pharmaceutical interactions.

It is the long-term support aspect of health care delivery coordinated across people and systems that will turn the tide on cancer. As discovery is accelerated through investments in bioinformatics, links must be made to the health care system to embed the discovery into usable guidelines and procedures. As advances in medical informatics are made, links must be drawn to the individual patient, to be sure that the patient is supported over a lifetime of health information decision-making.

4.3. Emphasize Universal Design

Creating an intelligent health environment must also mean creating an environment that is equally supportive of all members of the population. Usability engineers refer to this as the concept of "Universal Design;" that is, designing features in the environment that will allow for maximum inclusion across varying levels of physical ability and across ranges of socioeconomic strata [60]. A common example in the physical world is the inclusion of "curb cuts" in sidewalks outside of buildings. Curb cuts are those indentations built into sidewalks that give people in wheelchairs easy access to the grocery stores, office buildings, and malls. Curb cuts are also useful to people who are physically able, as they can be used as paths for shopping carts, baby strollers, bags on "wheelies," and bicycles. The feature is a universal design, since it can be used by anyone and does not get in the way of normal ambulation.

Software engineers have been working behind the scenes to build curb cuts into computer designs as well. An example is the ability to adjust visual perspective or "zoom" in graphical user interfaces. Size adjustments make it easy for people with differing levels of visual acuity to adjust the size of objects on the screen (say words or numbers) for ease of viewing. Another way of approaching universal design is to create systems that adapt easily to differing levels of experience or technical sophistication [61]. Staging a web site so that information of universal interest is contained within the first few layers, while providing well-marked paths to the more sophisticated technical information lying underneath, is a straightforward way of accommodating a multiplicity of audience types.

Work being done in the health care arena must pay particularly close attention to the informational messages given to patients across all channels. All messages, from instructions given by an advice nurse to the directions listed on a prescription label, must serve as road signs to direct the patient's health-motivated behavior through an unfamiliar health care environment. Evidence from the area of health literacy suggests that messages given to patients are often disconnected, fragmented, sometimes discordant, often highly technical, and typically difficult to understand [49]. Attention to principles of universal design in cancer care will create an intelligent health care environment that, like a well-marked highway, will lead all users down the road to cancer free lives.

5. Conclusion

It has been over three decades since Congress first declared war on cancer. Since that time, the nature of the battle has changed considerably but the pitch of the battle has remained strong. An expanding team of biomedical researchers, clinical practitioners, behavioral scientists, information engineers, and oncologists have been laboring unceasingly to push back the tide of cancer-related death and suffering. Although the increase in age-adjusted deaths due to cancer increased steadily through most of last century, the tide did turn in 1990 and has been decreasing ever since. Much of the success in cancer control can be attributed to victories within the early windows of opportunity in the disease process. Three decades of public health efforts in anti-smoking campaigns has decreased the rate of lung cancer in men, with similar decreases in women not far behind. Successful use of early detection programs in breast and cervical cancer, prostate cancer, and colorectal cancer have cut back rates of mortality on each of those fronts.

Coincidentally, the new war on cancer is being fought with a technology that was developed at the height of the cold war: distributed informatics computing. The NCI is now pushing the envelope of informatics technologies by expanding investments in areas of bioinformatics, medical informatics, and consumer informatics. The result should be to create a future in which the invisible college of science is made more expansive and productive; in which the benefits of that science are carried into the "healing relationships" of a transformed health care system; and in which individuals are empowered with the information and tools they need to lead cancer-free lives. More importantly, as envisioned by NCI's direct Dr. Andrew von Eschenbach, the future will be one in which death and suffering from cancer will be nonexistent.

References

[1] Institute of Medicine, 2001. *Crossing the quality chasm: A new health system for the 21st Century.* National Academy of Science Press, Washington DC.

[2] U.S. Department of Health and Human Services, June 21, 2004. The Decade of Health Information Technology: Delivering Consumer-centric and Information-Rich Health Care: A Framework for Strategic Action. HHS Fact Sheet–HIT Report At-A-Glance, available at http://www.hhs.gov/news.

[3] 92nd Congress. National Cancer Act of 1971, December 23, 1971. Public Law 92–218.

[4] Reed, S.I., 2005. Cell cycle, in V.T. DeVita, S. Hellman, & S. Rosenberg (Eds.) *Cancer: Principles and practice of oncology, 7th Ed.* Lippincott Williams & Wilkins, Philadelphia, pp. 83–104.

[5] Yuspa, S.H. & Shields, P.G., 2005. Etiology of cancer: Chemical factors, in V. T. DeVita, S. Hellman, & S. Rosenberg (Eds.) *Cancer: Principles and practice of oncology, 7th Ed.* Lippincott Williams & Wilkins, Philadelphia, pp. 185–191.

[6] Colditz, G.A. & Fisher, L.B., 2005. Etiology of Cancer: Tobacco Use, in V.T. DeVita, S. Hellman, & S. Rosenberg (Eds.) *Cancer: Principles and practice of oncology, 7th Ed.* Lippincott Williams & Wilkins, Philadelphia, pp. 193–199.

[7] Ullrich, R.L., 2005. Etiology of cancer: Physical factors, in V. T. DeVita, S. Hellman, & S. Rosenberg (Eds.) *Cancer: Principles and practice of oncology, 7th Ed.* Lippincott Williams & Wilkins, Philadelphia, pp. 201–215.

[8] Fidler, I.J., Langley, R.R., Kerbel, R.S., & Ellis, L.M., 2005. Angiogenesis, in V.T. DeVita, S. Hellman, & S. Rosenberg (Eds.) *Cancer: Principles and practice of oncology, 7th Ed.* Lippincott Williams & Wilkins, Philadelphia, pp. 129–137.

[9] Stetler-Stevenson, W.G., 2005. Invasion and metastases, in V.T. DeVita, S. Hellman, & S. Rosenberg (Eds.) *Cancer: Principles and practice of oncology, 7th Ed.* Lippincott Williams & Wilkins, Philadelphia, pp. 113–127.

[10] Von Eschenbach, A.C., 2005. The national cancer program, in V.T. DeVita, S. Hellman, & S. Rosenberg (Eds.) *Cancer: Principles and practice of oncology, 7th Ed.* Lippincott Williams & Wilkins, Philadelphia, pp. 2788–2793.

[11] U.S. Department of Health, Education, and Welfare, 1964. Smoking and Health. Report of the Advisory Committee to the Surgeon General of the Public HealthService. PHS Publ. No. 1103, Washington, DC: U.S. Department of Health, Education, and Welfare: Washington, DC.

[12] Hiatt, R.A. & Rimer, B.K. 1999. A new strategy for cancer control research. Cancer Epidemiology, Biomarkers & Prevention, *Vol. 8,* 957–964.

[13] Wingo, P.A., Ries, L.A., Giovino, G.A., Miller, D.S., Rosenberg, H.M., Shopland, D.R., Thun, M.J., and Edwards, B.K. 1999. Annual report to the nation on the status of cancer, 1973–1996, with a special section on lung cancer and tobacco smoking. *J. Natl. Cancer Inst., 91*: 675–690.

[14] McGinnis, J.M., and Foege, W.H. 1993. Actual causes of death in the United States. *J. Am. Med. Assoc., 270*: 2207–2212.

[15] Harvard Report on Cancer Prevention. 1996. Volume 1: Causes of Human Cancer. *Cancer Causes Control, 7*: S3–S59.

[16] Devesa, S.S., Young, J.L., Jr., Brinton, L.A., and Fraumeni, J.F., Jr., 1989. Recent trends in cervix uteri cancer. *Cancer (Phila.), 64*: 2184–2190.

[17] Institute of Medicine, 2001. *Fulfilling the potential of cancer prevention and early detection,* National Academy of Science Press, Washington DC.

[18] Brody, J.E., February 1, 2005. How cancer rose to the top of the Charts. *New York Times.*

[19] Shenk, D. 1997. *Data smog: Surviving the information glut.* Harper Collins: New York, NY.

[20] Nelson D.E., Rimer B.K., Kreps G.L., Hesse B.W., Viswanath K.V., Croyle R.T., Willis G., Arora N., Weinstein N., Alden S. 2004. The Health Information National Trends Survey (HINTS): Development, Design, and Dissemination. *Journal of Health Communication. 9*: 1–18.

[21] Hesse, B.W., Nelson, D.E., Kreps, G.L., Croyle, R.T., Arora, N.K., Rimer, B.K., Viswanath, K. (accepted for publication, 2005). Trust and Sources of Health Information: The Impact of the Internet and Its Implications for Health Care Providers. Archives of Internal Medicine.

[22] Agency for Health Care Research and Quality, June 2002. Medical informatics for better and safer health care. *Research in Action, 6,* 1–12.

[23] Hesse, B.W., Sproull, L.S., Kiesler, S.B., and Walsh, J.P. 1993. Returns to science: Computer networks in oceanography. *Communications of the ACM, 36(8),* 90–101.

[24] Computer Science and Telecommunications Board, National Research Council, 2000. *Networking health* National Academy of Science Press, Washington DC.

[25] Science Panel on Interactive Communication and Health, April 1999. *Wired for Health and Well-Being: The Emergence of Interactive Health Communication.* US Department of Health and Human Services, US Government Printing Office: Washington, DC.

[26] National Committee on Health and Vital Statistics, November 15, 2001. *Information for Health: A Strategy for Building the National Health Information Infrastructure.* US Department of Health and Human Services: Washington, DC.

[27] The Lewin Group, March 2005. *Health Information Technology Leadership Panel: Final Report.* US Department of Health and Human Services: Washington, DC.

[28] Buetow, K., 2005. Bioinformatics, in V. T. DeVita, S. Hellman, & S. Rosenberg (Eds.) *Cancer: Principles and practice of oncology, 7th Ed.* Lippincott Williams & Wilkins, Philadelphia, pp. 43–50.

[29] Wulf, William. 1989. The National Collaboratory – A White Paper in Towards a National Collaboratory. Unpublished report of a NSF workshop, Rockefeller University, NY. March 17–18.

[30] Wulf, William A., 1993. The collaboratory opportunity. Science 261 (August): 854–855.

[31] Institute of Medicine, 2003. *Large-scale biomedical science: Exploring strategies for future research.* National Academy of Science Press, Washington DC.

[32] AHRQ Publication No. 01-P017, March 2001. Translating Research Into Practice (TRIP)-II. Fact sheet. Agency for Healthcare Research and Quality, Rockville, MD. http://www.ahrq.gov/research/trip2fac.htm.

[33] National Library of Medicine: Fact Sheet MEDLINE. 24 Aug 2004. http://www.nlm.nih.gov/pubs/factsheets/medline.html.

[34] President George W. Bush, State of the Union Address, January 20, 2004. Available at www.whitehouse.gov.

[35] Miller, R.A. 1994. Medical Diagnostic Decision Support Systems — past, present, and future. *J Am Med Inform Assoc.1:* 8–27.

[36] Shortliffe, E.H., Perreault, L.E., Wiederhold, G., & Fagan, L.M. 2000. *Medical informatics: Computer applications in health care and biomedicine, 2nd Edition.* Springer, New York.

[37] Hersh, W.R., 2002. Medical informatics: Improving health care through information. *J Am Med Assoc., 288(16):* 1955–1958.

[38] Zuboff, S. 1984. *In the Age of the Smart Machine: The Future of Work and Power.* Basic Books, New York.

[39] Teich, J.M., Merchia, P.R., Schmiz, JL, et al., 2000. Effects of computerized physician order entry on prescribing practices. *Arch Intern Med, 160,* 2741–2747.

[40] Overage, J.M., Middleton, B., Miller, R.A., et al., 2002, Does national regulatory mandate of provider order entry portend greater benefit than risk for health care delivery? *J Am Med Inform Assoc, 9,* 199–208.

[41] U.S. Department of Commerce. A Nation Online: How Americans are expanding their use of the Internet. U.S.D.C., February 2002: Washington, DC.

[42] Rice, R.E., 2001. The Internet and health communication: A framework of experiences. In R.E. Rice & J.E. Katz (Eds.), *The Internet and health communication: Experiences and expectations.* Sage Publications: Thousand Oaks, CA, pp. 5–46.

[43] Eysenbach, G., 2000. Recent advances: Consumer health informatics. *British Medical Journal, 320,* 1713–1716.

[44] Leventhal, H., Brissette, I., & Leventhal, E. 2003. The common-sense model of self-regulation of health and illness. In L.D. Cameron & H. Leventhal (Eds.), *The Self-Regulation of Health and Illness Behavior.* Routledge. London, UK.

[45] Freimuth, V.A., Stein, J.A., Kean, T.J. 1989. *Searching for health information: the Cancer Information Service model.* University of Pennsylvania Press: Philadelphia.

[46] Albers, M.J. *Communication of Complex Information: User Goals and Information Needs for Dynamic Web Information.* Lawrence Erlbaum. Mahwah, NJ.

[47] Marchionini, G. 1995. *Information Seeking In Electronic Environments.* Cambridge University Press: Cambridge, UK.

[48] Croyle, R.T., Smith, K.R., Botkin, J.R., Baty, B., Nash, J. 1997. Psychological responses to BRCA1 mutation testing: preliminary findings, *Health Psychology, 16(1)* 63–72.

[49] Institute of Medicine, 2004. *Health literacy: A prescription to end confusion.* National Academy of Science Press, Washington DC.

[50] Deering, M.J. 2002. Developing the health information infrastructure in the United States. In R.G. Bushko (Ed.), *Future of Health Technology*, IOS Press: Amsterdam.

[51] Neuhauser L., Kreps G.L. 2003. Rethinking communication in the E-health era. *Journal of Health Psychology, 8(1),* 7–23.

[52] Fox, S., & Rainie, L. 2002. *Vital decisions: How Internet users decide what information to trust when they or their loved ones are sick.* Technical Report from the Pew Internet and American Life Project: Washington DC: Pew Research Center.

[53] Pava, C. 1983. *Managing New Office Technology: An Organizational Strategy.* The Free Press: New York, NY.

[54] Coiera, E., 2004. Four rules for the reinvention of health. *BMJ, 328*:1197–1199.

[55] Garg, A.X., Adhikari, N.K.J., McDonald, H., Rosas-Arellano, M.P., Devereaux, P.J., Beyene, J., Sam, J., Haynes, R.B. 2005. Effects of Computerized Clinical Decision Support Systems on Practitioner Performance and Patient Outcomes: A Systematic Review. *J Am Med Assoc., 293*: 1223–1238.

[56] Koppel, R., Metlay, J.P., Cohen, A., Abaluck, B., Localio, A.R., Kimmel, S.E., Strom, B.L, 2005. Role of Computerized Physician Order Entry Systems in Facilitating Medication Errors. *JAMA, 293*: 1197–1203.

[57] Wears, R.L. & Berg, R. Computer Technology and Clinical Work: Still Waiting for Godot. *J Am Med Assoc., 293*: 1261–1263.

[58] Institute of Medicine, 2000. *To err is human: Building a safer health system.* National Academy of Science Press, Washington DC.

[59] Zuboff, S. & Maxmin, J. 2002. *The support economy: Why corporations are failing individuals and the next episode of capitalism.* Viking, New York, NY.

[60] Hesse, B.W. 1995. Curb cuts in the virtual community: Telework and persons with disabilities. *Proceedings of the 28th Annual Hawaii International Conference on System Sciences, 28,* 418–425.

[61] Shneiderman, B., 1998. Designing the User Interface: Strategies for Effective Human-Computer Interaction: Third Edition, Addison-Wesley Publ. Co., Reading, MA.

Future of Intelligent and Extelligent Health Environment
R.G. Bushko (Ed.)
IOS Press, 2005

Future of Anti-Addiction Vaccines

Thomas R. KOSTEN, M.D.
Professor of Psychiatry and Medicine,
Yale University School of Medicine, New Heaven, CT, US

Abstract. The medical rational for using anti-drug antibodies in the serum as a treatment is to reduce drug levels in the brain and to bind drug before it enters the brain. Drugs of abuse are small molecules that can readily cross the blood brain barrier, while antibodies are larger molecules that cannot get into the brain. Thus, any drug that is bound to antibody also cannot cross the blood brain barrier and cannot enter the brain. Active anti-drug vaccines stimulate the body to makes its own antibodies, but the small size of abused drugs prevents them from stimulating an immune response. Thus, individuals do not ordinarily produce antibodies to abused drugs, and vaccines to stimulate antibodies are made by chemically linking these abused drugs to toxins such as cholera toxin. Alternatively, passive immunotherapy uses monoclonal antibodies that are generated in a laboratory and then administered via intravenous injection. Antibodies can be used to treat drug overdose; to reduce drug use relapse; or to protect certain at risk populations who have not yet become drug dependent. The advantages of anti-addiction vaccines are that antibodies target the drug, not the drug's sites of action in the brain and antibody binding inactivates the drug. These vaccines can complement behavioral and other medical therapies with minimal side effects and are not addictive like some chemical agonists. Technology advances in manufacturing and delivery systems will improve future anti-addiction vaccines, but social acceptance of anti-addiction vaccines will depend on substance abuse program staff and the families of substance abusers, who have some values that oppose medical solutions to addictive diseases and view addictions as moral problems.

1. Introduction

Nearly 200 years ago Jenner first used vaccination (active immunization) for the prevention and treatment of human disease, and over these 200 years only clean water may have provided a greater impact on worldwide public health. By stimulating an immune response to disease-related organisms vaccines have prevented illness or death in millions of individuals each year. Immunizations generate protective antibodies in the body fluids, which act as an early surveillance system to block or reduce the effects of an invading organism or substance, such as a toxin. Antibodies are continually produced and broken down (metabolized and inactivated) in the body. The most common type of antibody (IgG) has a half-life in blood of about 3 weeks [1]. That is, about half of the antibody produced on day 1 is eliminated by day 21. Blood levels of antibody after vaccination are maintained because new antibody is continually produced. After passive immunization with monoclonal antibodies, a steady decline in antibody level with a half-life of about 3 weeks is expected, so that repeated antibody doses every few months would probably be needed to maintain antibody levels in blood. Recently, we have begun to conceptualize abused drug as toxins that might also be treated and perhaps even prevented from developing into the disease of addiction by using immunotherapy.

Several advances in immunotherapy allowed us to consider manufacturing anti-addiction vaccines [2]. An early use of immunotherapy involved polyclonal antibodies in the form of specific immune serum to treat infectious diseases. These antisera effectively treated pneumonia and tetanus, but a serious adverse side effect was serum sickness, an allergic reaction resulting from the administration of animal antisera to humans. Thus, these animal antisera could only be used as a last treatment option. Later, human donors were immunized and human immune globulin collected for treatment, and these are still used to treat hepatitis B, tetanus and Varicella zoster. We can now produce monoclonal antibodies, which can be produced by large scale manufacturing techniques, without the use of animals or animal proteins and without the risk of transmitting human infectious agents such as HIV and hepatitis viruses.

2. What Are Anti-Addiction Vaccines?

The medical rational for using anti-drug antibodies in the serum as a treatment is to reduce drug levels in the brain and to bind drug before it enters the brain. Many small molecules such as drugs of abuse (molecular weights of 200–300 Daltons) can readily cross the blood brain barrier while larger molecules such as antibodies (molecular weights of about 150,000 Daltons) cannot [3]. Thus any drug that is bound to antibody also cannot cross the blood brain barrier and cannot enter the brain. In animals, immunotherapy reduces drug distribution to brain within the first few minutes after a single drug dose by up to 80% [4,5]. This is important because the rewarding effects of drugs are also greatest in the first few minutes after a dose. Thus, the drug binds to the antibody, and the rewarding or medically harmful effects of the drug are reduced or blocked. Because these therapies target only the drug, they are potentially safer than treatment with small molecule medications, which bind directly to important receptor systems in the brain and other organs.

Immunotherapies for drug abuse can be either active or passive. Active immunizations use drug vaccines to stimulate the body to makes its own antibodies and to create a long-term immunological memory for a more rapid future response to vaccine. An important consideration in this approach is that the small size of abused drugs prevents them from stimulating an immune response. Thus, individuals do not ordinarily produce antibodies to abused drugs, and even after effective vaccination continued drug use does not make more antibodies. This lack of immune stimulation by the abused drug alone contrasts with infectious disease vaccines where expose to the infectious agent will itself trigger a strong immunological response in a person who has been vaccinated and markedly increase the production of new antibodies. Like standard infectious disease vaccination, antibodies are not produced until several weeks after these active immunizations. Passive immunotherapy uses monoclonal antibodies that are generated in a laboratory and then administered via intravenous injection. In this case more antibody can be administered and the protection can be immediate, but it only lasts until the antibody is cleared and there is no immunological memory against the abused drug.

2.1. Active Anti-Addiction Vaccination

In active immunotherapy, the drug of abuse (called a hapten) is chemically coupled to an antigenic protein carrier like cholera toxin, and this combination is then used as a vaccine. Vaccines are currently being tested in humans for cocaine and nicotine [6,7]. Because stimulation of an immune response requires multiple interactions on the surface of an antibody forming B lymphocyte, a single, small drug molecule (like cocaine or nicotine) cannot produce cross-linking of cell surface antibodies on a B cell to activate it to produce more antibodies. For this reason, drug haptens must be irreversibly bound to their large protein carriers for use as vaccines. The molecular orientation and spacing of the drug haptens on the protein surface are critical factors that scientists must control for an optimal immune response. Thus, the antibody response will not increase if a vaccinated individual uses the abused drug, itself, and only the circulating antibody at the time of drug use will be protective. Because cross-linking of surface antibody on B cells is required to stimulate antibody production, the same drug hapten-protein vaccine must be used for making more antibody, called boosting the immune response, when the antibody levels fall to relatively low levels typically 4 to 6 months after the original vaccination series is completed. Periodic boosting with the vaccine is required to keep serum antibody levels high. The actual serum level of antibody is affected by the quality of the drug-protein vaccine, the dose of the vaccine, the frequency of vaccinations, the time interval between immunizations, and poorly understood genetic variations among individuals. Based on results from prior vaccine regimens it is anticipated that the immune response will not be adequate for at least 3–6 weeks after the start of vaccination, and booster immunizations will be required every 4–6 months to maintain a sufficient level of drug-specific antibodies. Improper timing of vaccinations could result in a poor response or a significant reduction in the amount of circulating antibody. Thus, the timing and duration of vaccinations will need to be carefully coordinated with patient needs and other medical interventions like counseling or behavioral modification programs.

2.2. Passive Monoclonal Anti-Addiction Immunotherapy

Passive immunotherapy does not vaccinate an individual to stimulate his/her antibody response, but administers pre-formed anti-drug antibodies to the person. This antibody medication could be polyclonal serum from an individual who has been vaccinated against a drug of abuse. However, a monoclonal antibody could be made with high affinity for a specific abused drug and be either a chimeric monoclonal comprised of 34% mouse protein and 66% human protein, a humanized monoclonal comprised of >90% human protein, or a fully human antibody. Currently, advanced biotechnological techniques have produced FDA-approved monoclonal antibodies for ten therapeutic and one prophylactic indication. For example, Synagis® is a monoclonal antibody approved for the prevention of serious lower respiratory disease caused by respiratory syncytial virus (RSV) in pediatric patients at high risk of RSV disease. This antibody is administered before and then monthly throughout the RSV season to maintain protective circulating antibody levels. Thus, passive immunotherapy with monoclonal is being successfully applied in a variety of medical areas and is beginning to be applied in chemical addictions.

Another technological development for monoclonal therapy has been new ways to make specific immunotherapies in relatively short periods of 12 to 18 months rather than the typical 15 years required for bringing a new medication to market [8–13]. These immunotherapies can be genetically engineered as new abused drugs are detected by emergency room admissions of overdoses, by police seizures from illicit drug dealers or by other early indicators of a new "designer drug" of abuse. Applying this technology to the immunotherapy of addictions would allow us to match the rapid proliferation of newly abused substances with an early-response system that can quickly treat new addictive disorders and potentially stop their epidemic spread. A similar rapid technology probably can be developed for developing the much less expensive active vaccines, since the initial development of both cocaine and nicotine vaccines has suggested that several carrier proteins derived from various bacterial toxins can be effectively coupled to drugs of abuse [7]. Extending this technology to other currently abused substances such as marijuana, amphetamine or ecstasy, as well as to new generations of "designer drugs" of abuse will be a tremendous opportunity to have new pharmacotherapies rapidly available before experimental abuse of a new substance develops into an epidemic.

3. How Might Anti-Addiction Vaccines Be Used in the Future?

3.1. Three Clinical Applications of Anti-Addiction Immunotherapies

Antibodies could potentially be used in drug abuse treatment for three clinical applications: to treat drug overdose; to reduce drug use relapse; or to protect certain at risk populations who have not yet become drug dependent [14]. Adolescent children of cocaine dependent parents might illustrate this third application. If these adolescents begin using cocaine, then preventative vaccination might be considered to protect these adolescents from becoming cocaine dependent with all its severe implications for psychosocial as well as developmental complications. Other special populations such as fetuses of drug abusing mothers might also warrant protective immunotherapy of the mother to prevent fetal exposure to the abused drug. Vaccination could potentially be used in all of these situations, except for drug overdose, where only monoclonals will be suitable, because the effect of the therapy must be rapid and cannot be delayed for several weeks. Monoclonal therapy might also be modified for special uses such as overdose. For example, antibody fragments, of a size that would be cleared by the kidney, could be used to treat overdose so that not only would the antibody bind the drug and lower the amount in the brain, but also, the drug-antibody complexes would be cleared quickly from the body. Depending on the particular setting, a combination of vaccination and monoclonal antibody therapy could be administered. In a drug abuse protection or relapse setting, where one would like to have significant antibody present over a long period of time, one could envision administering a loading dose of a monoclonal antibody along with active immunization (vaccination) with periodic repeat booster doses of vaccine to maintain the desired serum antibody concentrations. This combined approach of using active (vaccination) and passive (monoclonal) antibody therapy takes advantage of the relatively low cost of vaccination for long-term protection and the immediate efficacy of more costly monoclonal therapy. Monoclonal therapy can also be simply given repeatedly every couple of months. For example, Remicade® is given at 0, 2 and 6 weeks as a loading dose and then every 8 weeks thereafter for the treatment of rheumatoid arthritis. In summary, flexible combinations of vaccination and monoclonal immunotherapies can address a range of therapeutic challenges in the addictions, and the models for using immunotherapies are already being applied in other medical disorders.

3.2. Addressing Current Immunotherapy Limitations

While current immunotherapies have potential limitations, most of them can be addressed. Some of these limitations are technological, but others are challenges from the systems of medical care delivery and from social consequences of these therapies. Technological limitations differ for vaccines and monoclonals. One limitation for monoclonal antibodies involves their production, which is time-consuming and expensive. Furthermore, the development of a high affinity monoclonal anti-drug antibody is sometimes difficult to achieve. This discovery process of selecting an appropriate monoclonal antibody among the thousands that can be produced will led itself to high throughput screening, which has been very effectively applied to many aspects of the drug discovery process for small molecules such as antibiotics.

The technological challenges for vaccinations include the inadequate antibody response in some individuals. When an individual makes insufficient antibodies, then the blockade of the illicit drug will be ineffective or quite weak and easily overridden by increasing the amount of drug used. While biotechnology advances may address many biological reasons for such inadequate antibody responses, adherence rates for a wide range of treatment regimens have been far from perfect. For cocaine treatments lasting only 3 months dropout rates range from 15% to 79%, with an overall rate of 48% [15]. Adherence may be a particular problem for completing a series of three to five initial vaccinations over 2 to 3 months or for obtaining later booster vaccinations in substance abusers. Insuring behavioral adherence will require other social strategies beyond this paper, but are critical for the overall success of any anti-addiction vaccine program. However, a more optimistic view is provided in a recent intervention targeting over a thousand heroin addicts in Italy, 88% completed a full six-month hepatitis B vaccine series [16]. So high compliance is possible even in heavy drug-using populations.

Predicting who will develop adequate responses will be improved substantially as we develop better understanding of the genetic determinants of these responses. Individuals showing low antibody responses might then be treated more broadly for this relative immuno-deficiency by variations in gene transplantation and perhaps infusions of appropriate T and B type white blood cells to generate antibody responses, as well as being given cytokines and other small proteins that enhance immune responses. The importance of such treatments for their immune system is not simply to treat their inability to adequately respond to these anti-addiction vaccines, but also their diminished ability to fight a broad range of potential immune challenges such as infectious agents and large protein toxins. Improving vaccines by better adjuvants than the alum ones currently used, as well as by using concurrent cytokine treatments to enhance the antibody response are other potential technological fixes to these challenges of individuals' inadequate responses to immune stimulation. Vaccinations also may not produce antibodies in a timely fashion for proper integration with other medical interventions (*e.g.*, drug overdose). For overdoses, the obvious solution will be to develop monoclonal antibodies for passive use. For other applications, where such a rapid response is not essential, concurrent cytokine administration and sustained release formulations may accelerate the antibody response. Oral or even intranasal administration rather than injections of the vaccines may be another technological improvement for addictions like nicotine that sometimes are viewed more as lifestyle issues rather than immediately life threatening diseases.

3.3. Unexpected Social Consequences of Anti-Addiction Vaccines

Because in some cases the drugs of abuse are closely related in structure to either neurochemicals or approved medications (*e.g.*, nicotine replacement therapy for cigarette smoking), it is possible that the therapies could lead to unexpected adverse reactions or reduced effectiveness of other medications. This drug interaction is easily tested, however, and extremely specific because of the specificity of antibodies. Thus, this potential problem will be easily detected and of a very limited duration, since vaccines and monoclonals only maintain sufficiently high antibody levels to produce such effects for about 3 to 4 months without booster vaccination or re-infusion of the monoclonal. The duration of efficacy after an initial course of vaccination or active immunotherapy also raises ethical considerations about stigmatization, because of the potential for long-lasting immunologic memory to serve as a marker of past immunization for years or even a lifetime. Monoclonal antibodies, however, have a finite life span and several months following treatment would no longer be detectable.

Immunotherapies like all long-acting blockers also have special risks, because large amounts of drug could override the beneficial effects of immunotherapy. Effectiveness of the blockade will also decrease over time, but not at a predictable rate in a particular individual. Blockades that are completely effective either immediately from a monoclonal or progressively from a vaccine will both become progressively ineffective. As the level of blocking wanes over time following administration, there is no obvious signal to the patient that the blocking effects have diminished after weeks or months of sustained blockade. Toward the end of the "effective" duration of blockade the patient may ingest a relatively large amount of drug that previously had produced minimal effects, but now results in an overdose. Furthermore, immunotherapies will not reduce drug craving, and craving may increase as the blockade becomes weaker and the drug abuser feels a partial or delayed drug effect. This enhanced craving due to partial blockade when a modest amount of drug is used coupled with the diminished blockade of toxicities may enhance accidental overdose risk.

The success of any blockade strategy also assumes that the drug's pharmacological effects primarily drive drug use, but these effects are not the sole motive for drug use. In adolescents drug use may be a form of defiant behavior and attenuating the primary reinforcing effects of an abused substance such as tobacco or marijuana smoking may not deter the substance use. Furthermore, some harm stems from behaviors associated with drug use itself or from substances mixed in with the reinforcing drug that is blocked [17]. Those potential harms would be exacerbated if users sought to override immunotherapies' partial blocking by taking more of the drug or taking it more frequently. For example, the risk of lung cancer from cigarette smoke will be enhanced by greater use. Even if a vaccine intercepts the harmful effects of nicotine, tar and other carcinogen exposures will increase and damage the esophagus and lungs.

A related effect of relatively potent risk reduction strategies is increased engagement in these risky activities. Existing data support this unfortunate effect of risk reduction strategies. Smokers compensate for filters and low-tar tobacco by smoking more cigarettes, inhaling more deeply, or blocking the filter vents [18,19]. Similarly, Katz et al. [20] report that the percentage of San Francisco men who report unprotected anal sex increased from 24 percent to 45 percent between 1994 and 1999. The authors present correlations and anecdotal evidence linking this increase in risky sex to reduced fears of HIV since the advent of HAART, which can effectively treat AIDS. A survey reported by Ostrow et al. [21] also shows a correlation between unsafe sex and perceptions that HAART reduces the harmful consequences of HIV infection. In both these cases, some of the safety gains brought about by a reduction in the probability of harm given unsafe conduct have been offset by increases in the probability of that conduct.

For illicit drugs, adverse consequences of attempting to override the vaccines could extend beyond the drug user to other people, if immunotherapies increased the demand for drugs from drug dealers and black markets [17]. For example, crime committed by users to get money to buy drugs and conflict related to drug transactions, (e.g., disputes among dealers over drug money) account for more than 2/3 of drug-related crime. If immunotherapies increased market demand, they could yield a net increase in drug-related crime and violence.

3.4. Summary of Advantages for Future Anti-Addiction Vaccines

In spite of these various limitations, both active and passive immunotherapies have several major advantages over other approaches to treating drug dependence.

1. The antibodies target the drug, not the drug's sites of action in the brain.
2. The binding of drug to antibody inactivates the drug.
3. The antibody can be highly specific for the drug and/or the drug class.
4. These immunotherapies can complement conventional therapies (like behavioral modification) for a more comprehensive medical approach.

5.　The use of immunotherapy would not necessarily preclude the use of chemical agonists or antagonists for the brain receptors or transporters involved in the actions of the abused drug. An important exception is the combined use of a nicotine agonist therapy and anti-nicotine antibodies, although nicotine agonist therapy can be used during active vaccination without interfering with antibody production.
6.　Immunotherapy has a different pattern and generally minimal side effects compared to treatment with chemical agonists or antagonists.
7.　The antibodies are not addictive like some chemical agonists.

4. What Technological Advances Might Be Made in Immunotherapies?

Technology advances in manufacturing and delivery systems will improve future anti-addiction vaccines, as indicated above through several examples. Perhaps the most important will be a marked increase in the speed for discovering and bringing new treatments to market for abused substances, as new abused drugs constantly evolve and are spread among the youth of the world. Related advances will increase the stability and longevity of antibody blood levels and produce combination vaccines and monoclonal antibodies to simultaneously treat a variety of abused drugs. Delivery systems for vaccines can be improved. Current multiple injections can be converted to single injections in sustained release formulations to improve peak antibody levels and sustain those levels more effectively. Injections also can be converted to oral and intranasal administration forms. As our understanding of cytokines and other immune modulators improves, we will be able to add adjuvant agents to the basic vaccines that will markedly reduce the time for antibody production from several weeks to possibly several days. These adjuvants will also increase the peak antibody response and prolong the duration of these responses thereby enabling less frequent boosters. Monoclonal antibodies will be produced in more efficient plant-based systems rather than the significantly more expensive microbial incubator vats that now produce these molecularly engineered proteins.

5. Facilitating Adoption of Technology in Alcohol and Drug Treatment Services

Progress in the development of medications for the treatment of drug dependence will lead to little application of these therapies, if drug abuse treatment practitioners and programs are not ready, willing, and able to embrace medication technologies. Six broad sets of barriers to the diffusion and adoption of emerging technologies in drug abuse treatment settings were identified in the Institute of Medicine's [22] analysis of the linkages between research and practice:

- Structure – small programs with limited resources may be unable to afford the medical staff and training required to fully utilize medications;
- Financing – the multiple funding streams that support drug treatment may have unique rules and may not provide coverage for new therapies including medications;
- Education and training – in many programs training for staff relies more heavily on an apprenticeship (experiential training) emphasizing traditional approaches rather than the more theoretical and cosmopolitan perspective found in graduate education;
- Stigma – ignorance and prejudice about drug abuse contributes to inadequate training in graduate programs and medical schools, inhibits the construction and location of facilities, and reduces investments in technology development;

- Lack of knowledge about technology transfer – a lack of systematic research on the adoption of technology in drug abuse treatment settings slows the development of more effective dissemination strategies;
- Policy – local, state and federal policies sometimes restrict the types of services available and the individuals who receive those services.

These six issues that slow diffusion of any new medical therapy into substance abuse treatment may be complicated due to several unintended behavioral consequences of anti-addiction vaccines. These consequences can be divided into four potentially negative scenarios.

1. Users can attempt to override the therapy with larger doses.
2. One drug whose effects have not been blocked can substitute for another drug whose effects have been blocked. For example, amphetamine substituted for cocaine in a stimulant abuser taking a cocaine vaccine.
3. There may be an increased incidence and/or prevalence of drug use because of a perception of less risk involved with drug initiation.
4. Drug sellers losing sales may adopt aggressive actions in an attempt to move into new markets.

All of these scenarios emphasize how the intended recipients of intelligent health environments can defeat the benefits of these new technologies through unintended uses and distortions of technologies and their goals.

Although individuals seeking treatment and their families are the most direct beneficiaries of effective immunotherapy, they may not immediately buy in to these treatments or their benefits. Attitudes toward medications and beliefs about the efficacy and effects of medications will be critical in the adoption and diffusion of these new treatments. Moreover, because of the value of group support to recovery, there is a whole social system of individuals in recovery whose attitudes and beliefs could have substantial impact on the acceptability of these medications to the field of addictions treatment. Similarly, counselors communicate their beliefs and opinions to clients and as authority figures can potentially facilitate or inhibit the use of medications. Social and normative influences must be considered when assessing the cognitive factors that contribute to behavioral decisions, because much of what clients know about treatment comes from interactions with counselors and other clients. Therefore, a large part of the future for anti-addiction vaccines and immunotherapies will depend on substance abuse program staff and the families of substance abusers accepting these treatments as well as on the abusers themselves. Addressing this hurdle may require innovative new communication technologies to change some values within existing treatment delivery systems.

References

[1] T.A. Waldmann and W. Strober, Metabolism of Immunoglobulins, *Progress in Allergy* 13 (1969) 1–110.
[2] T.R. Kosten and D. Biegel, Therapeutic Vaccines for Substance Dependence, *Expert Review of Vaccines* 1 (3) (2002) 363–371.
[3] M.W. Bradbury and S.L. Lightman, The Blood-Brain Interface, *Eye* 4 (Pt 2) (1990) 249–254.
[4] B.S. Fox, K.M. Kantak, M.A. Edwards, et al., Efficacy of a Therapeutic Cocaine Vaccine in Rodent Models, *Nature Medicine* 2 (10) (1996) 1129–1132.
[5] P.R. Pentel, D. H. Malin, S. Ennifar, et al., A Nicotine Conjugate Vaccine Reduces Nicotine Distribution to Brain and Attenuates Its Behavioral and Cardiovascular Effects in Rats, *Pharmacology, Biochemistry and Behavior* 65 (1) (2000) 191–198.
[6] T.R. Kosten, M. Rosen, J. Bond, et al., Human Therapeutic Cocaine Vaccine: Safety and Immunogenicity, *Vaccine* 20 (7–8) (2002) 1196–1204.

[7] M. Haney and T.R. Kosten, Therapeutic Vaccines for Substance Dependence, *Drug Discovery Today: Therapeutic Strategies* (in press).

[8] T. Turpen, T.I. Cameron, S.J. Reinl, et al., Production of Recombinant Proteins in Plants: Pharmaceutical Applications. The Soc. Exper. Biol., Canterbury, UK, *Journal of Experimental Botany* 48 (Suppl) (12) (1997).

[9] G.P. Pogue, S. Garger, M. McCulloch, et al., From Dirt to Drugs: The Use of Viral Vectors to Make Pharmaceutical Grade Recombinant Proteins, *Fifth International Symposium on Positive Strand RNA Viruses,* 1998.

[10] R.B. Holtz and S. Garger. Commercialization of Recombinantly Derived Therapeutics from Tobacco Plants in a cGMP Facility: Division of Biological Chemistry, American Chemical Society National Meeting, 1999.

[11] R.B. Holtz. Purification Systems for Plant Derived Biologics. Invited Paper. *Plant Derived Biologics Seminar. Sponsored by FDA/CBER and USDA/APHIS.* Ames, Iowa, 2000.

[12] R.B. Holtz. Vaccine Production Using Plants as Bioreactors: Regulatory Issues and Opportunities. Invited Paper. *BIOPHEX.* San Jose, CA, 2002a.

[13] R.B. Holtz. Rapid Scale-up of Vaccine Production in Plants: Two Case Studies. Invited Speaker. *World Vaccine Conference.* Lyon, France, 2002b.

[14] H.J. Harwood and T.G. Myers, (eds.). New Treatments for Addiction: Behavioral, Ethical, Legal and Social Questions. The National Academies Press, Amsterdam, 2004. Committee on Immunotherapies and Sustained-Release Formulations for Treating Drug Addiction.

[15] M. Silva de Lima, G. Garcia de Oliveira Soares, A. Alves Pereira Reisser, M. Farrell, Pharmacological Treatment of Cocaine Dependence: A Systematic Review, *Addiction* 97 (8) (2002) 931–949.

[16] G. Quaglio, G. Talamini, F. Lugoboni, et al., Compliance with Hepatitis B Vaccination in 1175 Heroin Users and Risk Factors Associated with Lack of Vaccine Response, *Addiction* 97 (8) (2002) 985–992.

[17] R.J. MacCoun, P. Reuter Jr., C. Wolf, (eds.). Drug War Heresies: Learning from Other Vices, Times, and Places. Cambridge University Press, New York, 2001.

[18] J.R. Hughes, Applying Harm Reduction to Smoking, *Tobacco Control* 4 (1995) S33–S38.

[19] K. Stratton, P. Shetty, R.F. Wallace, S. Bondurant, Clearing the Smoke: Assessing the Science Base for Tobacco Harm Reduction, *Tobacco Control* 10 (2) (2001) 189–195.

[20] M.H. Katz, S.K. Schwarcz, T.A. Kellogg, et al., Impact of Highly Active Antiretroviral Treatment on HIV Seroincidence among Men Who Have Sex with Men: San Francisco, *American Journal of Public Health* 92 (2002) 388–394.

[21] D.E. Ostrow, K.J. Fox, J.S. Chmiel, et al., Attitudes Towards Highly Active Antiretroviral Therapy Are Associated with Sexual Risk Taking among HIV-Infected and Uninfected Homosexual Men, *AIDS* 16 (2002) 775–780.

[22] NIH Consensus Conference, Effective Medical Treatment of Opiate Addiction, *JAMA* 280 (1998) 1936–1943.

Future of Intelligent and Extelligent Health Environment
R.G. Bushko (Ed.)
IOS Press, 2005

Automating Addiction Treatment: Enhancing the Human Experience and Creating a Fix for the Future

David H. GUSTAFSON, Ph.D.[a], Tara E. PALESH[b], Rosalind W. PICARD, Sc.D.[c],
Paul E. PLSEK[d], Lynne MAHER, RGN, BSc Hons, MBA[e]
and Victor A. CAPOCCIA Ph.D.[f]

[a]*Research Professor of Industrial Engineering and Director of the Network for
Improvement of Addiction Treatment, University of Wisconsin, Madison, WI, USA*
[b]*University of Wisconsin, Madison, WI, USA*
[c]*Director, Affective Computing Research Group, MIT Media Laboratory,
Cambridge, MA, USA*
[d]*Paul E. Plsek & Associates, Inc., USA*
[e]*Head of Innovation & Acting Director for Improvement,
NHS Modernisation Agency, London, UK*
[f]*Senior Program Officer The Robert Wood Johnson Foundation, Princeton, NJ, USA*

Abstract. The country's system of providing treatment for people struggling with addiction requires a fundamental overhaul. To address these daunting problems, a group of experts from outside the addiction field met in an intensive retreat and envisioned a new future for addiction treatment that would use the latest available technology. Retreat leaders employed creative techniques to help free up thinking beyond incremental improvement ideas. Current and former addicts or alcoholics and family members also attended the retreat to provide the panelists with a real-world understanding of their lives. Through this process, the panelists generated eight idea categories that visualized future treatments for addiction using technology. They were: (1) Integrated System and Record; (2) Monitoring/Treatment; (3) Virtual Experiences; (4) Treatment Access and "One Stop Shop"; (5) Networks; (6) Tailored Media Campaigns; (7) Diagnostic Tools; and (8) Help for Family. Two stories illustrate how these ideas could help a heroin addict and an alcoholic. The sponsors plan another meeting to bring these visionary concepts closer to real application.

1. Introduction

It is the year 2020 in a large city. Scattered along the city's streets are booths that resemble the old public telephone booths that have long disappeared from the urban landscape. These booths cover a wide variety of health topics and people can talk to "virtual" counselors at the touch of a screen. Maria, a heroin addict, has passed these new public health booths a few times—perhaps on her way to rendezvous with her drug dealer. Today, she pauses for a closer look. Maria's boyfriend beat her up a few days before and she ended up in the emergency room. She is worried about her health.

At the booth, Maria enters some information about her background including telling the system that she is in her 20s. Then the booth's screen filled with an image of a young woman about Maria's age. The woman is friendly and draws Maria in with her easy-going manner. The young woman, who is a "virtual" substance abuse counselor named "Selene", talks about the difficulty of heroin addiction and says that she can help Maria through the process of quitting drugs. In fact, Maria can get started towards recovery today by stopping in any booth to talk to her virtually. Selene will be waiting for her. Maria pauses to listen.

This public health booth, where heroin addicts would be able to speak to a virtual substance abuse counselor, is just one way that technology may be able to provide critical support in some of the daunting problems facing this country's substance abuse treatment system. While many effective drug and alcohol treatment programs exist, they serve only a small fraction of those in need. According to the 2002 National Survey on Drug Use and Health, only 15% of an estimated 22.8 million addicts in the United States receive treatment. For every person who has been able to control this disease countless others are far less successful.

The Robert Wood Johnson Foundation (RWJF) supports research projects that focus on treating people with addiction disease. Two of the authors (Gustafson and Palesh) served in the national program office for the RWJF's Paths to Recovery Program, a program with a sister relationship to a federal government program called Strengthening Treatment, Access and Retention. The program was designed to improve administrative processes that prevent addicts from accessing and then staying in treatment. The program demonstrated substantial reductions in waiting time to receive treatment and in numbers of clients dropping out of treatment.

Even so, it quickly became apparent that improving the existing system would not substantially improve addiction treatment. The current system is not sustainable. Counselor salary levels are so low that it is difficult to prevent counselors from leaving the field for jobs that offer higher pay. Substantial increases in funding are unlikely in the foreseeable future. Yet the demand for services is almost certain to grow. The foundations of addiction treatment need to be rethought to take full advantage of the technology that is available today and that will be available in the future. With this in mind, RWJF funded a project to bring together creative thinkers in fields outside addiction to envision a new system that could effectively treat people struggling with addiction. The resulting ideas offer insights not only into the future of substance abuse, but in how to tap into the creative process to find solutions to some of the most daunting problems facing the health care system today.

2. The Creative Process

One of the difficulties in envisioning a new system of health care is that people doing the envisioning are often part of the system that is not working. When people are steeped in a current structure, it is daunting to think creatively about a new way of providing services. To remedy this ongoing problem, staff at Paths to Recovery looked for creative thinkers outside of the addiction field. The staff invited a small group of internationally respected experts in other fields to design an innovative and effective addiction treatment system. The experts represented fields such as nanotechnology, robotics, biomedical engineering, genetics, neurobiology, artificial intelligence, bio-informatics, social psychology, collaborative technologies and pharmacology. Facilitators had a few key criteria for those they wanted to invite. They needed people who:

- Had a sound grasp of the technology that will be ready for use by 2020
- Were not be encumbered by knowledge of the current system for treatment addiction
- Were creative, collaborative and communicative

In addition to the outside experts, the group included addiction experts and consumers of services (recovering addicts and alcoholics and family members) to provide a clear picture of the treatment system today. The consumers of addiction treatment services were vital to this project. They provided a first-hand, vivid portrait of their lives and their needs. In all, 28 experts gathered for an intense two-day retreat in November 2004 to envision a new substance abuse treatment system for alcoholics and heroin addicts.

Members of the expert panel

Futurists

- **Timothy Baker** – University of Wisconsin, clinical psychology.
- **Rena Bizios** – Rennesselaer Polytechnic Institute, biomedical engineering.
- **Patricia Brennan** – University of Wisconsin, nursing informatics.
- **Renata Bushko** – healthcare futurist.
- **Noshir Contractor** – University of Illinois, communication networks.
- **Juan de Pablo** – University of Wisconsin, nanotechnology.
- **BJ Fogg** –Stanford University, medical-informatics.
- **David Gustafson** – University of Wisconsin, medical informatics/technology innovation.
- **Thomas Kosten** – Yale University, pharmacology.
- **Dean Lea** – organizational development consultant.
- **Lynne Maher** – British National Health Service, Modernisation Agency
- **Jesper Olsson** – Swedish Federation of County Councils, medical-informatics.
- **Tara Palesh** – University of Wisconsin, systems engineering
- **Rosalind Picard** – Massachusetts Institute of Technology, human computer interfaces

- **Paul Plsek**, author and developer of DirectedCreativity
- **Victor Strecher** – University of Michigan, communications science
- **Peter Szolovits** – Massachusetts Institute of Technology, decision and computer science.
- **Sheila Wang** – social psychology.

Addiction Experts

- **Bret Shaw** – communication science.
- **Maria Levis-Peralta** – community activist.
- **Tom McLellan** – addiction services research.
- **Kristin Schubert** – Robert Wood Johnson Foundation, genetics.
- **Elaine Cassidy** – Robert Wood Johnson Foundation, evaluation.
- **Victor Capoccia** – Robert Wood Johnson Foundation, addiction treatment
- **Dwayne Proctor** – Robert Wood Johnson Foundation, communications systems.
- **George**, recovering alcoholic
- **James**, recovering heroin addict
- **Belle**, mother of a current heroin addict

---

3. Logistics

Coordinators paid close attention to the details of the meeting's location and ambience to help make the experience as positive as possible for the participants. A poor location or any unexpected travel inconvenience could have a severe impact on the creative thinking of the entire group. Planners chose a site that reflected the meeting's goals. It was a facility outside of Chicago in a location that was both relaxing and boasted the latest technology. The facility had ponds and streams with paths for walking as well as an extensive exercise facility, good food and easily accessible Internet connections throughout. Participants were provided with limousines to the facility and a cell phone number of a meeting organizer should any problems arise. With these preliminary arrangements, even the small glitches that did occur were addressed quickly. All of the participants arrived feeling well taken care of and ready to work.

To help the expert panel prepare for the retreat, facilitators developed a package for those who wanted more information on addiction prior to their arrival. Facilitators sent a copy of *Hooked: Five Addicts Challenge Our Misguided Drug Rehab System* by Lonny

Shavelson to each panel member. They also sent fact sheets about addiction and its treatment and stories of addicts and their families told in flow charts. However, the retreat did not hinge on panelists having done any background reading on addiction. Facilitators just asked the panelists to bring their creativity to the meeting and arrive on time.

4. Meeting

The first day of the meeting, facilitators gave participants their charge: to design an addiction treatment system that would involve no humans. They told participants that in the year 2020 all of the substance abuse treatment professionals had been killed by a virus. Addicts and their families would have to obtain help primarily through technology. This charge freed up thinking beyond incremental improvement ideas such as more training programs, more counselors, more clinics and more funding.

While facilitators felt that it was not important (and even counter productive) to understand the addiction treatment system of today, it was essential to understand how it feels to be an addict and the family member of an addict. One of the facilitators encouraged the development of a set of stories that described the life experiences of addicts and their family members. Another facilitator who had personal experience with addiction treatment (she is the daughter of an alcoholic) developed a prototype of a story. Instead of a story narrative, she wrote a flowchart. It was a concise, easy to follow format to present a large amount of information quickly. More important, it was an innovative way to break down the experience while highlighting key events and aspects of the disease. The team used that approach to develop three other flow charts that told the story of someone affected by addiction. Facilitators identified a recovering heroin addict from an inner-city ghetto (James), a recovering alcoholic CEO (George), and the mother of a 21 year-old current heroin addict (Belle).

4.1. Day 1

The morning of the first day of the meeting, a facilitator presented each of the flow charts. The consumers whose story was told in the flow charts were in the room. Provided with a rapid but detailed version of each consumer's life, the panel asked consumers questions about anything they did not understand or wanted more details about. Panelists said they found it powerful to have the four consumers depicted in the flow charts available to clarify any misconceptions and share more of their experiences. In fact, the question and answer phase was so useful that it took much longer than anticipated as panelists became deeply involved in the lives of their new "customers." The presentation of the flow charts and the in depth discussion they fostered encompassed the entire morning session rather than just a portion of it. However, during that time panelists were already placing ideas on post-it notes for future use (which had not been planned until the afternoon).

After lunch, the panel transitioned into the idea generation phase. The planning group had assembled a collection of creative thinking tools to prepare for the meeting. The idea generation tools were based on the "directed creativity" concepts of attention, escape, and movement. Innovative ideas are more likely to emerge in a group when people focus *attention* on something that they do not normally focus on, *escape* the current ways of thinking about the issue, and encourage free-wheeling mental *movement* to capture all ideas without censorship.[1,2,3] For example, in the *Future Tinkertoys™* tool, leaders helped generate escape

[1] de Bono, E. *Mechanism of Mind.* London: Penguin Books, 1969.

[2] Plsek, P.E. Innovative thinking for the improvement of medical systems. *Annals of Internal Medicine.* 131(6): 438–444. September 21, 1999.

[3] Plsek P.E. *Creativity, Innovation and Quality.* Milwaukee, WI: ASQ Quality Press, 1997.

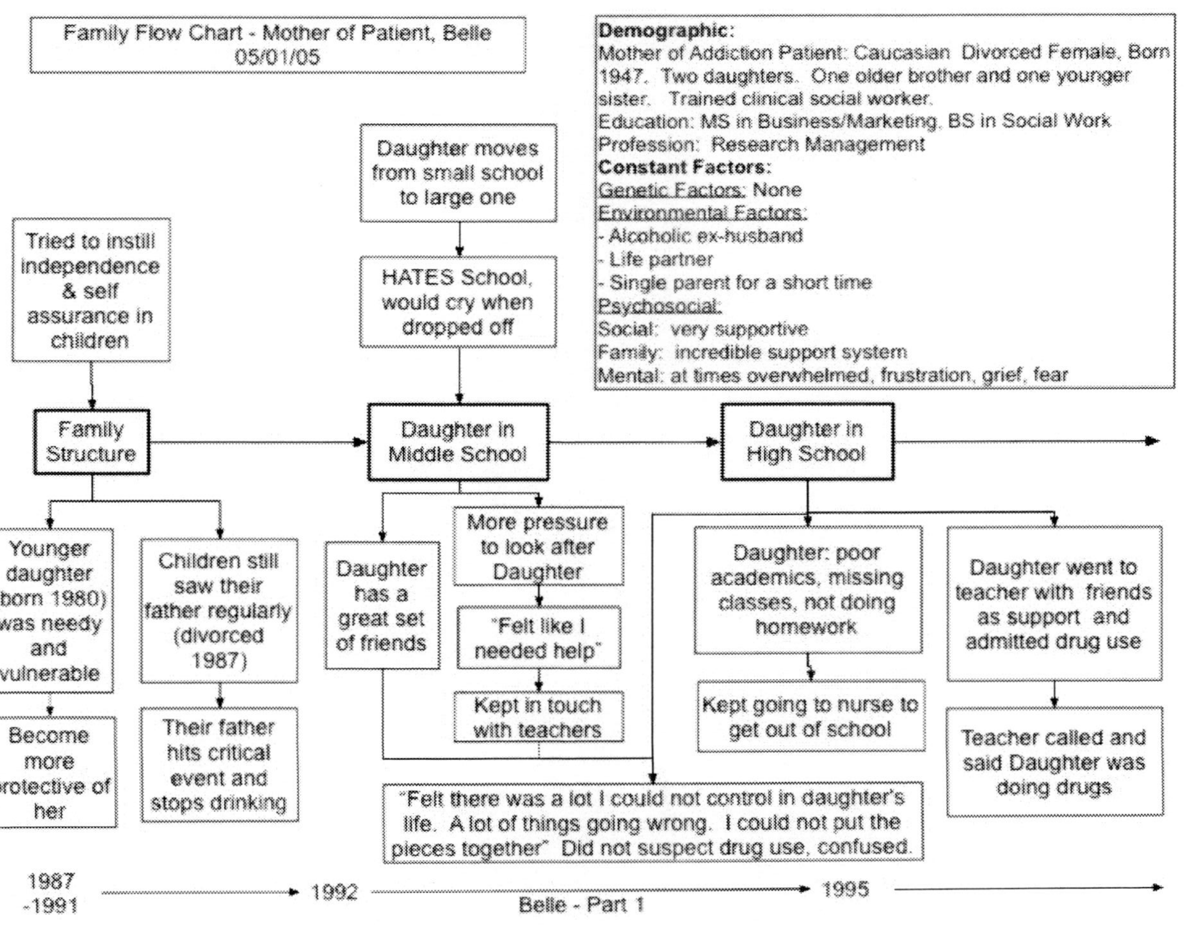

Family Flow Chart - Mother of Patient, Belle
05/01/05

Demographic:
Mother of Addiction Patient: Caucasian Divorced Female, Born 1947. Two daughters. One older brother and one younger sister. Trained clinical social worker.
Education: MS in Business/Marketing, BS in Social Work
Profession: Research Management
Constant Factors:
Genetic Factors: None
Environmental Factors:
- Alcoholic ex-husband
- Life partner
- Single parent for a short time
Psychosocial:
Social: very supportive
Family: incredible support system
Mental: at times overwhelmed, frustration, grief, fear

Tried to instill independence & self assurance in children

Daughter moves from small school to large one

HATES School, would cry when dropped off

Family Structure

Daughter in Middle School

Daughter in High School

Younger daughter (born 1980) was needy and vulnerable

Children still saw their father regularly (divorced 1987)

Become more protective of her

Their father hits critical event and stops drinking

Daughter has a great set of friends

More pressure to look after Daughter

"Felt like I needed help"

Kept in touch with teachers

Daughter: poor academics, missing classes, not doing homework

Kept going to nurse to get out of school

Daughter went to teacher with friends as support and admitted drug use

Teacher called and said Daughter was doing drugs

"Felt there was a lot I could not control in daughter's life. A lot of things going wrong. I could not put the pieces together" Did not suspect drug use, confused.

1987 -1991

1992

1995

Belle - Part 1

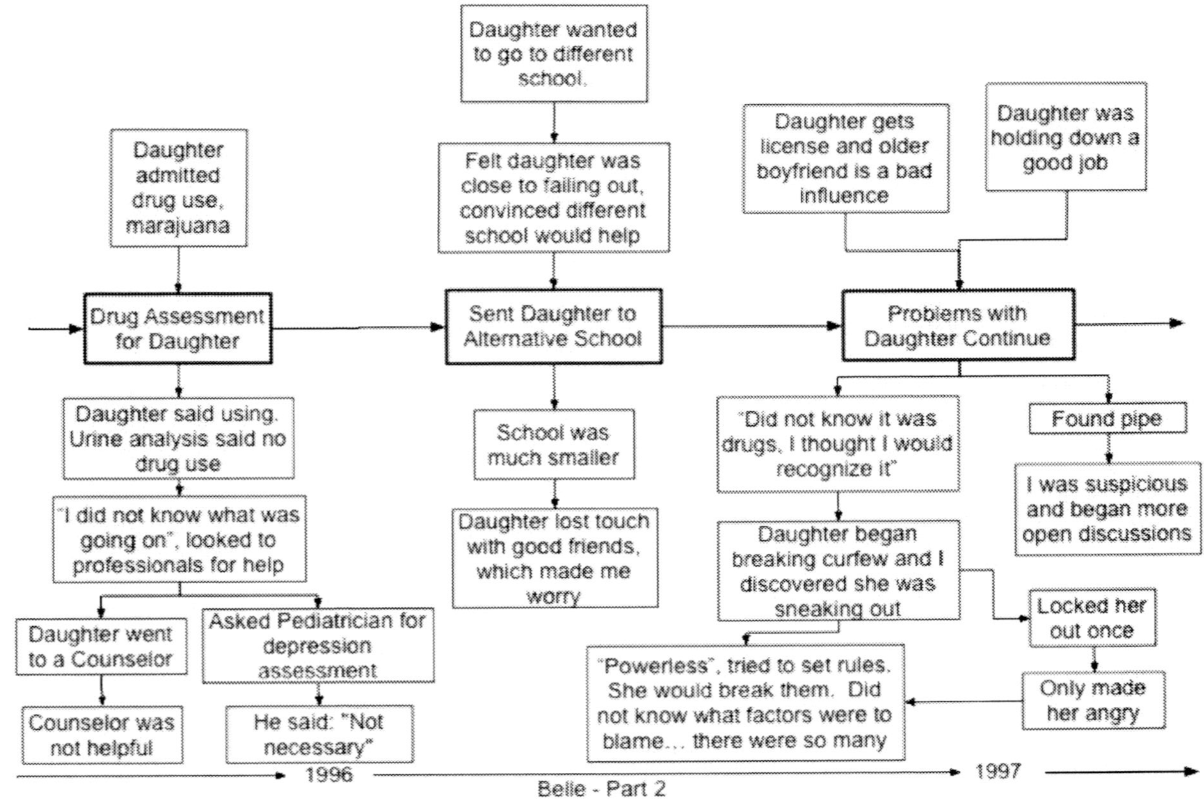

Daughter admitted drug use, marajuana
Daughter wanted to go to different school.
Felt daughter was close to failing out, convinced different school would help
Daughter gets license and older boyfriend is a bad influence
Daughter was holding down a good job
Drug Assessment for Daughter
Sent Daughter to Alternative School
Problems with Daughter Continue
Daughter said using. Urine analysis said no drug use
School was much smaller
"Did not know it was drugs, I thought I would recognize it"
Found pipe
"I did not know what was going on", looked to professionals for help
Daughter lost touch with good friends, which made me worry
Daughter began breaking curfew and I discovered she was sneaking out
I was suspicious and began more open discussions
Daughter went to a Counselor
Asked Pediatrician for depression assessment
Locked her out once
"Powerless", tried to set rules. She would break them. Did not know what factors were to blame... there were so many
Counselor was not helpful
He said: "Not necessary"
Only made her angry
1996
Belle - Part 2
1997

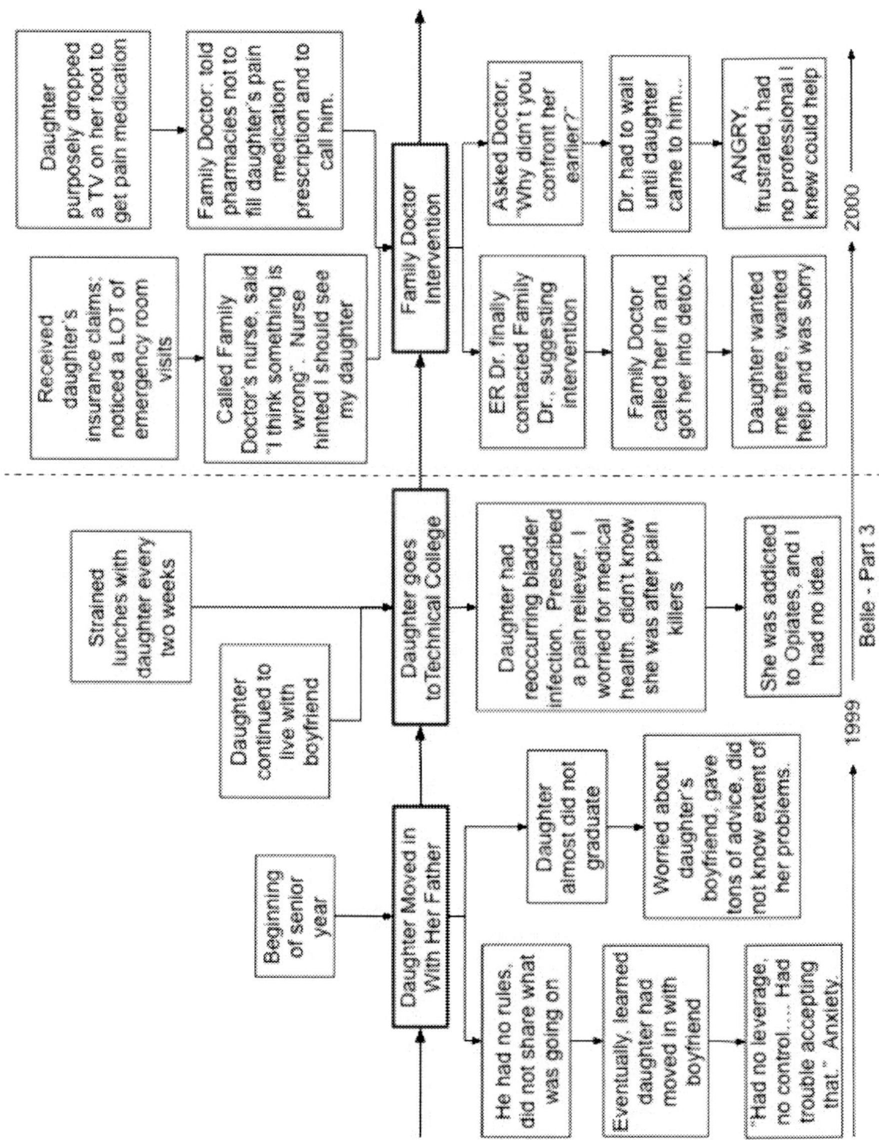
Daughter purposely dropped a TV on her foot to get pain medication
Family Doctor: told pharmacies not to fill daughter's pain medication prescription and to call him.
Family Doctor intervention
Asked Doctor, "Why didn't you confront her earlier?"
Dr. had to wait until daughter came to him....
ANGRY, frustrated, had no professional I knew could help
Received daughter's insurance claims; noticed a LOT of emergency room visits
Called Family Doctor's nurse, said "I think something is wrong". Nurse hinted I should see my daughter
ER Dr. finally contacted Family Dr., suggesting intervention
Family Doctor called her in and got her into detox.
Daughter wanted me there, wanted help and was sorry
2000
Strained lunches with daughter every two weeks
Daughter continued to live with boyfriend
Daughter goes to Technical College
Daughter had reoccurring bladder infection. Prescribed a pain reliever. I worried for medical health. didn't know she was after pain killers
She was addicted to Opiates, and I had no idea.
Belle - Part 3
Beginning of senior year
Daughter Moved in With Her Father
Daughter almost did not graduate
Worried about daughter's boyfriend, gave tons of advice, did not know extent of her problems.
He had no rules, did not share what was going on
Eventually, learned daughter had moved in with boyfriend
"Had no leverage, no control.... Had trouble accepting that." Anxiety.
1999

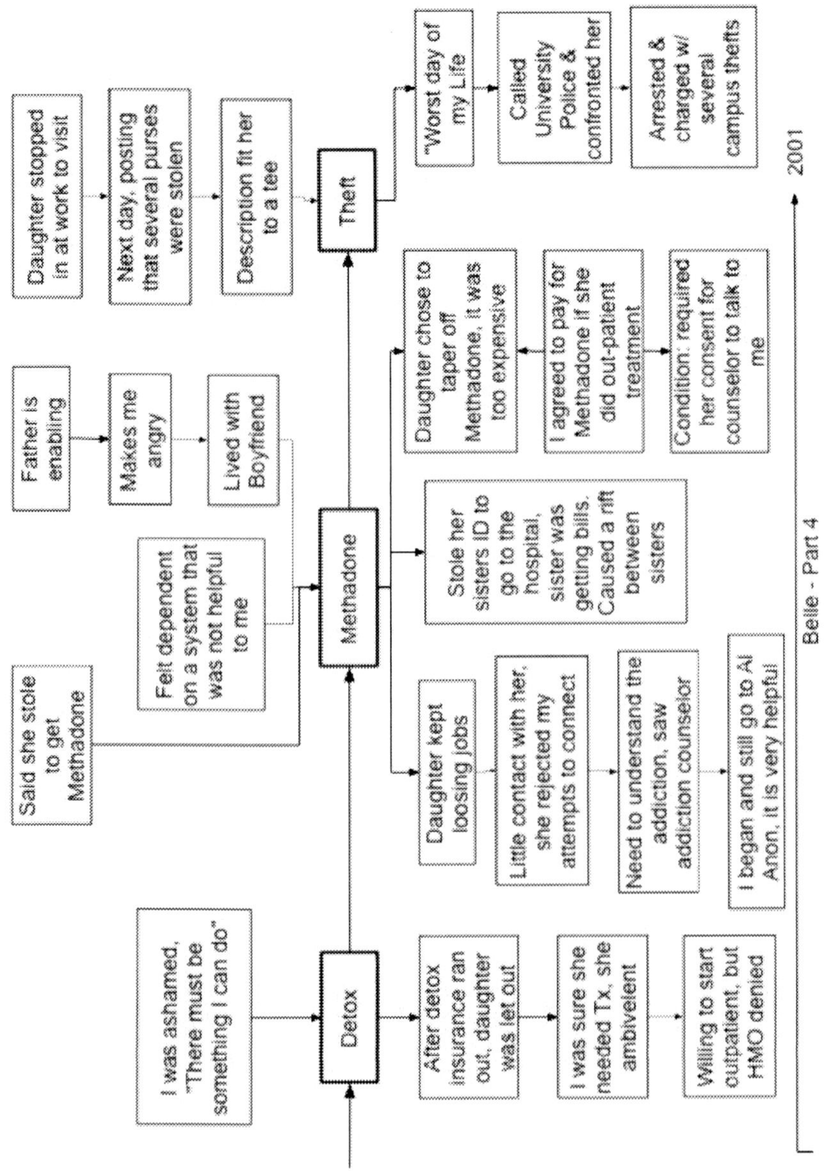
Daughter stopped in at work to visit
Next day, posting that several purses were stolen
Description fit her to a tee
Theft
"Worst day of my Life
Called University Police & confronted her
Arrested & charged w/ several campus thefts
Father is enabling
Makes me angry
Lived with Boyfriend
Felt dependent on a system that was not helpful to me
Said she stole to get Methadone
Methadone
Daughter chose to taper off Methadone, it was too expensive
I agreed to pay for Methadone if she did out-patient treatment
Condition: required her consent for counselor to talk to me
Stole her sisters ID to go to the hospital, sister was getting bills. Caused a rift between sisters
Daughter kept loosing jobs
Little contact with her, she rejected my attempts to connect
Need to understand the addiction, saw addiction counselor
I began and still go to Al Anon, it is very helpful
I was ashamed, "There must be something I can do"
Detox
After detox insurance ran out, daughter was let out
I was sure she needed Tx, she ambivelent
Willing to start outpatient, but HMO denied
2001
Belle - Part 4

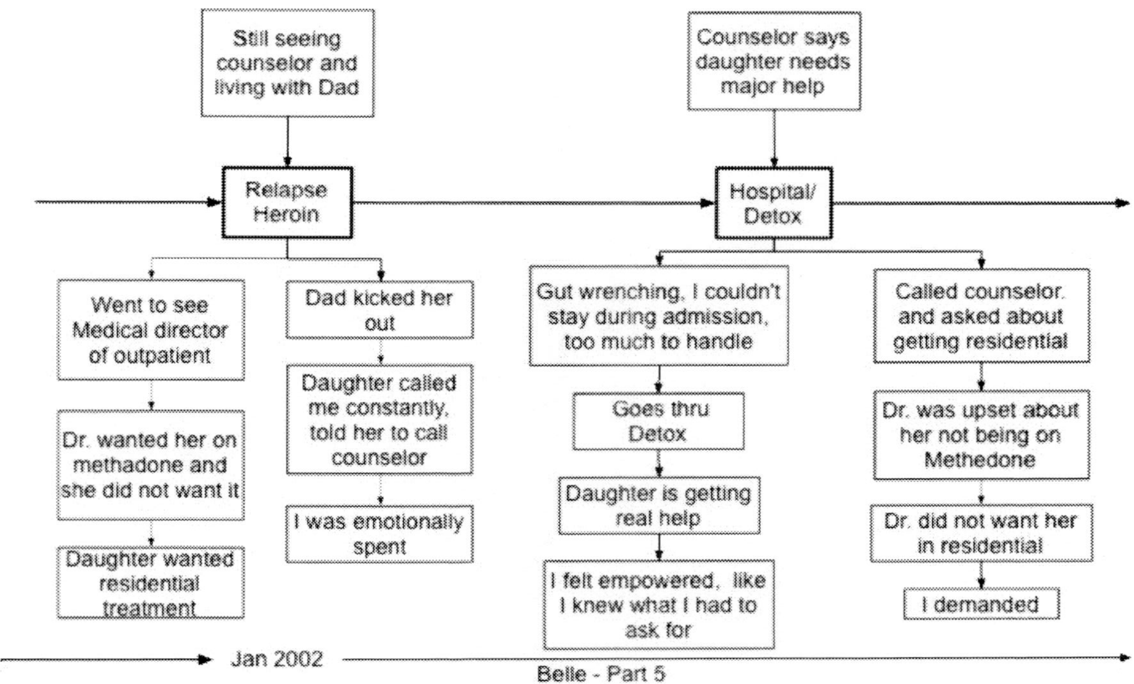
Still seeing counselor and living with Dad
Counselor says daughter needs major help
Relapse Heroin
Hospital/ Detox
Went to see Medical director of outpatient
Dad kicked her out
Gut wrenching, I couldn't stay during admission, too much to handle
Called counselor. and asked about getting residential
Dr. wanted her on methadone and she did not want it
Daughter called me constantly, told her to call counselor
Goes thru Detox
Dr. was upset about her not being on Methedone
Daughter wanted residential treatment
I was emotionally spent
Daughter is getting real help
Dr. did not want her in residential
I felt empowered, like I knew what I had to ask for
I demanded
Jan 2002
Belle - Part 5

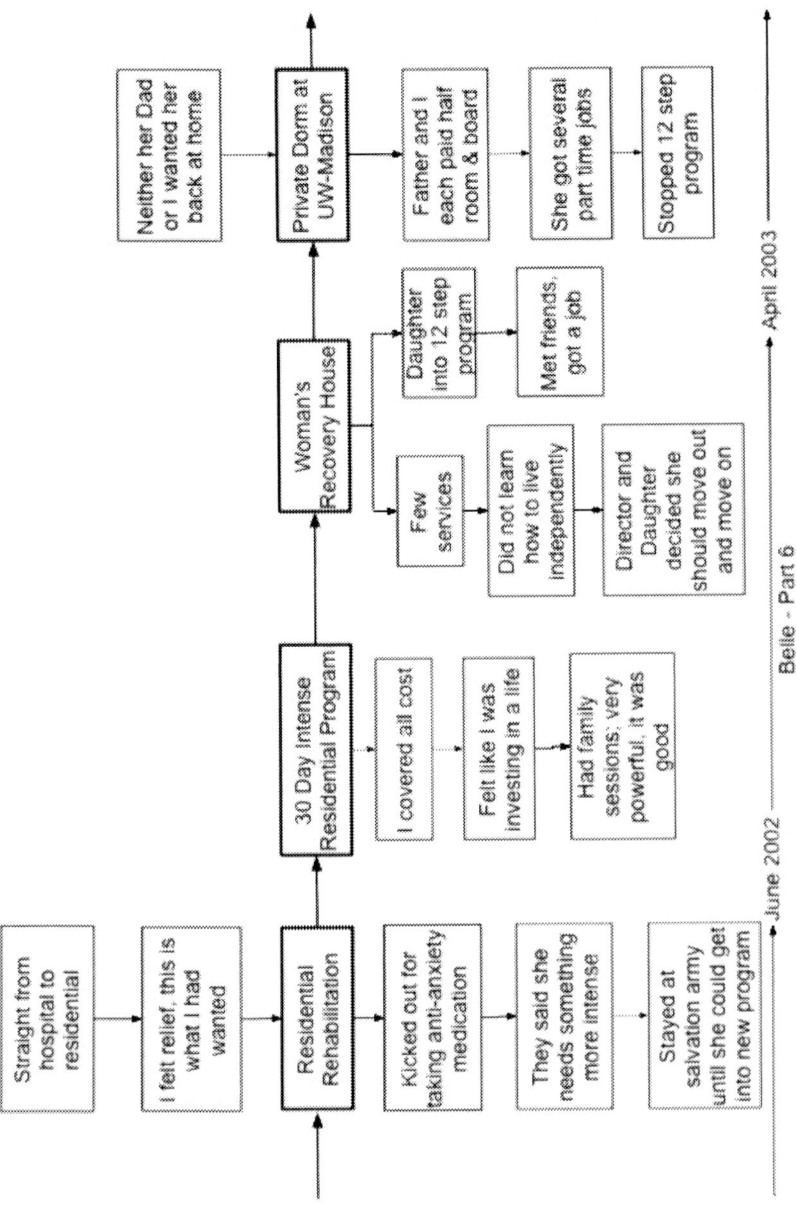
Straight from hospital to residential
I felt relief, this is what I had wanted
Residential Rehabilitation
Kicked out for taking anti-anxiety medication
They said she needs something more intense
Stayed at salvation army until she could get into new program
30 Day intense Residential Program
I covered all cost
Felt like I was investing in a life
Had family sessions; very powerful, it was good
Woman's Recovery House
Daughter into 12 step program
Met friends, got a job
Few services
Did not learn how to live independently
Director and Daughter decided she should move out and move on
Neither her Dad or I wanted her back at home
Private Dorm at UW-Madison
Father and I each paid half room & board
She got several part time jobs
Stopped 12 step program
June 2002
April 2003
Belle ~ Part 6

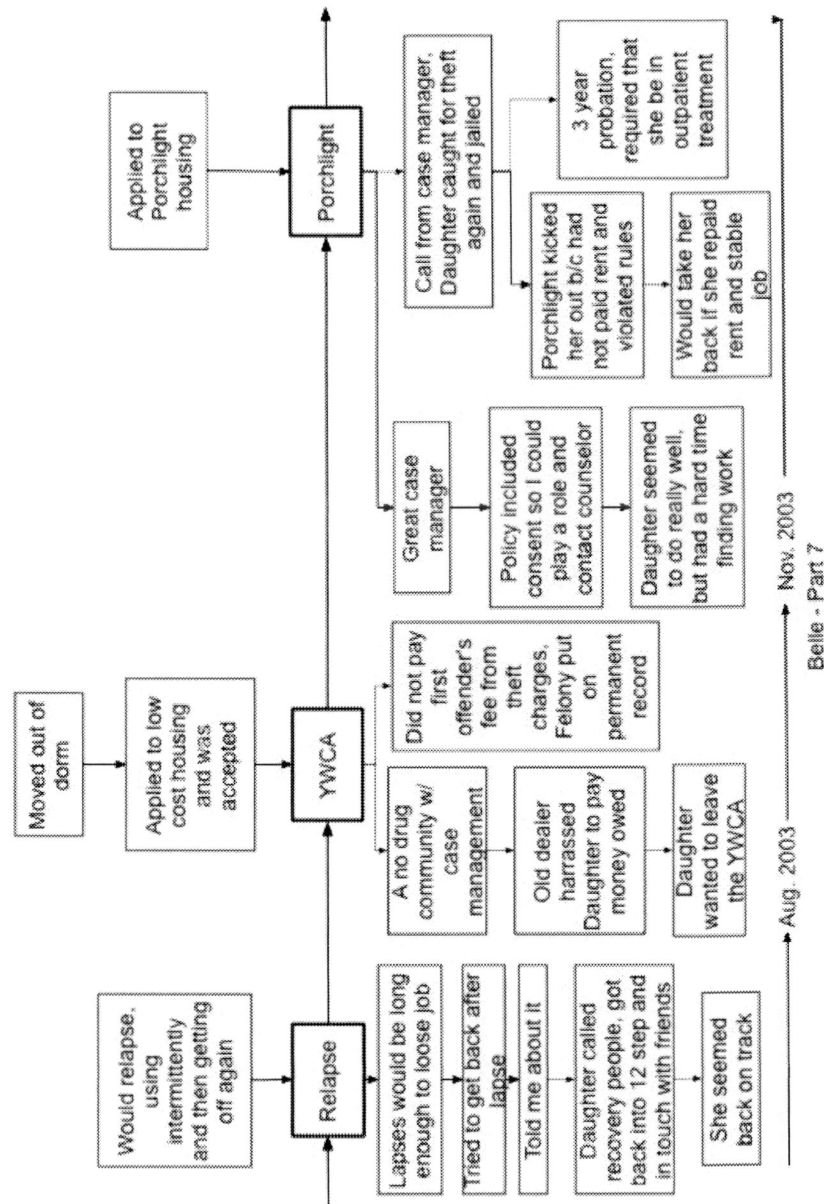

Applied to
Porchlight
housing

Porchlight

Call from case manager,
Daughter caught for theft
again and jailed

3 year
probation,
required that
she be in
outpatient
treatment

Porchlight kicked
her out b/c had
not paid rent and
violated rules

Would take her
back if she repaid
rent and stable
job

Great case
manager

Policy included
consent so I could
play a role and
contact counselor

Daughter seemed
to do really well,
but had a hard time
finding work

Nov. 2003

Belle - Part 7

Moved out of
dorm

Applied to low
cost housing
and was
accepted

YWCA

Did not pay
first
offender's
fee from
theft
charges.
Felony put
on
permanent
record

A no drug
community w/
case
management

Old dealer
harrassed
Daughter to pay
money owed

Daughter
wanted to leave
the YWCA

Aug. 2003

Would relapse,
using
intermittently
and then getting
off again

Relapse

Lapses would be long
enough to loose job

Tried to get back after
lapse

Told me about it

Daughter called
recovery people, got
back into 12 step and
in touch with friends

She seemed
back on track

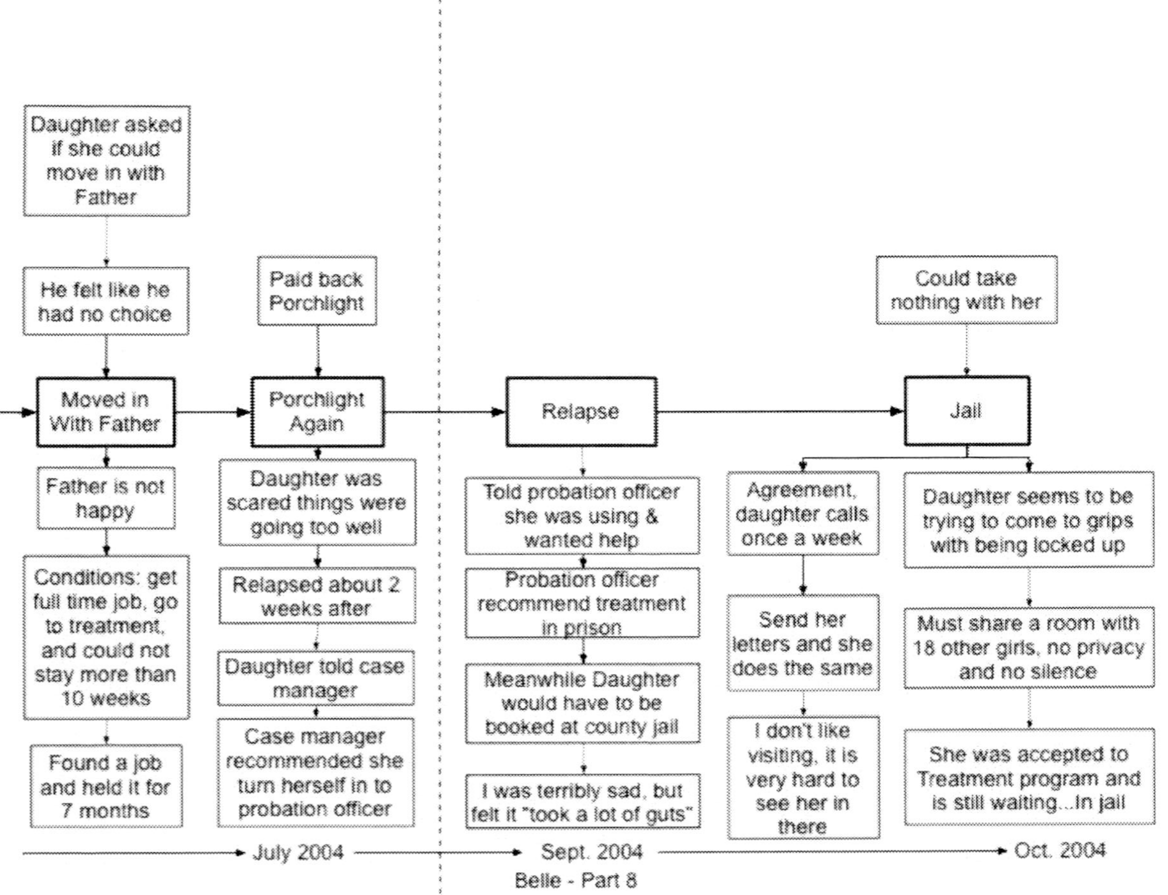

Daughter asked if she could move in with Father
He felt like he had no choice
Moved in With Father
Father is not happy
Conditions: get full time job, go to treatment, and could not stay more than 10 weeks
Found a job and held it for 7 months
Paid back Porchlight
Porchlight Again
Daughter was scared things were going too well
Relapsed about 2 weeks after
Daughter told case manager
Case manager recommended she turn herself in to probation officer
July 2004
Relapse
Told probation officer she was using & wanted help
Probation officer recommend treatment in prison
Meanwhile Daughter would have to be booked at county jail
I was terribly sad, but felt it "took a lot of guts"
Sept. 2004
Belle - Part 8
Could take nothing with her
Jail
Agreement, daughter calls once a week
Send her letters and she does the same
I don't like visiting, it is very hard to see her in there
Daughter seems to be trying to come to grips with being locked up
Must share a room with 18 other girls, no privacy and no silence
She was accepted to Treatment program and is still waiting...In jail
Oct. 2004

and attention by asking participants to identify attitudes, technologies, and devices that they expect to be commonplace in the year 2020. Ideas came in such a torrent that facilitators wrote furiously just to try and keep up. Participants often built upon one another's ideas—a demonstration that the panel was becoming comfortable with the notion of creative thinking and were working well together as a group. With that exercise as a start to future thinking the facilitators randomly assigned panelists to one of the four tables in the room. Each consumer joined a table so that they could answer any questions that arose during idea generation. Facilitators asked panel members to create as many ideas as possible related to the future treatment of addiction. The four groups began with simply throwing out ideas among themselves and then writing them all down. As expected, each of the four groups had a different method to generate ideas. The facilitators moved around the room reading the ideas and marking the ones that would need further explanation. In all the four groups generated 268 ideas. Facilitators compiled the ideas into an Excel sheet for further analysis. By the end of the first day, participants had begun to see a network of knowledge forming to focus on the future treatment of addiction.

4.2. Day 2

On the second day, the facilitators asked each of the four groups to select their top 10 ideas and then re-write those 40 ideas to ensure that they were explicit enough for anyone to understand. To help ensure that this did not become an opportunity for heated debate, each person was given 10 sticky dots with which to vote for their favorite ideas. If each person had several chances to vote, then the ideas that he or she believed in most strongly would end up among the top vote getters.

Once each group had chosen their top ideas, clarified each idea and placed them on a designated wall space, each panelist was asked to wander throughout the room and read all 40 ideas. This time they were given just seven sticky dots and told to vote on their favorite ones. Once all the dots had been placed, the ideas grouped into ones with many votes and ones with just a few. It was a visual process that made it easy to see the most popular ideas. Panelists also began to group together with others who had similar interests. In all, eight major idea categories emerged that visualized future treatments for addiction that used technology. Those idea categories were:

1) Integrated System & Record
   a. There would be a standardized, universal electronic health record with special attention to confidentiality and diversity issues. The integrated record would be linked across health and other systems and would be accessible from any location by those who have the right to access. Computers could take data from many different formats and put them into a common format. The records would form the foundation database upon which tailored plans of care would be created, delivered and monitored and which could be used for different research purposes.
2) Monitor/Treatment
   a. Devices would capture someone's mood, triggers and location that could put them at risk for using alcohol or drugs. For example, devices would monitor people's anxiety level (because anxiety had been a primary trigger for them to start drinking). When the anxiety reached a certain point, the devices could remind people to begin, for instance, deep breathing exercises that had been shown to help calm them in the past. The devices would detect mood and triggers through a sensor on someone's hand that monitored their skin perspiration, heart rate and other indications of stress that would be fed back to a computer.

b. A "relapse sensor" would provide early warning when a recovering alcoholic or addict was about to use alcohol or drugs again. For instance, a Global Positioning System might be programmed to detect when an alcoholic neared a bar where she used to drink and where many of her old friends hang out. If she entered the parking lot, the system might initiate a call from a virtual or real friend encouraging her to not go in. If she did go in it might initiate a rescue operation by alerting a close relative, such as her husband who is trained how to intervene.

c. A computer chip in blood vessel would sense drug use and release blocker medication from a depot stored in the body that would make the patient feel sick.

3) Virtual Experiences

A video game or virtual reality world would teach lessons about addiction, relapse and recovery. These could be accessed from a variety of sources such as smart phones, personal computers and public health booths where people could go at any time for help and information on addiction. Virtual "exposure" therapies would expose addicts to withdrawal symptoms, urges, and drug cues to allow addict to desensitize and practice coping in a safe context. The exposure could include music that tends to influence risk-taking behavior on the part of the user. Programs could also simulate encounters with drug pushers and teach how to resist such pressures.

4) Treatment Access and "One Stop Shop"

a. Patients would have many places to go for addiction services including "virtual" treatment centers on computer and public health booths. The sheer number of virtual treatment centers would reduce the stigma that patients often felt by going to just the one or two that were available and well-known in their area.

b. There would be automated distribution systems such as public health vending machines to obtain methadone-like medications and collect needed specimens to monitor drug use. Patients would be able to access methadone and other treatment by sensors that recognized their eyes or fingerprints. The machines might also be able to test whether the patients were "clean" in order to receive treatment.

5) Networks

a. Addicts and alcoholics would be able to use a computer program to get in touch with other people who were similar to them in age, race, background, personality and situation with whom they could talk, via computer, about their problems. A computer would also match addicts or alcoholics to a virtual support group to help address problems that a particular patient was experiencing at the moment. For example, one time someone might need to talk to fellow recovering addicts in a group. Another time he might be looking for spiritual counsel from clergy members.

6) Tailored Media Campaigns

a. Tailored multi-media campaigns would aim to de-stigmatize addiction for individuals. A multi-media campaign would sense the effect that it was having on someone and adapt it continually to be more effective. For instance, billboards might be equipped with miniature versions of a FMRI (functional magnetic resonance imaging system) that could detect how someone was responding emotionally to a message he received and adjust it to more closely match his emotional state.

b. A similar tailored system that would prevent or at least delay experimentation with drugs. People might have a Radio Frequency Identification (RFID), which is like a bar code that has information about them. A computer could read that information, see that the person was a risk for addiction, and begin sending messages to her aimed at dissuading her from drug or alcohol use.

7) Diagnostic Tools
   a. Patients could have a genetic analysis at birth or later on if they seem to be at risk for addiction because of their family history. That analysis could be passed on to a clinical team who would look it over and discuss with the parents or with the patient whether it would make sense to counteract the predisposition with gene replacement or other interventions.
   b. There could be computer-aided diagnosis that matched patterns in someone's history, such as symptoms, family background, gender and other factors to estimate the chance that the person will become addicted to a drug or alcohol. Once the computer collected all of the information, it could say that out of 100 people who have this constellation of clues, 78 will become addicts. The computer could also develop, transmit and monitor implementation of treatment plans.

8) Help for Family
   a. Computer based programs would include means to track the health and emotional status of family members. The programs would tailor the presentation of information to their health state, answer questions, and train family members how to intervene and practice the interventions. They would also provide on-line therapy, support healthy relating among family members, communicate with others facing similar problems, and provide advice from experts.[4,5]
   b. Programs would extend beyond standard health issues to address other dimensions of life (other health problems, economic and social) that might influence family members' ability to understand, cope and intervene effectively in the prevention or amelioration of addictions.

With the final ideas at hand, facilitators gave the panel their last task. They shifted participants into new groups and asked them to create and perform skits that demonstrated how the ideas could come together in a total system of care. Specifically, facilitators asked the panel to develop a news commentary (e.g. interview by a reporter of a drug addict who had used the new system or a brief vignette of how addiction would be handled in the future) that played out the important ideas collected by the group. The role playing was intended to meld the numerous ideas in a more rapid and fun approach than having a group write up a story. The future scenarios presented by the four groups were not only entertaining but insightful. They brought together the ideas and created a forum that can simplify communications to various audiences who need to hear about this work.

To illustrate in more detail how these future technologies might be able to help someone struggling with addiction, facilitators created several scenarios, two of which are presented below. They are based on the ideas generated by the participants in the meeting.

At the beginning of this chapter, we met Maria, a heroin addict who had happened by a public health booth that had a "virtual" counselor named Selene who talked with her about getting help. Here is the rest of Maria's story.

---

[4] Gustafson D., Hawkins R., Pingree S., et al. Effect of computer support on younger women with breast cancer. J Gen Intern Med 2001b; 16:435–445.
[5] Pingree S., Hawkins R., Gustafson D., et al. Can the disadvantaged ride the information highway? J of Broadcasting and Electronic Media 1996; 40:331–353.

Virtual Counselor Helps Young Woman Fight Heroin Addiction

At first Maria is not interested in talking to "Selene." But the next week Maria is stealing from family members to support her habit. She begins thinking about how far she has fallen. These are people she loves and she is violating their trust. Remembering the woman on the screen who claimed to be a former addict, Maria goes back to the booth looking for her. When she enters the booth, there are lots of characters on the screen – young and old, male and female and people of different races. Maria touches the image of a young woman, whose image suddenly fills the screen and greets her.

Selene is easy to talk to, and treats Maria with dignity and respect. Maria likes her and answers all her questions (some are just friendly getting-to-know-you, and others are more medically-oriented). The interaction is brief – perhaps 30 minutes. Before it ends Selene asks if Maria will come back to see her tomorrow. Maria agrees and they say goodbye.

Several weeks later Maria has visited Selene many times and discussed her heroin use and all the treatments she has tried. Maria is still using heroin but less than before. Selene has asked Maria permission to develop an online record of these interactions. On this day, she asks Maria for permission to give her an ID bracelet that can provide this information to any licensed treatment center she visits. Selene provides Maria with a list of local licensed treatment centers that provide care focused on her issues and background. The bracelet can be given out by any staff person – it does not require a physician to dispense and she doesn't have to have an appointment. Maria accepts the offer and picks up the bracelet at a local treatment center.

The bracelet brings up a web page immediately with all of Maria's treatment and medical history that treatment center professionals can access. It also contains sensors specific to her drug addiction and emotional history. These sensors watch for patterns between Maria's behaviors, stress, strong feelings, and drug use. The bracelet wirelessly transmits the sensor information to an Internet-based system that uses sophisticated analysis tools to detect patterns and suggest interventions. The suggested interventions are sent to a team of experts.

The team culls the computer's suggestions, and combines them with their theories and experiences, as well as with the computer's latest data about locally available resources to suggest appropriate interventions. These experts make recommendations about how to begin Maria's treatment. Then they feed the computer their plan, specifying parameters that would trigger calls to human experts. The computer could provide support in some areas, such as cognitive behavioral therapy, but would need to seek human professionals when it detected that the patient was in more distress than the computer was programmed to respond to. For example, if the computer detected that 60% of a patient's words reflected sadness it would send that information to a central resource, which would contact a professional to get in touch with the patient for further assistance.

Selene passes this treatment intervention plan to Maria but she is not ready to start yet. Meanwhile, Maria visits Selene regularly. She likes that she doesn't have to make an appointment and can stop in whenever she feels she needs to talk. Selene is sometimes kind of dumb; in fact, Selene jokes that she is more machine than human, and that she doesn't understand everything Maria says. Maria knows Selene is a software agent, not a human, and she knows sometimes there is a real person behind Selene but she still likes her, and finds some of her quirks endearing. The person behind Selene is a substance abuse counselor who acts as a backup for Selene.

In one visit, Selene detects signs of trust from Maria's answers. Selene has kept track of Maria's answers to her questions over time. Heroin addicts are notorious at lying and misleading people and Maria has done this to Selene. But lately Selene has detected a consistency in her answers that would be unlikely if Maria were lying to her. Because Selene has detected these signs of trust, she asks whether Maria has a cell phone. Maria does, and because she feels Selene cares about her and can be trusted, Maria shares her number with Selene. Selene asks how Maria would feel if she were to call her sometimes when Selene detects through the sensors that she is about to use heroin. Maria says that would be great. She is still trying unsuccessfully to quit even though her use has decreased somewhat since meeting Selene.

The next day, Maria's boyfriend dumps her. She is so stressed she heads immediately for something to kill the pain. Just across the street from her dealer, her phone rings. It is Selene who asks Maria if she's okay. The sensor in Maria's bracelet has alerted Selene that she is approaching a location where she has gotten drugs in the past. Maria breaks down crying. Selene says some comforting words to try to help Maria regulate her feelings. But Maria is still inconsolable. Selene's program tells her that she cannot provide the help that Maria needs right now. She asks Maria if she would be willing to talk to one of the women behind Selene. Maria says yes, and then hears a new voice (a hotline worker). Introducing herself as a "part of Selene," the hotline worker listens to what has happened to Maria and is empathetic. She learns Maria is about to buy drugs, and gets her to promise to head in the other direction. The worker encourages her by telling her that this is an opportunity to test some of the things she has learned through her conversations with Selene. Maria walks away without buying drugs. While Maria avoided using heroin that day she is still unwilling to enter treatment.

The turning point came on the worst day of Maria's life. Her beautiful 5-year-old daughter had been in and out of foster care as Maria struggled with addiction. Maria always thought she would get Lily back permanently someday. But that day the court had begun action to terminate Maria's parental rights. The only way Maria has a chance to see Lily again is to enter a treatment program immediately and remain clean for a year.

Maria asks Selene about starting treatment. Selene tells her about a program that will take her in and help her get off heroin for good. Maria enters the program and makes real progress in overcoming her addiction. In the program, she undergoes simulations of great stress and the strongest triggers she has ever experienced to use heroin. Some of these included unusual new technologies that put her in virtual spaces with people who looked just like those who caused her trouble. Many times these simulations drove her to extreme responses such as losing her temper and having panic attacks that had often preceded her drug use. Through repeated exposure, she started to respond better, and as a result, became more confident. She had relived all the old patterns that triggered her drive to take drugs, but this time without the drugs.

When Maria graduates, Selene calls to congratulate her. Maria knows that the real work begins now. She does well on her own for months with a new job and a new place to live. Then she is assigned a new work supervisor who makes her life miserable. She feels an escalation of frustration and stress. Because Maria is still wearing her bracelet, Selene notices and calls her. Maria hasn't heard from Selene in months. It is so great to talk to her even if she is just a machine. Selene suggests some things that Maria had forgotten but says she is going to try. Maria is able to regulate her feelings using some of these skills she had learned before. She just needed the reminder and the encouragement. Selene continues to check in when the sensors alert her that Maria is having a crisis.

Maria has been off drugs for a year now. She hears from Selene every now and then. It has been one of the hardest years of her life. Maria doesn't know if she might relapse in the future but she does know it is okay to call Selene anytime – night or day. Unlike calling some of the human workers at the rehab center, Maria never feels like she is disturbing Selene. Selene reminds Maria regularly of skills and responses she can use at this phase, which reinforces what she learned earlier and continues to give her hope for recovery and a better life.

A Lifelong Intervention for a Man Predisposed to Alcoholism

They knew they could be headed for trouble. When John was born, his parents worried because alcoholism ran in the family. At his birth, his physician offered John's parents an opportunity for a genetic test to see if their son had the alcoholism predisposition gene. A genetics counselor explained there was an Internet site to help them decide whether or not to have John tested. The counselor showed the parents how to access the site directly from their cell phone. The site contained a persuasive video played on the cell phone screen that explained the essence of genetics and the testing process. Because the test would be administered and analyzed by the parents through the use of a secure Internet they did not need to worry about confidentiality being compromised. The computer linked to their cell phone also helped them plan for what action they could take if the test was positive – and it was.

Genetic therapy was an option, but a still controversial one. Genetic therapy would modify John's genes so that he was no longer predisposed to alcoholism. But the therapy was still new and carried risks of modifying other genes that could cause John problems. The same computer program helped John's parents understand that option, and decide whether or not to proceed given the therapy's still-uncertain effectiveness. The program also helped them realize that, with care, there was good reason to believe that alcoholism could be prevented. The parents decided against genetic therapy and the genetics counselor introduced them to a virtual counselor ("Jennie") who offered to contact them annually to help them assess John's situation. Jennie counselor offered to work with them on prevention strategies that had been proven effective in children with similar backgrounds. Jennie also pointed out that extensive research on alcohol and alcoholism was underway. She offered them an opportunity via computer to access the latest research results whenever they were interested, and to do so with a translator that would help them understand the results and implications in layperson's terms. In fact, Jennie tailored the translator so that it would only point out research that was relevant to John's situation. She also noted that the tailoring would change to match John's growth and development.

By age ten, John was beginning to manifest some signs suggesting emotional distress. His father had died in an automobile accident the year before and John had become withdrawn. His school performance was declining, and he began to reject his friends. Jennie and John's mom had been interacting about this problem for several months. Using a computerized diagnostic program called the problem knowledge coupler the results strongly suggested that John was suffering from clinical depression. The coupler was able to draw upon the universal medical record that had been tracking John's life for the last ten years. Years earlier, the parents had given a release for this device to access and track John's records. The computer helped Jennie and John's mother examine different options for treating the depression and matched John's characteristics to a particular treatment plan.

John's mom was happy to learn that a program on the home computer could provide effective cognitive behavior therapy in a game format appealing for a child his age. He would not have to see a psychiatrist or behavioral health professional. Moreover, his emotional condition could be tracked by having John wear a sensor on his skin. The senor relayed the information over the Internet to the medical record. The resulting analyses allowed Jennie and John's mom to determine the events that tended to pull John down emotionally, as well as those that lifted him up. Jennie was always available to help John's mom understand the treatment and John's progress throughout it. John seemed to regain and maintain his emotional balance. Things were looking much better.

During his adolescence, John hit his stride. He was a star soccer player and took great pride in his physical conditioning. He did not want to use alcohol and risk getting impaired, especially when he was driving. The memory of his father's fatal car accident at the hands of a drunk driver was still fresh. He had developed his own relationship with Jennie whom he had begun to trust. Jennie checked in every few months through e-mail. At times he would initiate more of a personal contact using the video chat room function on his cell phone.

Life continued well for John until the war. By this time, John had graduated from the Air Force Academy, and had distinguished himself as a skilled pilot of a newly-designed helicopter. During the war, John's helicopter was shot down. Captured and imprisoned for two years, he was tortured unmercifully. While he was eventually freed, the experience left an indelible mark on a man who once held so much promise.

His mother had died while he was in prison and he had no other relatives. "Jennie" had contacted him via e-mail on several occasions to check in and had encouraged him to get help for the severe post-traumatic stress disorder he was experiencing. However in John's view, his help lay in alcohol. Before long, John was living on the streets of New Orleans and drinking himself into oblivion.

One day he was arrested and jailed for breaking into a liquor store. Since this was his first offense, he was sent to drug court. The judge gave John three choices. He could spend six months in jail followed by a two-year relationship with a parole agent. He could be placed under six months of house arrest, and wear a Global Positioning System (GPS) bracelet around his ankle followed by a two-year probation. His final option was to have a chip inserted into his arm that had a GPS as well as a sensor that would assess his emotional condition and would report any use of alcohol to a treatment facility with ties to his probation officer. He would not be under house arrest, but he would need to agree to satisfactorily complete a two-year program of study at a virtual university for drug and alcohol addicts. The program was designed to help recovering addicts and alcoholics learn more about alcoholism, its causes, treatments and practice ways to avoid alcohol abuse. If he were successful and had no further run-ins with the law, his arrest record would be erased. Even though the judge warned him that this would be a highly interventional option, John chose option three.

John was surprised to find the university experience was centered on a smart phone and a pair of glasses. With the glasses, he could look at his smart phone, a much more sophisticated cell phone of today, and see a computer screen the size of a 17-inch LCD monitor The glasses and the smart phone meant he could access the university from any location. The university was flexible. John found that it offered learning experiences in all aspects of life. He learned how to search for a job, how to manage his money, how to interact with people and more.

There were many other helpful services. John found that he could get short answers to hundreds of frequently asked questions about addiction and other issues concerning him at the moment, read hundreds of articles (many of which were translations of scientific studies), talk anonymously with a support group of recovering alcoholics, ask questions of experts, think through key decisions he was facing, plan changes in his life, learn how to relate to others and receive virtual psychotherapy via the computer.

But the most impressive aspect was how sophisticated the computer was. First, it was able to read that chip in his arm so it knew how he was doing emotionally by tracking his anxiety level. And it tailored the information it provided so that it responded to how John was feeling that day. For instance, on bad days the computer might suggest that John start by doing some mindfulness exercises to calm himself before he tried to practice any new skills. Second, when he would learn a skill, he would practice it in a virtual reality. For instance, one time he practiced ways of resisting offers to drink. The experience was so real. He honestly felt like he was right there at a cocktail party. His responses prompted the computer to take him in different directions. It taught him how to gracefully decline such an invitation (either to the party in the first place or to have a drink). It also showed him how to fake a drink by adding olives to a soft drink to appear to be drinking a martini. John was interested in how the computer seemed to know him so well. The computer told him that the program used something called "persuasion technology" where it monitored his emotional status and immediately sent messages on the smart phone that, for him, had a powerful influence.

The support groups were also helpful. Any time he needed to talk with someone, they were there online. And it was not the same group every time. Depending on his needs, the computer recruited a different set of people to help. One day it might be a group of recovering alcoholics; another day it might be two Buddhist monks who helped him deal with his stress and his spiritual journey. All of these were real people who had some background or expertise to help John. These sessions could be formed on the fly to respond to issues he struggled with right then.

Of course, things were not always easy. John had gotten a job as a private helicopter pilot for wealthy and demanding clients. One day, one of his clients screamed at him in a way that brought him flashbacks to his captors in prison. John was shaken. At the end of that day, John was driving home, and approached a part of town where he used to have a lot of drinking buddies. He longed to see them again and decided to "just drive by" the bar where they hung out. As he turned the corner to the bar, his smart phone rang. It was his virtual counselor (Jennie) whom he had not heard from in several months. She said that information from his chip indicated he was having a rough day and the GPS system suggested he was driving toward danger. The computer was programmed to recognize parts of town where he was not permitted to go. She cautioned him to turn around. He didn't. He drove by the bar and recognized cars of two old friends. He drove by another time and another.

Finally, he pulled into the parking lot. As he did so, he received a call from his probation officer reminding him of the risk he was about to engage in. On the line also was his girlfriend begging him to not go in. Finally, the navigation system in the car (which had access to soothing technologies) started a set of relaxation interventions such as soft music and an offer to go through a guided meditation that helped him calm himself. He drove away and as he did so, Jennie called again to congratulate him. She mentioned that if he had gone in, he would not have been able to start the car when he came out.

John was drained. Sometimes the urge to drink felt overwhelming. He was humiliated that he had let this client get to him and he was a little frightened that it seemed so easy to send him to close to drinking again. The experience brought back the fears and vulnerability he had while in captivity. He felt weak and helpless.

The next day, John received a call from his probation officer who pointed out how close he had come to serious consequences. The officer also told John that a recently-developed medication was available. The medication required only one annual injection. The long-acting injected drug would make John sick if he drank alcohol. It would be activated by a device called a "bot," a tiny sensor injected into his blood stream. John thought about it for a few days, and decided it might be good to do.

The two years passed quickly. John was succeeding. He had a job, a wife, and a set of resources that could help him for the rest of his life. Because he had completed the requirements of the virtual university for drug and alcohol addicts, the record of his conviction had been erased. While he could have removed the chip at that time, he decided that life was too precious to take that chance.

The meeting detailed above was just the beginning. This is an initiative to fundamentally improve the process of caring for patients and their caregivers. Technology exists today that can help addiction. Developments now on the horizon can help even more. Rather than struggling to play catch-up as inventions surface on the market, the facilitators' goal was to collaborate with the inventors to develop feasible ideas that could shape the treatment world of the 21st century. The meeting also demonstrated an exciting approach to creatively envision a new way of providing health care. Facilitators chose experts who knew nothing about addictions because they wanted the panelists to look at the system with fresh eyes. To help these experts understand some of the issues facing people seeking treatment, facilitators brought in consumers rather than providers. This enabled the focus to be truly on the customers rather than the treatment system. Facilitators also used techniques that would support the experts in thinking creatively. They provided exercises to help them move from conventional thinking and challenged them to deal with unreasonable constraints—such as designing a system that included no human beings as treatment professionals. They did not want the participants to fall back on easy solutions. The meeting facilitators also used stories as a way to communicate. Stories and skits are helpful because they force people to test and reflect on the consistency and flow of ideas. Seeing them told or acted out makes it clear what is unclear and needs to be clarified or adapted.

5. Further Analysis

After the meeting was concluded facilitators integrated all 268 ideas into groups of ideas that relate to one another. The technology used in the scenarios will be further analyzed and enhanced to understand which aspects can be used today and which will require more basic research and development. A second meeting is being planned to focus on how the "future" can meet the present. While the earlier panel was composed primarily of visionary technologists the next one will include visionary addiction treatment providers, technologists and people from other fields (e.g. ethics, spirituality and other payers of healthcare). The goal will be to move these visionary concepts closer to real application.

Acknowledgements

The authors gratefully acknowledge the members of the meeting for their input, advices and consultation.

Long Life Era –
Extending Human Life-Span and
Future of Caring for Elders

A Strategy for Postponing Aging Indefinitely

Aubrey DE GREY, Ph.D.
Department of Genetics, University of Cambridge, Cambridge, UK

Abstract. It may seem premature to be discussing approaches to the effective elimination of human aging as a cause of death at a time when essentially no progress has yet been made in even postponing it. However, two aspects of human aging combine to undermine this assessment. The first is that aging is happening to us throughout our lives but only results in appreciable functional decline after four or more decades of life: this shows that we can postpone aging arbitrarily well without knowing how to prevent it completely. The second is that the typical rate of refinement of dramatic technological breakthroughs is rather reliable (so long as public enthusiasm for them is abundant) and is fast enough to change such technologies (be they in medicine, transport, or computing) almost beyond recognition within a natural human lifespan. Here I explain, first, why it is reasonable to expect that (presuming adequate funding for the initial preclinical work) therapies that can add 30 healthy years to the remaining lifespan of healthy 55-year-olds will arrive within the next few decades, and, second, why those who benefit from those therapies will very probably continue to benefit from progressively improved therapies indefinitely and thus avoid debilitation or death from age-related causes at any age.

1. Introduction

The approach to postponing aging that I shall describe in this essay is one of maintenance and repair. Those who like to claim that aging is intrinsically immutable are often inclined to start by asserting, ex cathedra, that living organisms are qualitatively unlike machines and therefore cannot be maintained beyond their "warranty period" in the way that typical machines can. Even leaving aside the absence of any justification of the "therefore" in that assertion, there is a conspicuous fragility in the idea that organisms (even humans) are in any relevant way unlike machines. The property of living organisms that is most often suggested as distinguishing them from machines is their capacity for self-repair, and indeed that is undoubtedly something at which organisms are vastly superior to any machine currently in existence. But to consider it a qualitative difference is clearly incorrect: as a simple example one need only consider household robots that plug themselves into the mains when their batteries run low, or photocopiers that suspend operation to clean their wires when they automatically detect the need.

The pessimist often retorts that, even if this is not a qualitative difference, the difference of degree is so astronomical that the practical feasibility of maintaining an organism as one does a machine is far too distant to be worth considering. But here again we see a crass logical error, because the idea is to *augment* our natural maintenance systems: thus, the fact that they are so good already means that there is that much *less* for us to do to make them good enough to work indefinitely. There is much more to this question, as will emerge below, but the crux of the argument is as just stated.

In the next section I will describe in rather abstract terms the sort of maintenance that I believe we should be working towards in the quest to postpone aging as much as possible as soon as possible. In the following section I will go into more concrete biological detail, giving an overview of the specific types of maintenance and repair that humans need to do better in order to maintain our health and youth for a lot longer and the methods already under development to implement those required improvements. The concrete and detailed nature of those prospective interventions leads me to the view that we are potentially within only a decade of developing them all in laboratory mice, and that once we have done so we have perhaps a 50% chance of developing them in humans within only 15 years thereafter. Then, in the final section I will explain why this should be enough to put us beyond "life extension escape velocity" – the point at which we are improving these technologies faster than the remaining imperfections in them are catching up with us. Once we reach that point, and presuming we can stay there (which, I will argue, is virtually certain), no one need die of old age ever again, whatever age they attain.

2. The Lag Phase of Aging: Our Window of Opportunity

What is aging, actually? It is often suggested that aging is very hard to define. That is true if one requires a definition that suits all purposes, but when discussing interventions an altogether uncontroversial definition is easily found. A typical one is as follows:

> Aging is the set of side-effects of metabolism that alter the composition of our bodies over time to make it progressively less capable of self-maintenance and thereby, eventually, less functional.

This definition allows us to identify three very distinct strategies for postponing aging and thereby extending healthy and total lifespan. Curiously (at least in retrospect), only two of them have historically been pursued. They are depicted in Fig. 1, in which the flat-headed arrows are used in the conventional genetics sense to mean "inhibits".

Putting Fig. 1 into words: the gerontology approach is pre-emptive, seeking to diminish the side-effects of metabolism mentioned above and thereby to slow down the rate at which metabolism changes the composition of our bodies, whereas the geriatrics approach is reactive, seeking to delay the functional decline (i.e., pathology) that those changes in composition cause. The changes in composition themselves, in Fig. 1, are simply denoted by the term "damage": they are no more nor less than the accumulation of that damage. It is important to stress that I will use the term "damage" in this very precise sense throughout this essay: for present purposes it is defined as the entire set of changes of bodily composition that (a) are side-effects of metabolism and (b) are eventually pathogenic. In particular, the reader should not infer any implication concerning how this damage is laid down, such as whether it could reasonably be called "wear and tear".

What is the prognosis for the gerontology and geriatrics approaches, in the foreseeable future? It is easy to see that the geriatrics approach is short-termist almost by definition: as damage accumulates, its natural pathological consequences become progressively harder to avert. Besides, even if we could in principle develop geriatric medicine so sophisticated that pathology was slowed, that would be a somewhat mixed blessing, as it would constitute an extension of the frail period of life.

The gerontology approach initially seems much more promising. If one can retard the rate at which metabolism lays down damage in the first place, one will certainly extend the healthy part of life, which would seem unambiguously desirable. (Possibly the frail part would be extended too, but probably less so.) However, it has two daunting shortcomings.

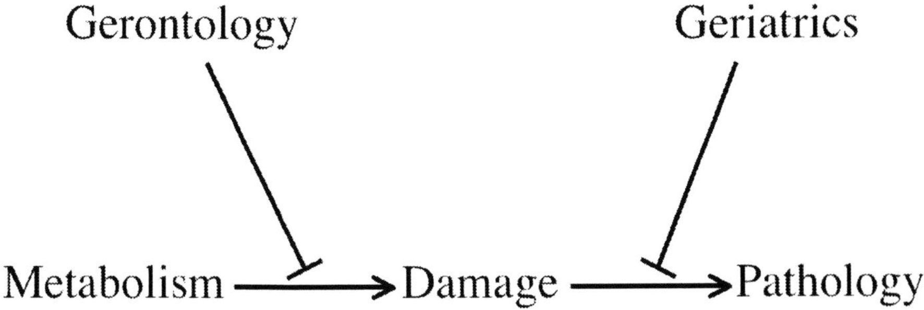

Figure 1. The two traditional approaches to postponing aging.

Firstly, damage that has already been laid down before the treatment begins will not be affected: hence, those who already have enough of it to be starting to suffer functional decline will not have that loss of function restored by such therapies. Secondly, the practicality of the gerontology approach is determined by the extent to which we understand metabolism, because altering the workings of a system that we understand only very poorly tends either to have no effect at all on its behaviour or to do more harm than good. And unfortunately, that is the case with metabolism: though we certainly understand far more about it than we did only a few decades ago, we are regularly reminded by the discoveries of fundamental new aspects of metabolism (such as RNA interference, discovered only a few years ago [1]) that in reality we have still hardly scratched the surface of its complexity. This bleak conclusion is reinforced by the failure of the rational but evidently over simplistic approaches to extending mammalian lifespan that gerontologists have attempted over the past 50 years: it remains the case that, apart from a scattering of reports that were never reliably reproduced, the only way to extend mammalian lifespan is to elicit a response that metabolism already has available to it, namely the intensification of repair and maintenance that results from moderate deprivation of nutrients [2]. (This is no longer the only way to elicit that response – genetic manipulation has done it too [3,4] – but it is still essentially the same response.)

If we wish to postpone aging any time soon, therefore, it seems clear that we must seek a third way – something radically different from the gerontology and geriatrics approaches. Just such an approach has been the focus of my work since 2000 and has become known as "Strategies for Engineered Negligible Senescence" or SENS [5,6]. It can best be explained by embellishing Fig. 1, as shown in Fig. 2.

The key feature of the SENS approach is that it intervenes early enough to avoid being a "losing battle" like the geriatrics approach, but at the same time it does not attempt to improve the already indescribably complex and well-honed machine that is our metabolism, but rather to clean up after it. In short, the SENS approach does not attempt to interfere in processes – neither the process whereby metabolism causes damage, nor that by which damage causes pathology. Rather, it seeks to remove the damage that metabolism lays down, at least as fast as it is laid down, and thereby to prevent it from ever translating into pathology at all.

The SENS approach relies on a frequently overlooked aspect of aging which is mentioned in the definition I gave earlier: that even though metabolism causes damage all the time, throughout our whole life, damage only *eventually* causes functional decline. If you live and eat essentially as your mother told you to, and if you are not particularly unlucky in terms of genetics, you will probably be able to run and think more or less as fast at the age of 40 as you could when you were 20. This tells us that there is a threshold level of damage

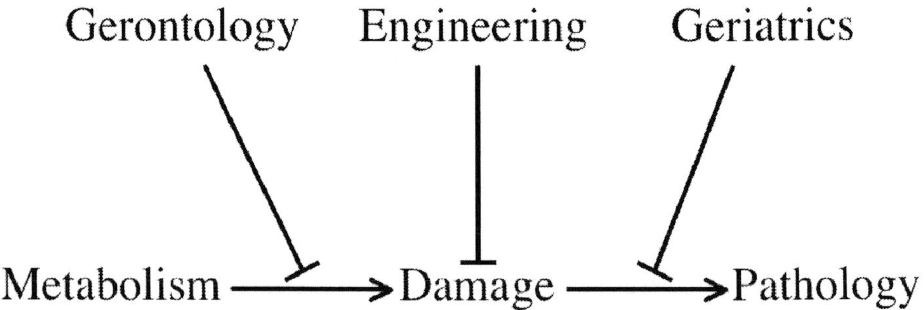

Figure 2. How the engineering (SENS) approach to postponing aging relates to the two traditional approaches.

beyond which trouble starts but below which metabolism copes without degradation of performance, rather as a roof carries on keeping the rain out if only a couple of isolated slates are dislodged, or as a car continues to work if it has acquired just the odd patch of rust. A machine is only as dependable as its weakest link, of course, so there may be a variety of types of damage, all of which must be kept below the threshold, but that does not alter the logic.

Perhaps the most obvious initial objection to the SENS approach, and certainly a common one heard from biogerontologists, is that it "must" be impossibly infeasible simply because it seeks to reverse age-related decline. The idea here is that reversing a process is intuitively far harder than slowing it down, and we have made precious little progress (even in mice, let alone humans) in slowing aging down. There are two main errors in this logic. The first is that reversing a process is only necessarily harder than retarding it if one restricts oneself to using the same methods for reversal as one would for retardation and doing them so well that the retardation outstrips the progression. In reality, there are other approaches to reversing a process that do not act in this "head-on" way. Consider the predicament of a person in a small rowing-boat in the centre of a large lake, which has sprung a leak. The person has two fundamentally different options for keeping afloat until rescue arrives: he can try to plug the leak, thereby retarding the rate at which water enters, or he can bail water over the side, counterbalancing the influx. The latter process constitutes a reversal of the accumulation of the problem, but by a method that (unlike forcing the water back through the hole!) is technologically no more challenging than plugging the leak.

The other error in the idea that reversal is inherently far harder than retardation is equally important. If one has few tools available, one may only be able to plug the leak rather imperfectly, so that some water continues to enter and one will prolong one's survival but not indefinitely. In the case of bailing, by contrast, a sufficient but finite rate of removal of water will suffice to keep one afloat for as long as may be required. This has especially profound implications in the longer term, as will be explained below.

3. From Boats to Biology: Is the Analogy Valid?

Analogies are all very well for showing that an idea makes sense in principle, but what about putting it into practice? In order to demonstrate that the SENS approach is truly foreseeable, it is necessary to describe in concrete terms what the "damage" is that SENS must repair, and also to propose specific biotechnological approaches to that repair for each type of such damage. Moreover, the proposed approaches must embody sufficient detail to give confidence that we can get there from here in a meaningfully predictable timeframe.

Table 1. The seven "deadly things": types of damage that SENS seeks to combat and the dates when they were first suggested by gerontologists to contribute to mammalian aging.

Type of age-related damage	Suggested by, in
Cell loss, cell atrophy	Brody, 1955 [7]
Senescent/toxic cells	Hayflick, 1965 [8]
Oncogenic nuclear mutations/epimutations	Szilard, 1959 [9]; Cutler, 1982 [10]
Mitochondrial mutations	Harman, 1972 [11]
Intracellular aggregates	Strehler, 1959 [12]
Extracellular aggregates	Alzheimer, 1907 [13]
Extracellular crosslinks	Monnier and Cerami, 1981 [14]

Without further ado, then, I offer in Table 1 what I claim is an adequately complete list of the types of side-effect of metabolism that can be considered to qualify as "damage" by the definition being employed in this essay – that is, changes that there is some reason to believe contribute to age-related pathologies of one sort or another. By "adequately complete" I mean that it includes all types of change in our molecular and cellular composition that may contribute to tissue dysfunction in a currently normal lifetime; I acknowledge that other types of such change, such as nuclear mutations that do not affect the cell cycle, may be pathogenic when we reach ages considerably exceeding our existing lifespan.

The suggestion that this list is indeed adequately complete is a bold one and is routinely challenged. However, there are two strong arguments for this contention. The first concerns the dates noted in the right-hand column, the most recent of which is 1982. The analytical sophistication available to biologists has advanced very considerably since then, so the fact that this list has not been extended as a result constitutes a strong circumstantial argument that no "eighth sin" will be discovered in the future either (except, as noted above, in those who reach ages that the seven problems listed above currently prevent anyone from attaining).

The second argument that the above is a complete list is perhaps more attractive to the biologist: it is that the list can be derived from first principles by examining our biology systematically. The starting-point for doing this is to note (a) that the list is of types of damage, not of processes that cause that damage (which would be a much longer one – indeed, one that certainly could not be confidently completed with current knowledge) and (b) that, by definition, damage can only accumulate in long-lived structures. Intracellular proteins, for example, vary somewhat in half-life but never survive for more than a small fraction of the human lifespan: thus, any deleterious modifications that they suffer are eliminated when they are destroyed. With these two points in mind, we can then ask: what are we made of? The first-level answer is: cells and stuff between cells. Cells of a given type can become more or less numerous with age: when this is deleterious we have the first two of the seven types of aging listed in Table 1. Within cells there are only two types of long-lived molecule – DNA (which of course is long-lived in an unusual way, because it is synthesised by replication) and garbage, i.e. indigestible substances that are sequestered indefinitely, usually in the lysosome. That accounts for items 3, 4 and 5 in Table 1. In the extracellular space, similarly, there are just two types of long-lived molecule: complex proteinaceous structures such as the lens of the eye and the artery wall that can become chemically and thus physically modified over time (item 7), and garbage, again of different composition in different tissues but collectively termed amyloid (item 6).

So far, so good: we have a satisfactorily complete description of the problem. What about solutions? Table 2 summarises the current state of play as I see it.

The first point to emphasise about Table 2 is that, of the seven therapies listed, two are not strictly *repair* strategies (reversing the accumulation of the specified type of damage) but rather *obviation* strategies that make the phenomenon no longer capable of causing pa-

Table 2. Foreseeable approaches to repair or obviation of the seven types of damage listed in Table 1.

Type of damage	Proposed repair (or obviation)
Cell loss, cell atrophy	Stem cells, growth factors, exercise [15]
Senescent/toxic cells	Ablation of unwanted cells [16]
Oncogenic nuclear mutations/epimutations	"WILT" (Whole-body Interdiction of Lengthening of Telomeres) [17,18]
Mitochondrial mutations	Allotopic expression of 13 proteins [19]
Intracellular aggregates	Microbial hydrolases [20,21]
Extracellular aggregates	Immune-mediated phagocytosis [22]
Extracellular crosslinks	AGE-breaking molecules [23]

thology, and thus make it cease to classify as "damage". These are items 3 and 4 in the list, addressing nuclear and mitochondrial mutations respectively. For nuclear mutations, the proposal is a treatment for cancer that does not stop cells from accumulating the mutations that allow them to divide uncontrollably, but instead gives them a time-bomb – telomere shortening – which they cannot defuse even by the hypermutation that makes cancers so versatile in eluding all contemporary therapies. For mitochondrial mutations the suggested strategy is to make such mutations harmless by allotopic expression – introducing copies of the 13 protein-coding genes of the mitochondrial DNA into the nucleus, with modifications such that they will still encode the correct amino acid sequence when translated on cytosolic ribosomes and will then be targeted to and imported into mitochondria by the pathway already employed by the thousand-odd naturally nuclear-coded mitochondrial proteins. These proteins would maintain mitochondrial function in the presence of any mitochondrial mutation.

How far away are the therapies listed in Table 2? In order to answer that question one must ask it somewhat more precisely, by specifying two additional things: how well the therapies must work, and in what organism. Here we encounter an slightly paradoxical pair of comparisons: initial, relatively modest progress will certainly occur sooner in shorter-lived mammals (specifically mice) than in the relatively long-lived human, but longer-term and more dramatic advances will occur in humans first – indeed, they will quite probably never occur in mice. The latter will be the topic of the next section; in this section we consider more modest, more near-term advances.

There are two main reasons why the first substantial steps in extending healthy lifespan with late-onset interventions will occur in mice sooner than in humans: firstly there is the biological reality that organisms with longer lifespans are already avoiding aging rather well and thus are harder to improve by copying ideas (genes, in particular) from even longer-lived species, and secondly there is the sociological reason that society mostly considers the deaths of rather large numbers of mice in the quest to perfect a therapy to be much more acceptable than the death of even one human in that quest. Neither is likely to change any time soon, so we first address the extension of mouse lifespan.

As noted, we must also specify a degree of progress that can be considered an appropriate milestone. The one that I have championed in recent years, with the moniker "Robust Mouse Rejuvenation" (RMR) [24], is to treble the remaining average lifespan of a cohort of naturally long-lived mice that are already 2/3 through their natural lifespan before any intervention (whether genetic, pharmacological or dietary) is begun. Long-lived mouse strains typically live to three years of age on average, so this means initiative a protocol on such mice at the age of two years and giving them an average age at death of five years.

So to the timeframe for interventions. The last two items in Table 2 are the ones in which we are furthest advanced at present. In 1996, a small molecule was revealed which restored elasticity of rat tail tendons to a remarkable degree [25]; subsequent work from the same group has demonstrated the restoration of youthful elasticity in a biomedically more significant tissue, the artery wall [23]. Likewise, in 1999, a mouse model of Alzheimer's disease was shown to exhibit a dramatic reversal of the accumulation of senile plaques, the main extracellular feature of the disease, in response to vaccination against their major constituent, the Abeta peptide [22]. Both these discoveries are only the start in developing comprehensive reversal of their respective "sins", but they are both promising enough to have progressed in only a few years to clinical trials. In both cases the main work remaining to be done in mice is to apply the same principles to other major types of (respectively) crosslink and amyloid than the ones which these pioneering therapies address, but in fact it may transpire that these initial treatments, though currently restricted to one category of crosslink and one amyloid-accumulating tissue, will address a sufficient proportion of their respective categories of damage to deliver RMR (so long, of course, as the therapies for the other five classes of damage are also up to scratch).

Compensation for cell loss is also going rather well. Many tissues that lose cells during normal aging or in the context of disease are the subject of intensive research into cell replacement using growth factors or stem cell therapy, some of which has also reached the clinic [26–28]. This work lags behind the two SENS strands just discussed only insofar as the differences between therapies for different tissues are probably more challenging, relying as they currently do (at least in the case of stem cell therapies) on rather precise ex vivo "pre-differentiation" of initially over-versatile stem cells that are otherwise prone to develop not only into the desired cell type but also into a variety of unwanted ones.

Elimination of supernumerary cells in rodents varies greatly in difficulty depending on the type of cell to be eliminated. The simplest is visceral fat, which can be surgically removed from the abdominal cavity of rats and results in the abrupt alleviation of previously advanced diabetes [16]. Potentially there is also the possibility of converting the cells in question to a benign form, but no systematic method to identify such an intervention is yet evident. There are two attractive options that do qualify as "rationally designed", however, both exploiting the identifiability of the problematic cells by their excessive expression of particular genes. In the first method, "suicide" genes [29] are introduced by somatic gene therapy: these typically enter cells of many cell types, but the gene is placed under the promoter of the excessively-expressed gene so that it is only expressed in the cells that one wishes to eliminate. In the second approach, the undesired cells are removed by the immune system as a result of stimulation by appropriate vaccines and adjuvants [30]. However, none of these strategies has yet reached the clinical trial stage.

The remaining three SENS strands may be considered the "critical path" towards RMR, as they are all some way from implementation even in mice. Allotopic expression of the mitochondrial proteins from nuclear transgenes may be closer than it seems in vitro, as recent work gives considerable confidence that the only remaining requirement is to identify amino acid changes to these proteins' transmembrane domains which makes them a little less hydrophobic and thus more readily importable by the mitochondrial protein import apparatus [19,31]. The remaining issue for RMR in regard to mitochondrial mutations is delivery of these genes to affected cells, and the current state of somatic gene therapy in mice is such that this may be only moderately challenging, especially in view of the fact that introduction of these genes into mitochondrially healthy cells should be harmless.

The runner-up in the difficulty stakes for RMR is probably the removal of intracellular aggregates. Indigestible material progressively impairs cell function, not least by impairing the degradation of other substances that the cell was hitherto able to process efficiently. An approach to this problem that I introduced in 2002 [20] and which has since enjoyed increasing interest [21] is to identify microbial enzymes that can break down such compounds (or convert them to ones that mammalian metabolism already handles). Exploration of the microbial ecology of contaminated environments has proven so extraordinarily successful in bioremediation that there is widespread optimism for the corresponding strategy in respect of material that accumulates in the environment of our bodies. However, the challenges that will arise in the later stages of implementing such a therapy – such as the avoidance of toxicity, the retention of function in the mammalian cell and the management of any immune response – mean that "lysosomal enhancement" is realistically up to a decade away even in mice.

Finally we come to nuclear mutations, and specifically those which promote cancer. The energy with which cancer has been fought by the biomedical research community over recent decades, especially since Nixon's initiation of the "War on Cancer" in 1971, is matched only by that effort's lack of success in coming close to the rate of progress predicted by many leading cancer specialists at that time. This sobering reality led me to introduce recently [17,18] a proposed anti-cancer strategy, termed WILT (Whole-body Interdiction of Lengthening of Telomeres) that is as ambitious as it is audacious: the use of both ex vivo and somatic gene therapy to delete the genes for telomerase and (as and when they are identified) ALT (Alternative Lengthening of Telomeres) from as many of our cells as possible. This will have deleterious side effects that are obvious and daunting: telomere shortening will irresistibly eliminate the stem cell pools that maintain all our continually-renewing tissues, such as the blood, the gut and the skin. My proposal is to avert these consequences by periodic replenishment of our stem cell pools with new cells that also lack genes for telomere elongation but have had their telomeres extended ex vivo to normal lengths with exogenous telomerase. This is a decidedly tall order, and is only even worthy of contemplation because it appears that the frequency of such replenishment may not need to exceed once a decade in humans. However, WILT is for many reasons exceptionally difficult to test in mice and may thus need to be developed in less convenient species. It is this, above all, that makes it the hardest SENS strand to develop. In a sense this could be argued to be irrelevant to RMR, because many of the anti-cancer therapies that have had such modest success in humans actually work extremely well in mice, quite possibly well enough to achieve the RMR milestone. However, ultimately the purpose of working towards RMR is to achieve the corresponding advance in humans thereafter, so there is a certain inadequacy in that line of reasoning.

4. Escape Velocity: When Humans Become Easier than Mice

Once RMR is achieved, I am convinced that society's attitude to the postponement of human aging will become unrecognisable. I have therefore predicted that there is a 50% chance of our achieving a comparable advance in human life extension within 15 years after we achieve RMR. This human milestone, which I rather unimaginatively term "Robust Human Rejuvenation" or RHR, is not in my formulation precisely proportional to RMR: rather than a trebling of the remaining lifespan of people who are already 2/3 of the way to the prevailing average age at death, I define it as only a doubling. This means roughly 25–30 years of extra healthy life for people who are perhaps 55 when treatment begins.

Why have I chosen a relatively toned-down version of RMR to define as RHR? Simply, because 25–30 years is a familiar duration in the history of technology, and specifically in that part of the history of many technologies which, in respect of life extension, I will now discuss. How long does it take, following some fundamental technological breakthrough, for that technology to progress by incremental refinements to a stage beyond that which the architects of the original breakthrough could reasonably have contemplated? The answer seems rather reliably to be in the 20–30 year range. Lindbergh flew the Atlantic 24 years after the Wright brothers' first flight. Commercial jetliners first flew 22 years after that, and supersonic airliners 20 years after that. In computing, the personal computer arrived about 28 years after the first electronic computer and the first convenient laptops arrived about

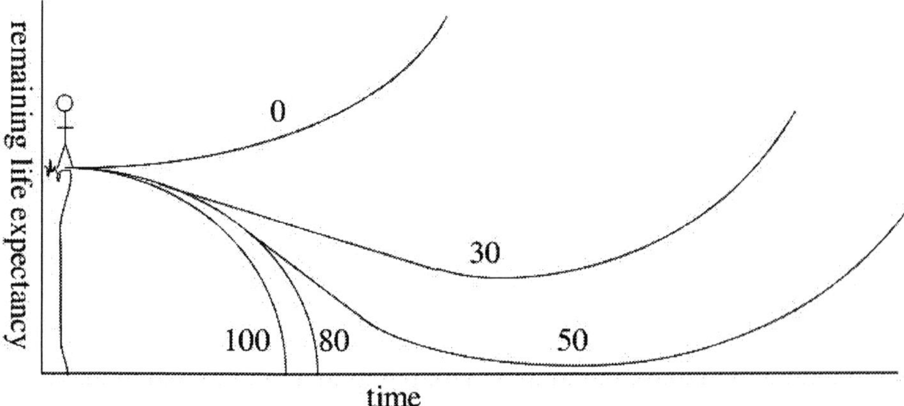

Figure 3. Plausible trajectories of "biological age" for typical individuals of the specified ages at the time RHR arrives, presuming access to the best therapies at any time.

20 years later. In medicine, the discovery of antibiotics followed the publicising of the germ theory by about 30 years and was in turn followed, after another 25 years, by the development of methods to manufacture vaccines specific for a particular disease.

The implications of this pattern for the lives of people who are in middle age or younger at the time that RHR is achieved is clear, but no less dramatic for that. Put simply, there is a very high probability that the 25–30 years of good health conferred on its recipients by the first-generation panel of rejuvenation therapies (defined as those which achieve RHR) will suffice for the development of much more thorough and comprehensive therapies, capable of delivering more like a century of extra life to those who are in relatively good health at the time those therapies arrive. This is where the longevity escape velocity (LEV) concept [24] arises. The recipients of the *first*-generation therapies – the ones that gave only around 30 years of extra healthy life – will, at least if sociopolitical pressures do not intervene, mostly *also* be among the beneficiaries of the *second*-generation ones, since they will be in the same degree of health at that time as they were when the first-generation therapies arrived. The same logic of course applies indefinitely into the future, just so long as the rate of progress in improving the comprehensiveness of the therapies continues to outstrip the rate at which the remaining imperfections in those therapies allow the accumulation of eventually pathogenic damage. It should now be clear why the correspondingly dramatic extension of mouse lifespan may in fact be much harder than for humans (indeed, maybe impossible) – since mice age so fast, new age-related problems will kill mice rather soon after they are discovered, too quickly for those problems to be addressed by scientific advances.

What does this add up to for lifespan? Clearly the life spans of those who live their entire lives in a period when progress is faster than LEV will be indefinite, since a given individual's risk of death at any adult age will be less than at earlier adult ages. What is less immediately clear is how to estimate the life spans of those already alive (and at various ages) at the time RHR arrives. My estimates are depicted (for actual numbers are too speculative to estimate) in Fig. 3. To summarise: I estimate that 50-year-olds who are in average health at the arrival of RHR and who are, thereafter, able to benefit from the latest and best rejuvenation therapies, will have at least a 50/50 chance of reaching their own personal escape velocity – that is, of being restored to a truly youthful state with a very low mortality risk. Most of those who are only 30 at that time will never reach a state of age-related frailty. Moreover, elite individuals – those who would naturally live to 100 or more even in the absence of these therapies – will have that 50/50 chance even if they are already in their 70's when RHR arrives.

A key corollary of the above considerations is that there will be a stunningly sharp "cusp" in the increase in life spans of those born in successive years. One way to quantify this is that the first 1000-year-old is probably only about ten years younger than the first 150-year-old. Another, possibly of more relevance to those who do not consider themselves inherently likely to live exceptionally long, is that a whole generation will be, in the words of the Australian writer Damian Broderick [32], the "last mortal generation" – a cohort who live roughly as long as those born in 1900, but whose offspring mostly live indefinitely and die only of causes unrelated to age. The sociopolitical implications are highly unpredictable but it seems inescapable that they will be unprecedentedly profound.

5. Conclusion: We Know Not What the Future Brings, but We Must Hasten It Anyway

I have attempted in this essay to outline the methods by which humanity will in due course defeat its greatest remaining scourge. Much of what I have written is plainly speculative in the extreme, yet I have stuck my neck out and given estimates of timeframes, with probabilities attached to them. Some feel that speculations of this sort are irresponsible, engendering unwarranted optimism about the rate of progress. I take the diametrically opposite view: I am convinced that it is irresponsible to remain silent on such matters, because doing so engenders unwarranted pessimism: the public are predisposed to presume that nothing can be done about aging and thus do not agitate for efforts to hasten progress, and that will only change if their sights are raised [33]. Accordingly, I have no compunction in setting out (here and elsewhere) a scenario that, after much consideration, I consider the most likely way in which, and rate at which, we will move to a post-aging world.

References

[1] A. Fire A et al., Potent and specific genetic interference by double-stranded RNA in *Caenorhabditis elegans*, *Nature* 391 (1998) 806–811.

[2] A.D.N.J. de Grey, The unfortunate influence of the weather on the rate of aging: why human caloric restriction or its emulation may only extend life expectancy by 2–3 years, *Gerontology* 51 (2005) 73–82.

[3] K.T. Coshigano et al., Deletion, but not antagonism, of the mouse growth hormone receptor results in severely decreased body weights, insulin, and insulin-like growth factor I levels and increased life span, *Endocrinology* 144 (2003) 3799–3810.

[4] M. Holzenberger et al., IGF-1 receptor regulates lifespan and resistance to oxidative stress in mice, *Nature* 421 (2003) 182–187.

[5] A.D.N.J. de Grey et al., Time to talk SENS: critiquing the immutability of human aging, *Annals of the New York Academy of Sciences* 959 (2002) 452–462.

[6] A.D.N.J. de Grey, An engineer's approach to the development of real anti-aging medicine, *Science of Aging Knowledge Environment* 2003 (2003) vp1.

[7] H. Brody, Organization of the cerebral cortex III, *Journal of Comparative Neurology* 102 (1955) 511–556.

[8] L. Hayflick, The limited in vitro lifetime of human diploid cell strains, *Experimental Cell Research* 37 (1965) 614–636.

[9] L. Szilard, On the nature of the ageing process, *Proceedings of the National Academy of Sciences USA* 45 (1959) 35–45.

[10] R.G. Cutler, The dysdifferentiation hypothesis of mammalian aging and longevity. In: E. Gicobini et al. (eds.), The Aging Brain: Cellular and Molecular Mechanisms of Aging in the Nervous System. Raven Press, New York, 1982, pp. 1–19.

[11] D. Harman, The biologic clock: the mitochondria? *Journal of the American Geriatrics Society* 20 (1972) 145–147.

[12] B.L. Strehler et al., Rate and magnitude of age pigment accumulation in the human myocardium, Journal of Gerontology 14 (1959) 430–439.

[13] A. Alzheimer, Uber eine eigneartige Ehrankung der Himrinde, *Allgemeine Z Psychiatr Psychish-Gerichtliche Medizin* 64 (1907) 146–148.

[14] V.M. Monnier and A. Cerami, Nonenzymatic browning in vivo: possible process for aging of long-lived proteins, *Science* 211 (1981) 491–493.

[15] M.S. Rao and M.P. Mattson, Stem cells and aging: expanding the possibilities, *Mechanisms of Ageing and Development* 122 (2001) 713–734.

[16] N. Barzilai et al., Surgical removal of visceral fat reverses hepatic insulin resistance, *Diabetes* 48 (1999) 94–98.

[17] A.D.N.J. de Grey et al., Total deletion of in vivo telomere elongation capacity: an ambitious but possibly ultimate cure for all age-related human cancers, *Annals of the New York Academy of Sciences* 1019 (2004) 147–170.

[18] A.D.N.J. de Grey, Whole-body interdiction of lengthening of telomeres: a proposal for cancer prevention, *Frontiers in Bioscience* 10 (2005) 2420–2429.

[19] S.J. Zullo et al., Stable transformation of CHO Cells and human NARP cybrids confers oligomycin resistance (oli^r) following transfer of a mitochondrial DNA-encoded oli^r ATPase6 gene to the nuclear genome: a model system for mtDNA gene therapy, *Rejuvenation Research* 8 (2005) 18–28.

[20] A.D.N.J. de Grey, Bioremediation meets biomedicine: therapeutic translation of microbial catabolism to the lysosome, *Trends in Biotechnology* 20 (2002) 452–455.

[21] A.D.N.J. de Grey et al., Medical bioremediation: prospects for the application of microbial catabolic diversity to aging and several major age-related diseases, *Ageing Research Reviews*, in press.

[22] D. Schenk et al., Immunization with amyloid-beta attenuates Alzheimer-disease-like pathology in the PDAPP mouse, *Nature* 400 (1999) 173–177.

[23] D.A. Kass et al., Improved arterial compliance by a novel advanced glycation end-product crosslink breaker, *Circulation* 104 (2001) 1464–1470.

[24] A.D.N.J. de Grey, Escape velocity: why the prospect of extreme human life extension matters now, *PLoS Biology* 2 (2004) 723–726.

[25] S. Vasan et al., An agent cleaving glucose-derived protein crosslinks in vitro and in vivo, *Nature* 382 (1996) 275–278.

[26] M. Tuszynski et al., A phase 1 clinical trial of nerve growth factor gene therapy for Alzheimer disease, *Nature Medicine* 11 (2005) 551–555.

[27] E.A. Ryan et al., Five-year follow-up after clinical islet transplantation, *Diabetes* 54 (2005) 2060–2069.

[28] O. Lindvall and A. Bjorklund, Cell therapy in Parkinson's disease, *Neurorx* 1 (2004) 382–393.

[29] R.N. Felmer and J.A. Clark, The gene suicide system Ntr/CB1954 causes ablation of differentiated 3T3L1 adipocytes by apoptosis, *Biology Research* 37 (2004) 449–460.

[30] D. Berd, M-Vax: an autologous, hapten-modified vaccine for human cancer, *Expert Reviews on Vaccines* 3 (2004) 521–527.

[31] A.D.N.J. de Grey, Forces maintaining organellar genomes: is any as strong as genetic code disparity or hydrophobicity? *BioEssays* 27 (2005) 436–446.

[32] D. Broderick, The Last Mortal Generation: How Science Will Alter Our Lives in the 21st Century, New Holland Publishers, London, 2000.

[33] A.D.N.J. de Grey, Resistance to debate on how to postpone ageing is delaying progress and costing lives, *EMBO Reports* 6 (2005) S49–S53.

Future of Intelligent and Extelligent Health Environment
R.G. Bushko (Ed.)
IOS Press, 2005

Future of Caring for an Aging Population: Trends, Technology, and Caregiving

Stephan G. WIET, Ph.D.
Director, McNeil Consumer & Specialty Pharmaceuticals, Ft. Washington, PA, USA

Abstract. Demographic trends clearly indicate that the US population aging patterns will continue to skew increasingly older for decades to come. Driven largely by healthcare and environmental improvements, the average life expectancy in the industrialized world has increased almost 30 years in the last century, allowing people to routinely live well into their 70s and beyond. A concomitant trend has also emerged as a result of increased longevity – the increased number of family caregivers responsible for managing the diverse needs of an elderly spouse or parent. This chapter reviews these emerging trends and their ramifications in more detail. It will also provide insights into some of the issues facing family caregivers as they attempt to balance this added responsibility along with other demands in their lives. Finally, this chapter will outline some of the technology-driven, needs-based solutions that are necessary for maintaining the quality of life for both the family caregiver and the care recipient.

1. The Aging Population – Is America Prepared?

The U.S. population is graying. Growth of the US population 65 and older is affecting every aspect of our society – especially our families – and challenging health care companies and providers alike. Projections by the U.S. Census Bureau show a significant rise in growth of the population age 65 and older through the year 2050, with people over 85 years demonstrating the fastest growth segment [1,2]. Entering the 21st century, approximately 13% (35 million people) of the U.S. population was 65 or older. This percentage is ten times greater than evident at the turn of the last century. In just 5 years, the "baby boom" generation will begin turning 65, and in 25 years, it is projected that one in five Americans will be 65 or older. This trend is depicted in Table 1.

A marked increase in the upper age segments of the US population has a significant impact on the healthcare system, in part due to the incidence of chronic illnesses common among aging Americans. Major chronic physical illnesses like arthritis, hypertension, cancer, and heart disease will continue to plague older Americans (Table 2). As the US population ages, higher incidence of memory impairments (Table 3), and psychiatric disorders like depression (Table 4) are evident. Finally, limitations in mobility and movement are reported in a large percentage of older Americans (Table 5).

Despite these illnesses and limitations, older Americans are attempting to maintain good health, largely through diet, exercise, and routine medical care. In fact, an extremely large number of older individuals report having good to excellent health (Table 6).

Taken together, it is apparent that there will be an ever-increasing demand on our present health care system to respond to the needs of the growing aging population, be it maintaining the well being of older Americans, or managing the health-related problems associated with aging.

Table 1. Age trend of Americans, 65 or older, by age group – 1900–2050.

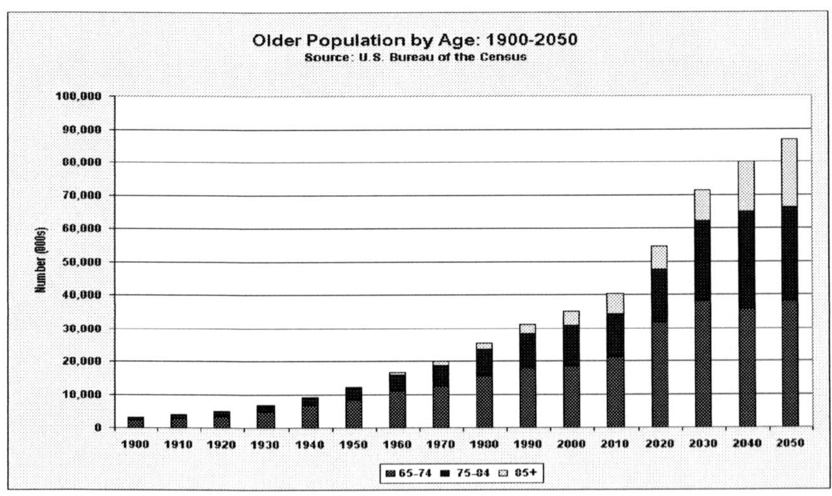

Table 2. Incidence of select chronic physical ailments by gender – 1984 & 1995.

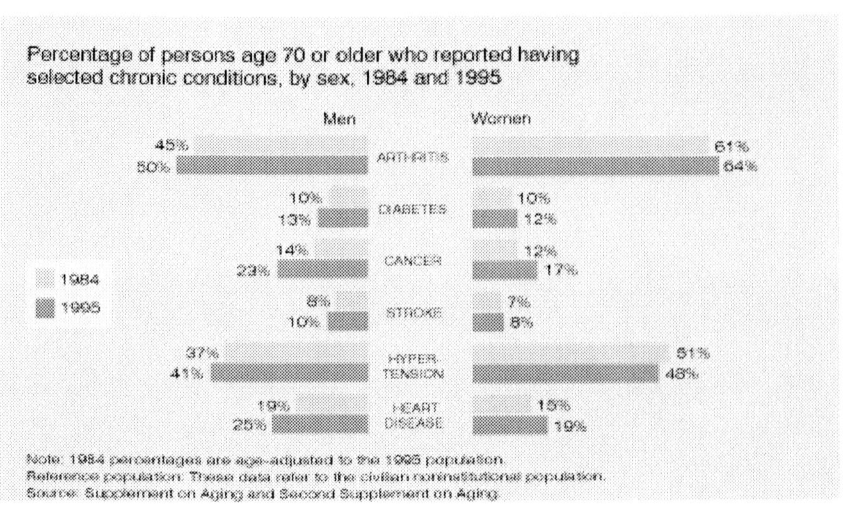

Table 3. Percentage of population 65+ with memory impairment – 1998.

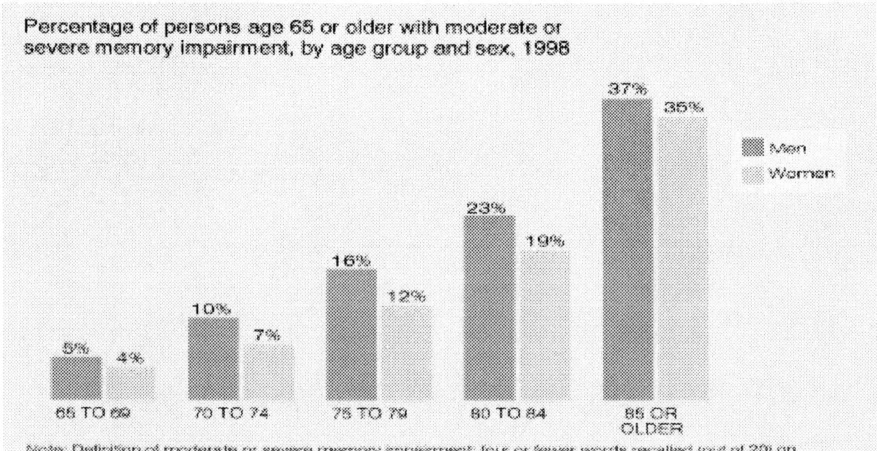

Table 4. Percentage of population 65+ with severe depression – 1998.

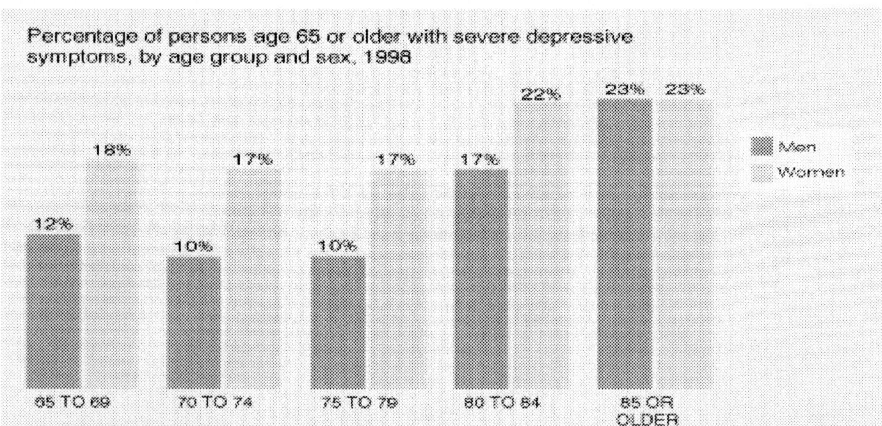

Table 5. Percentage of population 70+ with mobility impairments – 1984 & 1995.

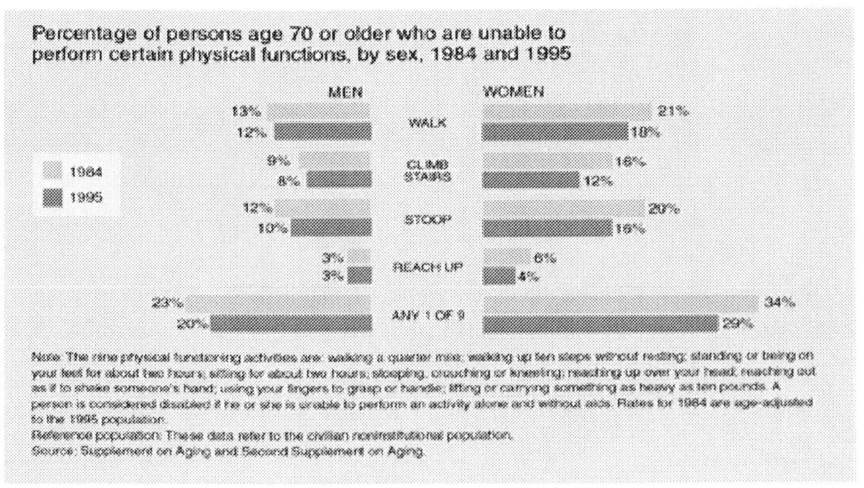

Table 6. Percentage of population 65 + reporting good to excellent health – 1994–1995.

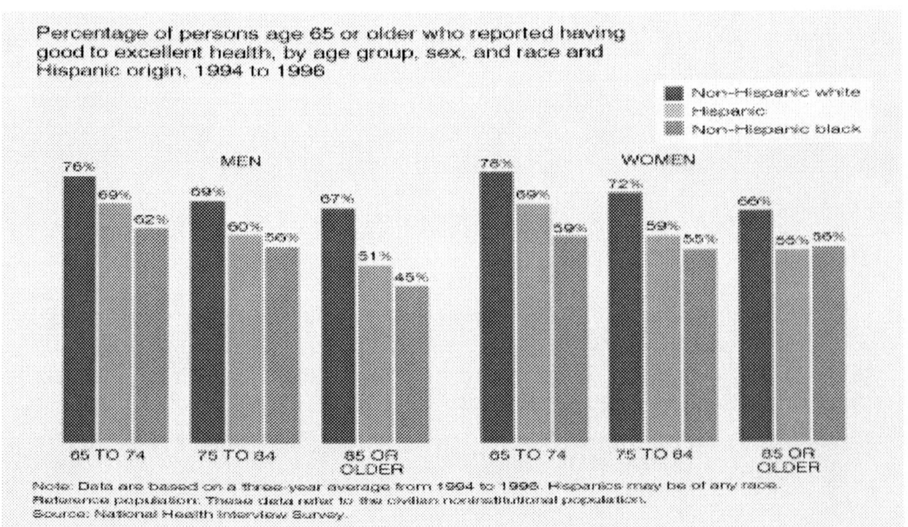

2. Healthcare Trends – Are We Ready for the Disruption?

How will the future of healthcare handle the growing needs of an aging population? Current trends indicate that the care and diagnosis of medical problems will continue to shift from more centralized to less centralized locations, and from more skilled to less skilled care providers. This implies that a greater emphasis is being placed on parents, family members, and patients themselves to provide care, diagnose illnesses, and receive treatment in locations outside of the hospital or the doctor's office. This includes self-help options such as kiosks, and home-based alternatives.

In addition, the healthcare system is placing greater emphasis on the prevention and early detection of illnesses rather than managing and treating diseases that are more clearly manifest. This shift from an "after-the-fact" treatment model to a "before onset care" model further reinforces the transfer of healthcare responsibility onto the shoulders of patients and their caregivers. Together, the goal of the future of healthcare is to have the aging population stay healthy and stay home.

In order to accomplish this goal, the healthcare system must rely on a number of enabling technologies for older Americans to maintain their health, as well as get the necessary, critical information when they need it, regardless of their location. One area that is presently well positioned to offer these capabilities is the telecommunication industry. The connectivity to outside resources provided by wired and wireless infrastructures like the internet, telephone, and cable television can be utilized to form the backbone of a 2-way "personal medical advisor." This advisor can offer such critically important healthcare aids such as:

- Home monitoring
- Home diagnostics
- Personalized healthcare and medical information
- Personalized medical records
- Smart medicine cabinets
- Mobility assistants
- Medication reminders and auto dispensers

While these innovations can all assist the aging American to stay healthy and stay home, it is inevitable that caregivers will become an important source of support for an aging population. Despite different alternatives to receiving care, it will be the family caregiver that will take on the greatest burden of responsibility both near term and long term.

3. Preparing America for Care

Former First Lady Roselynn Carter is attributed the quote "There are only four kinds of people in the world – those who have been caregivers; those who are currently caregivers; those who will be caregivers; and those who need caregivers." As the healthcare system is changing, the vital role of the family caregiver is receiving national attention.

Presently, there are approximately 44.4 million family caregivers in the US [4]. This represents 23% of the adult population. The "typical" family caregiver is a 49-year-old married female with a family of her own (approximately 35% of family caregivers are men). Two-thirds hold a job outside of the house. Family caregivers provide on average over 20 hours of care per week to a spouse or parent. Each caregiving episode lasts for an average of 5.2 years, with many caregivers having more than one caregiving episode in their lives. With the ever-increasing number of older Americans, the pool of family caregivers is dwindling [5]. In 1990, there were 11 potential caregivers for each person needing care. In 2050, that ration will be 4:1.

Family caregiving has both positive and negative aspects. Interviews with caregivers indicate there is a strong sense of duty and pride in supporting a parent as they age, a reciprocation of the love, care, and nurturing provided them when they were younger. Many report a strengthening of the bond between them and the care recipient. However, the negative impact of caregiving often far outweighs the positive aspects. These can be felt financially, physically, and emotionally.

Table 7. Formal home care, nursing care, and informal caregiving expenditures as a function of total national health expenditures – US.

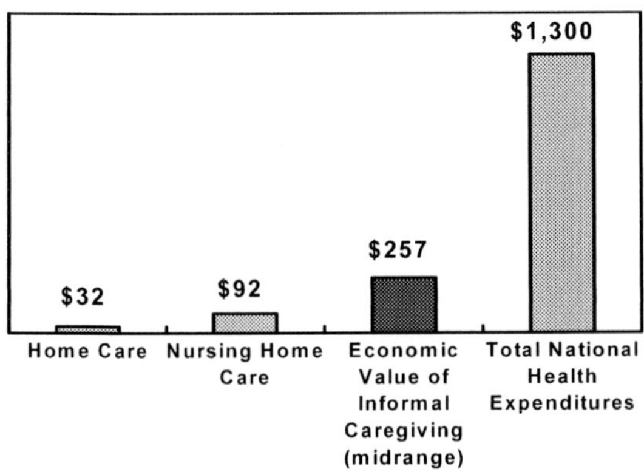

Table 8. Key activities provided by caregivers.

Activity	% Involved	Activity	% Involved
Transportation	94%	Bathing	76%
Housekeeping	92%	Dressing	68%
Shopping	91%	Walking	65%
Fixing Meals	88%	Getting in/out of car	64%
Schedule Health Care	88%	Using Bathroom	53%
Money Management	84%	Eating	45%
Taking Medicine	84%	Other	26%

The economic consequences of family caregivers are significant. The economic value of informal caregiving is approximately one-fifth ($257 billion dollars) the total national health expenditure, and significantly greater than formal home care and nursing home care expenditures combined (Table 7). In addition, it has been recently reported that American businesses lose between $11–$29 billion dollars each year due to employees' need to care for loved ones 50 years of age and older [5]. Over the course of the typical caregiving situation, the caregiver gives up approximately $600,000 in lost wages, pension, and social security [5]. Further, they spend about $170 a month out of their own pockets to pay for things required for the care recipient. This includes medicines, groceries and consumer products, and home modifications. Considering the additional financial responsibilities that caregivers have toward their immediate families, it is clear that the added monetary investment in caring for a loved one places great burdens on families.

In addition to financial burdens, caregiving also places enormous demands on one's time and attention. Table 8 summarizes the results from 1,000 caregivers surveyed as to the types of activities they help manage for their care recipients [2]. The overwhelming majority handles basic assistance of everyday living such as transportation, shopping, scheduling appointments, taking medication, and performing housekeeping duties. Half of all caregivers, however, also provide more critical help in the areas of bathing, walking, dressing, eating, and bathroom assistance. These data clearly indicate that caregiving manifests itself in different ways. There is often a clear progression in the nature of activities underlying caregiving over time, especially in cases where caring for an older parent or terminally ill family member is concerned. In these cases, caregiving typically starts with performing household management tasks, and then progresses to more physically involved personal care ac-

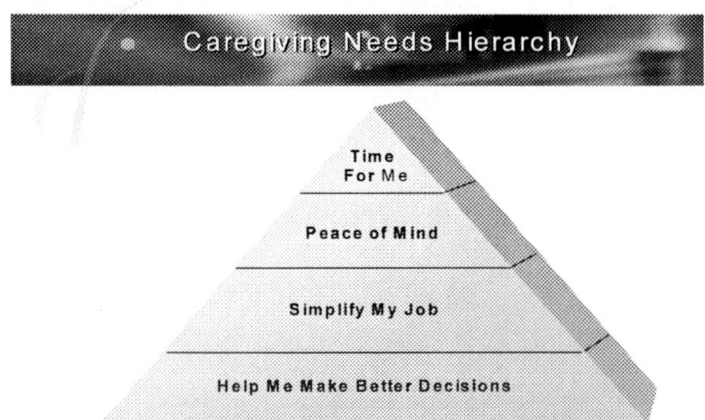

Figure 1. Caregiving Needs Hierarchy.

tivities. Once these activities become too overwhelming for the caregiver, additional activities in seeking outside assistance and formal services come into play. In time, caregivers must often give consideration of nursing home placement when in-home services cannot be maintained.

Termination of caregiving does not stop when a care recipient is placed into a nursing home. In fact, the level of responsibilities often increase as attention must be given to both the recipient and the nursing home staff in insuring that the recipient is being provided with proper care in their absence. Termination of caregiving occurs upon the death of the care recipient, however, a caregiver may often repeat this cycle for another parent, relative.

Finally, caregiving takes a heavy toll on the physical and emotional well being of individuals. Stress and anxiety are common symptoms afflicting caregivers, and often lead to physical ailments such as heart disease and high blood pressure. The extent to which emotional and physical ailments manifest are largely determined by the level of care being provided and the extent to which the caregiver had a choice in providing care. It has been reported that on average, approximately 50% of all caregivers state that their own health is poorer as a result of providing care [4].

4. Caregiving Needs – How Technology Can Help

Caregivers have a multitude of unmet needs. These needs are multidimensional and target solutions aimed at the both the care recipient and the caregiver directly. Caregiver needs can be categorized into several key themes. These themes can best be visualized using the needs hierarchy depicted below. The pyramid grows from tangible solutions aimed at simplifying or improving the quality and level of care being provided, to higher-order needs aimed at the physical and emotional well being of the caregiver specifically. These levels and possible solutions will be briefly discussed next.

4.1. Help Me Make Better Decisions

As caregivers inherit greater responsibilities, the decisions they must make on behalf of the care recipient grow in terms of number, frequency, and complexity. There is a tremendous need to access information that is customized to the unique needs of the care recipient. This can include diverse issues ranging from understanding medication side effects to identifying local assistance programs. This information needs to be accessible when they need it,

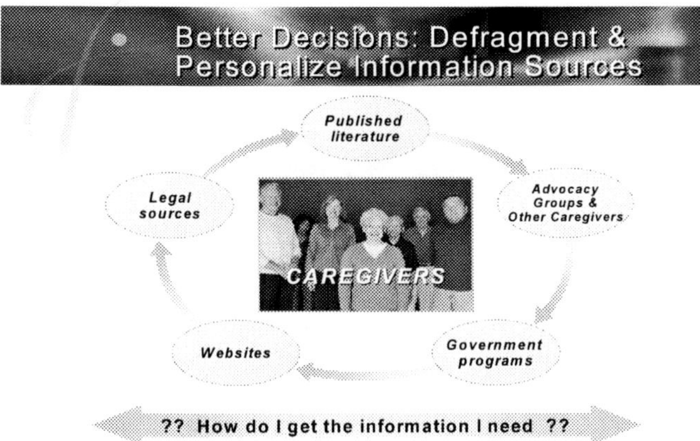

Figure 2. Better Decisions: Defragment & Personalize Information Sources.

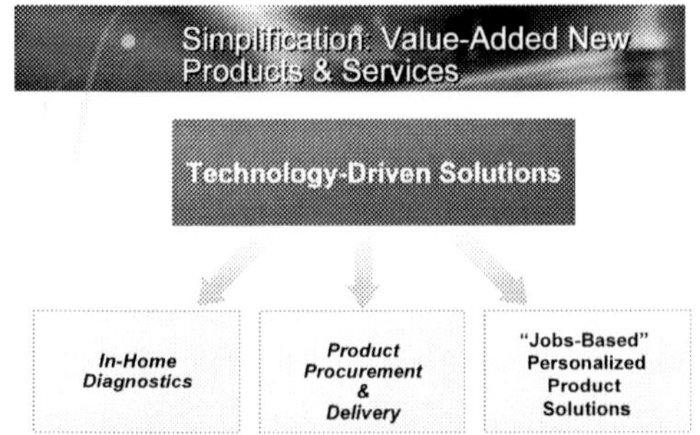

Figure 3. Simplification: Value-Added New Products and Services.

where they need it, and in a format that answers their questions quickly and effectively. It must not only provide information on current needs, but also prepare them for future issues they will likely face.

The types of information that benefit caregivers come from a variety of sources. These include websites, legal services, published literature, advocacy and support groups, and government programs. Given the time constraints that caregivers face, there is a tremendous need to defragment this information, simplify its format, and offer greater personalized content that addresses the unique needs of each caregiver. While the internet is a likely solution, the vast majority of websites dedicated to caregiving offer a tremendous amount of diverse content – most of which is generic in nature. While valuable, caregivers have limited time to find the answers most relevant to them. Future systems must get smarter in their ability to identify the individualized needs of each caregiver, and provide content more tailored to their unique set of caregiving issues. These smart systems must be affordable, easily accessible, portable, and capable of providing both content as well as a human interface if needed. This model closely resembles true "concierge" service.

4.2. Simplify My Job

The many jobs a caregiver performs require greater simplification. This results in greater time efficiency, reduces stress and physical fatigue, improves the balance between work

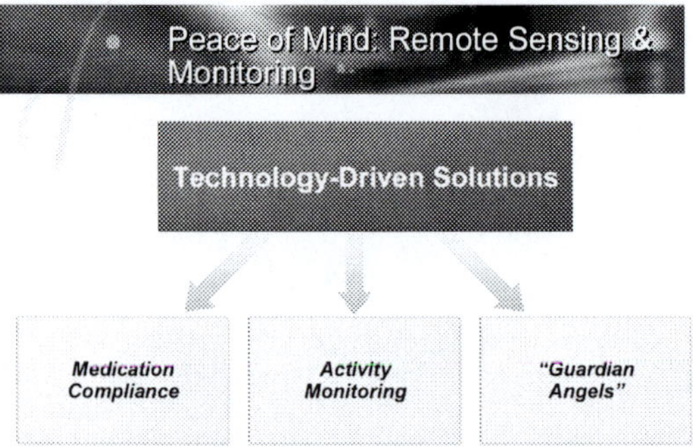

Figure 4. Peace of Mind: remote Sensing and Monitoring.

and caregiving, and enhances the "quality time" a caregiver can spend with the care recipient. Three areas that can be simplified through technology are in-home diagnostics, product procurement and delivery, and value-added product solutions.

Diagnosing illnesses or assessing the therapeutic benefits of medications usually requires visits to medical facilities. This requires extra time, coordination, and planning on the part of the caregiver. Technology-driven solutions are being sought to enable caregivers to perform a greater array of tests in the home, such as determining infections – with fast results available either directly or through interfaces that connect to remote sites via the internet.

Technology-based solutions are also becoming available that will enable caregivers to obtain healthcare supplies more easily and conveniently, thereby reducing the need to visit traditional grocery stores and pharmacies. Product procurement and delivery services can be accessed via computers, wireless hand held remote units, and via the television.

Finally, innovative product improvements are required that simplify and enhance the caregiver's ability to perform tasks aimed at maintaining good personal hygiene of the care recipient. This includes improved delivery systems for applying medicated creams and lotions to maintain healthy skin, innovative solutions for maintaining good oral care without the need to brush teeth, dry cleansers that will effectively "wash" the body and hair, and easy to use cleaning products to be used following bowel movements and occasions of urinary incontinence.

4.3. Peace of Mind

As mentioned previously, caregivers provide approximately 20 hours of care each week to a parent or spouse. Only a small percentage of family caregivers provide continuous, round the clock care. While it is clear that the activities performed by caregivers can create great stress and emotion, equally stressful is the time when the caregiver is not present. Questions concerning the care recipient's health and well being while away can be ever present. One solution is to better "connect" the caregiver with the care recipient throughout the day to provide greater peace of mind and insure the caregiver that critical events are taking place in their absence. Three technologies appear useful in maintaining this connection.

The first area concerns medication compliance. Devices are currently being marketed that enable caregivers to know when and if medications are being taken according to schedule. Feedback is typically provided via the telephone if a scheduled dosing time is not met. Wireless communication methods will likely be seen in second-generation pill dispensing devices.

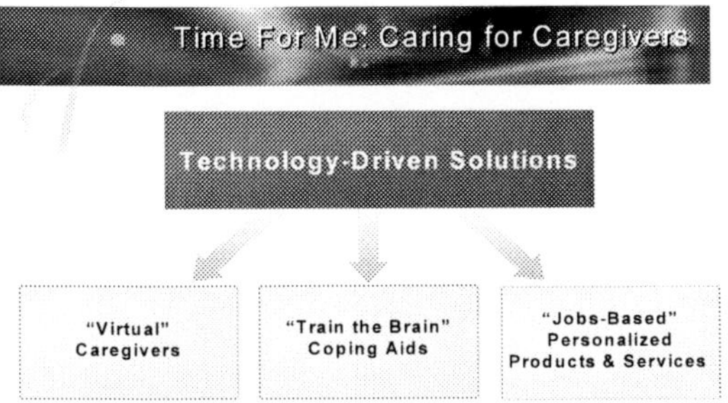

Figure 5. Caring for Caregivers – Technology Driven Solutions.

A second area for providing a remote connection between caregiver and care recipient is activity monitoring. Sensor technology and GSP systems enable movement patterns to be monitored from great distances. These technologies will be helpful in enabling caregivers to insure that care recipients are safe and performing necessary tasks as required.

Perhaps a more futuristic idea is the notion of a "guardian angel." This technology would rely on robotics and sensors to virtually duplicate many of the supervisory behaviors, reactions, and activities that caregivers provide. The robotics field is making great strides in developing robots with greater human tendencies. First generation prototypes suitable for certain caregiving activities should be available soon.

4.4. Time for Me

The greatest unmet need among caregivers is finding personal time [2]. Among 1000 caregivers surveyed, 98% indicated they needed more help managing their emotions. In addition, 94% stated they needed more help in finding time for themselves. Certainly, the opportunity to give personal time back to caregivers results in healthier, more emotionally stable care providers. A net positive effect on the care recipient is also likely to occur. While products are available that offer temporary respite, such as warm baths, aromatherapy candles, and a variety of sleep aids, future technologies targeting the caregiver directly can dramatically enhance the overall well being of this target group. Several areas, some rather far reaching, come to mind.

Advances in biofeedback and biotelemetry will enable future caregivers to quickly "escape" into alternate mind states using sophisticate "train the brain" technologies. These "escapes" may resemble mini-vacations.

Similarly, the ability to received customized pampered care without having to leave the care recipient is a business model yet to be exploited.

Finally, can technology create a "virtual caregiver" – providing care recipients all the necessary assistance and comforts that caregivers offer personally? Perhaps this ideas is a bit far fetched, however, virtual reality technologies coming out of the gaming world may have some usefulness in other non-obvious areas.

5. Conclusions

It is apparent that America is in a crisis. The demographic trends clearly indicate that the U.S. will be increasingly relying on a dwindling supply of family caregivers to assist an ever-aging population. Presently, lifestyles are fast-paced and growing increasingly more complex. Time is becoming more precious. In order to provide for the needs of aging family members, while at the same time attending to the needs of immediate family members, we will be placing a greater reliance on technology to address the many day-to-day responsibilities that underlie caregiving. This will only be successful through innovation and partnerships formed between the technology-driven worlds of academia, technology industries, and government.

References

[1] Older Americans 2000: Key Indicators of Well-Being. Federal Interagency Forum on Aging-Related Statistics, 2000, www.agingstats.gov/chartbook2000.
[2] L.J. Kotlikoff, S. Burns, The Coming Generational Storm: What You Need to Know About America's Economic Future, MIT Press, Cambridge, MA, 2004.
[3] R. Eder, A. Alexander, Underserved at Retail, Overtaxed Caregivers Cite Need for Help Among Chief Concerns, Drug Store News, November, 12–19, 2003.
[4] Caregiving in the U.S. National Alliance for Caregiving and AARP, April, 2004, www.AARP.org.
[5] National Family Caregivers Association, 2005, www.nfcacares.org.

Future of Intelligent and Extelligent Health Environment
R.G. Bushko (Ed.)
IOS Press, 2005

231

Promoting Safe and Comfortable Driving for Elders[*]

Elizabeth VAN RANST, M.S.S.S.[a], Nina M. SILVERSTEIN, Ph.D.[b]
and Alison S. GOTTLIEB, Ph.D.[c]
[a]*Research Fellow, Gerontology Institute, University of Massachusetts Boston,
Boston, MA, USA*
[b]*Associate Professor of Gerontology, College of Public and Community Service,
University of Massachusetts Boston, Boston, MA, USA*
[c]*Research Fellow, Gerontology Institute, University of Massachusetts Boston,
Boston, MA, USA*

Abstract. Americans are life-long drivers. It is imperative that aging drivers remain on the road safely. This chapter addresses one strategy for achieving this end, namely the utilization of low-tech vehicle modifications for addressing challenges with driving due to functional deficits that normally occur with aging. It focuses primarily on the selection of useful features to be demonstrated in a video intervention in a research project to assess whether watching the video would increase elders' awareness of and likelihood of using the features. The features were chosen with the assistance of a panel of experts in transportation, aging, rehabilitation, and related fields plus a focus group of older drivers. Selecting the features, developing survey instruments, and producing the video constitute Phase I of the study. Phase II investigates whether watching a video would increase older drivers' awareness of such features and motivate them to use any of them. This chapter also includes an overview of Phase II and some comments with respect to high-tech features and the future of automobile travel.

1. Introduction

Baby boomers are rapidly approaching their later years. By 2030, the 65+ population in the United States will number 70 million, twice what it is today; one of every five Americans will be elderly [1]. In 2001, one of every ten licensed drivers in this country was age 70 or older [2]. This number is expected to rise dramatically not only because of the sheer numbers of aging baby boomers, but also because they will remain more independent and active than previous generations. Coughlin projects that "baby boomers who have grown up with the car are likely to be even more wedded to the automobile... in the future than were their parents" [3, p. 20].

People experience physical and cognitive changes as they age. For example, aging often leads to reduced height, strength, and flexibility; decreased peripheral vision and increased sensitivity to glare, and a slower processing of information. Such changes in physical, vis-

---

[*] Research results will appear in "Use of a Video Intervention to Increase Elders' Awareness of Low-Cost Vehicle Modifications to Enhance Driving Safety and Comfort" in the 2005 Transportation Research Record series (Journal of the Transportation Research Board).

ual, and cognitive conditions can affect driving ability. While some changes are temporary side effects of medications, others are permanent. Though safe driving may seem relatively straightforward, it is in fact a complex task requiring precise coordination of numerous physical, visual, and cognitive abilities.

1.1. Accidents and Injury

How safe are older drivers? According to the Department of Transportation, they are "not a significant risk to others" [1, p. 2]. However, they are at risk to themselves. Elder drivers, according to the American Medical Association, have the highest fatality rate per mile driven except for drivers under age 25. Based on estimated annual travel, "the fatality rate for drivers 85 and older is 9 times higher than the rate for drivers 25–69 years old" [4, p. 2]. Further, the AMA claims "motor vehicle injuries are the leading cause of injury-related death among 64–74-year olds and are the second leading cause (after falls) among 75–84-year olds" [4, p. 2]. The driver fatality rate per 100 million vehicle miles traveled begins increasing after age 60, and increasing sharply about age 75. The Insurance Institute for Highway Safety and Johns Hopkins University attribute this high death rate to the frailty of elders [1]. In fact, the situation is so serious that the safety of older drivers is now being called a public health issue by the American Medical Association [4].

1.2. Consequences of Driving Cessation

Driving has long been a symbol of independence – being able to go where one wants, when one wants. The private car is the preferred mode of transportation in this country. Even after giving up driving, riding as a passenger in a private car is the next favored means of transport. More than 80 percent of those age 65 and older drive or ride in automobiles [3]. This percentage is likely to increase when the boomers turn 65.

While alternate modes of transportation such as mass transit buses and trains, human service transportation programs, and/or taxicabs may exist in some communities, in others they do not. Even where they are available, there are numerous reasons why such alternatives may not be as well accepted by elders as the private car. For example, it may be impossible for elders to walk to the service, the vehicles may be inaccessible, trips may need to be scheduled several days ahead, or the service may have limited geographical coverage. Elders may be fearful for their physical safety (security) or find the fare excessive. Moreover, some former drivers do not wish to burden friends and family by asking for rides, so they keep their requests to a minimum. In most communities, only the private vehicle regularly meets the "ice cream cone standard" as described by Coughlin [5]: One can get in the car and go out for an ice cream cone whenever one wishes. Inherent in this standard is the element of spontaneity. This is the minimum criterion that needs to be met to ensure that quality of independence usually provided only by a private auto.

Having to stop driving is difficult both physically and emotionally for people who are accustomed to having the freedom to travel as they please. Driving cessation can lead to a diminished quality of life, including social isolation and depression. Indeed, giving up driving has been found to be one of the strongest predictors of depressive symptoms in elders [6,7]. Hence, it is important to keep safe drivers on the road as long as possible.

1.3. Strategies to Consider Prior to Driving Cessation

Although driving cessation is one means of reducing elders' injuries and fatalities, less drastic alternatives can achieve the same goal. First, the rate of accidents can be reduced by improvements in street design and roadway signage, enforcement of traffic laws, driver education and retraining, and use of vehicle modifications (the strategy addressed in this project). Second, injuries to vehicle occupants and pedestrians, when accidents do occur, can be reduced by changing vehicle design. Third, emergency medical care can be provided more quickly through the use of emergency call and vehicle tracking systems. All these methods are expected to play a role in decreasing the high rates of injury and death on the road for everyone, regardless of age.

For most elders, driving cessation will be a gradual process. This gradual process might include the use of vehicle modifications designed to keep drivers safely on the road [8,9]. Although numerous helpful vehicular features are currently on the market, they are not well known by the general public. More education is needed about vehicle modifications and features that may help people with a range of specialized requirements continue to drive safely.

1.4. One Strategy for Increasing Elders' Awareness of Low-Tech Features

The specific goal of this project is to examine one method, the development and use of a video, to increase public awareness of low-tech features that may be helpful in driving. These products may help to compensate for the effects of functional deficits commonly occurring in aging. Many of these features have been known to the disabilities community for some time, and it is the authors' contention that it is important that such features become known to the population at large. These features can be beneficial for people of all ages with either long-term or temporary impairments much in the same way that universal design has been helpful in housing and public buildings. By developing a method for disseminating information about these features, it is hoped that the project will empower older drivers to take steps to stay on the road more safely than they would otherwise for as long as they can drive.

The project includes two phases. Phase I encompasses determination of the functional deficits, driving challenges, and features to be demonstrated in a video, development of data collection instruments, and production of the video. Phase II includes showing the video to elderly drivers in an educational setting and evaluating the effectiveness of the intervention. This chapter primarily addresses Phase I but also touches on Phase II, which was in process when this chapter was submitted for publication.

A video was selected as the means to demonstrate the chosen features for three reasons: First, a video models behavior; that is, it would show the participants the features being used by drivers similar to themselves, thus making use of a powerful tool for behavioral change [10]. Second, a video is a convenient way for elders to see and hear about what is currently available that may be helpful for them to keep driving safely and in comfort. Third, a video can be widely distributed to reach many individuals, elders, their family members, and professional care providers. Accordingly, a video was developed that demonstrated about a dozen features potentially helpful to older drivers. It was hypothesized that the post-video assessment questionnaires would show that the participants' awareness of the demonstrated features had increased, that the telephone survey several weeks later would reveal that the awareness had lasted, and that many participants had, in fact, taken action steps toward using one or more of the features regularly.

2. Method

2.1. Literature Search and Discussions

The first step was to ascertain expert opinion on three factors related to elders' driving:

- *Functional deficits* – problems or impairments that prevent normal functioning, for example, reduced peripheral vision due to changes in the eye.
- *Driving challenges* – problems or difficulties with driving caused by functional deficits, for example, increased difficulty seeing vehicles in adjacent lanes and parking due to reduced peripheral vision.
- *Features* – products or items that can be used to address the driving challenge caused by the functional deficit, for example, convex side- and rear-view mirrors that enable the driver to see to the side and rear without depending on peripheral vision.

To determine what content to include in the video, the researchers consulted with experts in the driver rehabilitation and van conversion fields, thus producing a general baseline of vehicle modifications for individuals with more serious disabilities than the target population. Several databases were searched, and occupational therapists were consulted about their experiences with low-tech, low-cost vehicle modifications useful to their clients. The literature search and discussions yielded numerous functional deficits and consequent driving challenges commonly found in the older demographic group as well as over 50 features for possible inclusion in the video.

2.2. Initial Selection of Functional Deficits, Driving Challenges, and Features

Selecting functional deficits, driving challenges, and features for the video was a fluid process. In some instances, the functional deficit was chosen first; in others, the driving challenge or the feature was selected first. The researchers' judgment played an important role.

To guide the researchers in reducing the 50 features to a smaller, more manageable number to include in the video demonstration, the following criteria were developed:

- *Currently available* – The feature may be found in new cars or could be installed in older ones.
- *Affordable* – The feature is affordable to most elder drivers, thereby ruling out most of the high-tech features.
- *Effective* – There is some evidence-based research indicating that the feature significantly addresses a specific problem resulting in increased safety, or the feature is endorsed by rehabilitation professionals.
- *Comfortable* – Something that is really uncomfortable is not likely to be used. If a safety feature, such as a safety belt, is not used, it is not effective. Thus, making the safety belt comfortable to wear is extremely important.
- *Convenient* – The product is easy to use. If, for example, a safety belt is not convenient to use, it may not be used, and if it is not used, it cannot be effective.
- *Easily understood* – The feature can be effectively demonstrated within the time constraints of a video.
- *Common* – The feature is common enough that elders would not be reluctant to try it.
- *Safe* – The feature is considered safe and would not put users at risk.

The first-round selections for professional review included 17 typical functional deficits, 20 associated potential driving challenges, and 30 features proposed to address the corresponding driving challenges. Table 1 provides examples of how the factors interrelate. The Appendix displays all the factors and their relationships.

Table 1. Examples of Functional Deficits, Potential Driving Challenges, and Features for Addressing the Challenges.

Functional Deficit	Potential Driving Challenge	Feature
Physical Reduced flexibility in torso and arms	Reaching safety belt	Ribbon on safety belt for easier reach
Vision Reduced peripheral vision	Seeing merging vehicles	Convex side-view mirrors to help eliminate blind spots
Sensory-Tactile Reduced sensitivity to pressure and touch in foot	Foot may slip of pedals, especially when wet	Pedals with non-slip surfaces (or hand controls)
Cognitive Reduced ability to accurately assess distance	Judging distance to curb when parking	Curb feeler makes noise when car is close to curb

2.3. Outside Comment

Comment was sought from additional people outside the project team to provide additional validation for the selection of features for the video. The researchers first solicited comment from a panel of experts in transportation, safety, law enforcement, aging and related fields and then from a focus group of drivers age 70+.

2.3.1. Professional Panel

A rating tool was sent along with a copy of a table similar to that in the Appendix (functional deficits, potential driving challenges, and features) to 16 professionals in transportation, safety, law enforcement, aging and related fields. These experts were asked to rate on a scale of 1 to 5 how detrimental each of the driving challenges may be to driving safely and how well each feature alleviates the corresponding driving challenge.

Ten of the experts completed the rating tools. Opinions varied greatly, and numerous items were not rated. Some respondents outside the disabilities field were hesitant to rate the driving challenges and features, suggesting that they might be less familiar with them than people in disabilities' fields. The average rating score was calculated for each driving challenge. Table 2 lists the driving challenges rated from the most to the least detrimental to driving safely. As with their ratings for the driving challenges, the experts did not fully agree in their ratings of the features proposed for addressing the challenges. The average rating score was calculated for each feature; Table 3 displays the results in descending order.

Upon further investigation, the researchers found that a number of items that were highly rated by the expert panel did not actually meet the selection criteria. The side air bags, pretensioner, and load limiter were original market items so would not be appropriate as add-on installations after purchase of a car. The sonar for backing up seemed too high tech and costly for the target audience, so it, too, was eliminated. One of the experts strongly cautioned against elders' using the small diameter power steering wheel since it would be very different and more powerful than steering wheels to which elders would be accustomed. It was also dropped for safety reasons. Several features were deleted because there was not much interest in them among the experts; the control switches were dropped because they might not show up well in a video. One feature, fleece on the safety belt, was

Table 2. Ratings of Driving Challenges by Professional Panel with type of functional deficit.

	Driving Challenges*	Functional Deficits
	Increased likelihood of injuries and fatalities resulting from crash	Physical
**	Backing up, looking for merging vehicles and vehicles in adjacent lanes	Vision
**	Backing up, looking for merging vehicles and vehicles in adjacent lanes	Physical
**	Pressing on foot pedals	Physical
**	Seeing the road clearly and making out vehicles, people, animals, signage (glare)	Vision
	Reaching/turning steering wheel and/or holding onto it for long periods	Physical
	Foot slipping off the pedals, especially when wet	Sensory-Tactile
	Seeing the road clearly and making out vehicles, people, animals, signage (wet windshield)	Vision
**	Reaching, securing/releasing the safety belt	Physical
**	Seeing the road may be obscured by the steering wheel	Vision
	Judging distance when backing up	Cognitive
**	Seat belt being too high or low	Sensory-Tactile
**	Seat belt creating pressure on chest	Sensory-Tactile
**	Discomfort when wearing seat belt due to skin sensitivity	Sensory-Tactile
	Opening and closing car door from inside the car	Physical
	Judging the distance from the wheels to the curb when parallel parking	Cognitive
	Reduced dexterity when using control knobs and buttons on dashboard	Physical
**	Turning and getting into and out of car	Physical
**	Putting the ignition key behind the steering wheel; turning it in the ignition	Physical
	Finding radio controls confusing due to information overload	Cognitive
	*The challenges are listed in descending order with those rated most detrimental to driving safely appearing first. **These driving challenges were included in the video.	

subsequently added by the researchers because it met the selection criteria and was another product in the sensory-tactile category, an area with few available features. A list of 12 features was finalized for presentation to the focus group.

2.3.2. Focus Group

The focus group consisted of 11 current drivers age 70 or older, nine women and two men. Most were alumni of the Frank J. Manning Certificate in Gerontology program, University of Massachusetts Boston, and were well suited to evaluating survey forms, having participated in action-research projects as part of their gerontology certificate requirements. At the first meeting, the focus group members completed and critiqued a draft pre-test survey form. Questions on this instrument specifically addressed the members' level of familiarity with and likeliness of using each of the designated features. Listed below are the 12 features presented to the focus group in the draft questionnaire:

- *Convex side-view mirrors*
- *Improved rear-view mirror* (later became convex rear-view mirror)
- *Seat cushion*

Table 3. Ratings of Features by Professional Panel and types of functional deficits they address.

	Features*	Functional Deficits
	Side air bags with head, torso, and pelvic protection	Physical
**	Seat rise – cushion	Vision
**	Convex side-view mirrors	Vision
**	Safety belt extender	Physical
**	Convex side-view mirrors	Physical
**	Clip-on rear-view mirror	Physical
	Pretensioner	Sensory-Tactile
**	Key extender	Physical
**	Assist strap or handle	Physical
**	Safety belt adapter	Sensory-Tactile
**	Ribbon	Physical
	Control switches	Physical
**	Pedal extender	Physical
	Hand grip/knob on standard steering wheel	Physical
	Load limiter	Sensory-Tactile
	Sonar for backing up	Cognitive
	Pedals with non-slip surfaces	Sensory-Tactile
	Large inside door handle (similar to grab bar)	Physical
**	Visor clip-on extension	Vision
	Contoured sun visor	Vision
	Windshield tinting	Vision
	Self-dimming mirrors	Vision
	Sun shield	Vision
**	Inflatable safety belt; soft cloth or fleece	Sensory-Tactile
	Wider wiper blades	Vision
	Curb feeler	Cognitive
	Anti-glare windshield styling stripe	Vision
	D-ring (adjustable)	Sensory-Tactile
	Small diameter power steering wheel	Physical
	Simpler radio	Cognitive
	Safety belt material	Physical
	*The features are listed in descending order with those rated most effective appearing first. **These features plus two others not on this table were demonstrated in the video.	

- *Steering wheel knob* (later dropped)
- *Safety belt extender*
- *Ribbon on shoulder harness* (later changed to ribbon on safety belt)
- *Pedal extender*
- *Key extender*

- *Ceiling hand grip*
- *Non-slip pedal* (later dropped)
- *Fleece for safety belt* (later became safety belt pad)
- *Visor clip-on extension* (later designated visor extender)

The language used in naming the features for the focus group was carefully selected to give the elders a reasonable chance of understanding what the features were even if they were not familiar with them. Experience has shown that presenting respondents with questions containing unfamiliar technical terms tends to yield unreliable responses.

Several focus group members had no idea what many of the features were. This was consistent with the researchers' own premise of the general public's lack of awareness of these features. The group did, however, make numerous comments that were instructive to the research team. One member said people might not even know what features are in their own cars because they do not read the entire owner's manual. The focus group members also noted that not all auto features are demonstrated during the test drive or in the showroom.

They mentioned having difficulty using side-view mirrors due to limited neck motion and keeping their feet from slipping off the pedals occasionally. The focus group members also raised driving issues that were not addressed by any of the designated features. Several members mentioned having a problem with the glare from oncoming car lights, especially the Xenon (blue) ones, at night. A couple of people reported being disturbed by headlights behind them, particularly those of sport utility vehicles, reflecting off their mirrors. Interestingly, one of the major concerns was the attitude of other drivers. Members felt that when they were seen as being elderly, other drivers would act differently towards them, making assumptions that were not necessarily accurate, that is, displaying an ageist attitude. However, addressing these matters was beyond the scope of the current project.

2.4. Final Selection of Features for the Video

Further alterations were made in the list of features that had been presented to the focus group. The research team eliminated the knob on the steering wheel since it had not been popular with the Professional Panel and because it might be too closely associated with disability and scare away the target audience. Moreover, one or two of the experts felt a pedal with a non-slip surface would be labor intensive to prepare for the video, but more important, believed that if a driver's foot were slipping off the pedals, it was probably time to switch to hand controls for safety. Hence, the non-slip pedal was eliminated. Three additions were made, however. A support handle was brought to a filming session and, being an instant success, was added to the list. A trash bag (or silk scarf) used on the seat to help the driver slide in and out of the car was initially going to be mentioned as a possible alternative to the ceiling handgrip but was not going to be filmed. When filming time came, however, it was discussed while the camera focused on an empty car seat. The third item was a safety belt tension adjuster, which was filmed because it had been very highly recommended by an expert. It was demonstrated for two purposes.

After filming, one expert who viewed a draft video questioned the use of the safety belt tension adjuster on the shoulder harness to reduce pressure from the shoulder harness on the chest and in the neck area, that is, for comfort. If it were too close to the safety belt anchor on the wall of the car, the belt might not retract as intended to pull the occupant into the correct position before deployment of the front air bag during an accident; it might also interfere with the air bag's operation. Although strong opinions were voiced on both sides of this matter, the research team felt prudence should prevail and decided not to demonstrate the adjuster for comfort. Consequently, it was shown in the final video only as a means of positioning the belt for easy reach down near the floor rather than having to reach up the inside wall of the car. As an additional precaution, a caveat was displayed at the bottom of the screen when this feature was being demonstrated: "Caution: Have a professional recommend proper placement."

The features demonstrated in the final video are as follows:

- *Visor extender* – reduces glare from the sun
- *Convex side-view mirrors* – help to eliminate blind spots
- *Convex rear-view mirror* – helps to eliminate blind spots
- *Seat cushion* – raises the driver to have an obstruction-free line of sight
- *Pedal extenders* – put pedals closer to the driver so a short person can reach the pedals; (cushion may result in legs being higher up so cannot reach pedals)
- *Support handle* – portable handhold helps when getting in and out of the car
- *Ceiling hand grip* – helps when getting in and out of the car—use arm strength to move in and out of car, especially if weakness in lower body
- *Safety belt extender* – facilitates fastening of the safety belt by raising the receptacle; also good for large people
- *Ribbon for safety belt* – used to pull the safety belt over the shoulder
- *Safety belt adjuster* – positions the safety belt for easier reach
- *Safety belt pad* – soft cloth or fleece that covers a portion of the safety belt for a more comfortable fit
- *Key extender* – useful in inserting the key into ignition and turning, for people with arthritic hands
- *Trash bag/silk scarf* – for use as a seat cover for sliding in and out.

These 13 features are associated with eleven common driving challenges that are also covered in the video. These challenges are noted in Table 2.

2.4.1. Making the Video

A 23-minute video was produced, with a well-known Boston television health reporter giving the introduction and closing for the video. Hers is a familiar face on the evening news that many elders watch, and it was anticipated that her presence would lend further credibility to the video. The main content of the video was a certified driver rehabilitation specialist demonstrating the features to three older drivers, all volunteers from the Gerontology Institute, University of Massachusetts Boston. The producers hoped that using "real people" rather than professional actresses in the video would increase its appeal and make it more acceptable. In fact, these individuals were facing some of the driving challenges themselves. The video was shown at a second meeting of the focus group for comment and underwent numerous edits. The final product included a recap of the features with pictures and resources for additional information.

3. Phase II

Phase II of this research project included showing the video and evaluating the video's effectiveness. The video was seen by about 150 drivers age 70+ at seven Councils on Aging/Senior Centers in eastern Massachusetts. The participants completed written questionnaires immediately before and after they watched the video; several weeks later most of them responded to a telephone follow-up survey. Early indications are that the video intervention has been effective in increasing participants' awareness of the features and in motivating some to try one or more features, particularly the support handle (for help in getting in and out of the car), the seat cushion (to raise the driver for a clear line of sight), and the visor extender (to help reduce glare). Data analysis, report preparation, and dissemination of findings will be completed by January 2005. The final report will be posted on the University of Massachusetts Boston Gerontology Institute website, www.geront.umb.edu.

4. Discussion

This project focused on existing low-tech features that may enable elders, or anyone, to continue driving safely. The selected features are fairly simple to understand and use, and they are priced such that most drivers can afford them. The results of this research will demonstrate whether a video is an effective method for promoting their use.

The process of developing an effective video that accurately presented common driving challenges faced by elders and low-tech features that might address these challenges was instructive. The researchers found that it was important to bring both professionals and older drivers into the planning process. The panel of experts, who represented a range of disciplines, provided differing perspectives on the driving challenges for older drivers and features for addressing them. Some experts outside the rehabilitation field were hesitant to complete the rating tool, claiming insufficient knowledge. Thus, knowledge about the existence of vehicle modifications that may be useful for older drivers was limited among both professionals and older drivers themselves.

The opinions of focus group members represented the perspective of practicing older drivers. Elders in the focus group had numerous concerns about driving that were not related to the driving challenges or features identified by experts or represented in the video. Elders reported that glare caused by the headlights of oncoming cars, especially blue Xenon lights, or by sport utility vehicles following their cars was particularly troublesome. Interestingly, one of the major concerns voiced was the ageist attitude of other drivers. However, the researchers did not have effective features for addressing these glare problems, and correcting the ageist attitude was beyond the scope of this project.

Although the researchers had anticipated that developing a video would be straightforward, based on substantial consensus on challenges and features, the project revealed the complexity associated with identifying driving challenges and appropriate safety features. Developing a video that represents consensus and demonstrates features that meet the gold standard of usability is challenging. Individual differences in experience, perspective, and need, were found across professional disciplines and within groups of older drivers. Although the resulting video represents a cross-section of driving challenges and features, the researchers believed it was important to emphasize in the video that features other than those depicted might be more appropriate for some people.

Finally, for the video and evaluation tools to be effective, it was important to include elders in the process of critiquing the driving challenges and vehicle features, including how they were presented in the video and worded in the evaluation materials. Preliminary feedback from elders who saw the video was very positive.

5. Post Script on High-Tech Features for Safety

The present research is limited to low-tech automobile features. However, many more technically sophisticated features are now available, and others will be in the near future. Some examples are provided in this section. They are most often found on luxury models, as standard or optional equipment. Many of these features would be beneficial for elders or anyone needing or wanting a little extra help. Virtually all of them are designed to help reduce accidents or protect occupants during crashes, thereby saving lives and preventing injuries.

If a driver has difficulty reaching the foot pedals, it will be more difficult to use them in an emergency situation; if a driver sits too close to the steering wheel, deployment of the front air bag can result in injury. Since people tend to become shorter in their later years due to skeletal changes, they and younger people who are short may particularly benefit from the following vehicle modifications. Electronically adjustable foot pedals that enable people with different leg lengths to drive the same vehicle are now appearing in some cars. Augmenting or substituting for adjustable foot pedals is a telescoping steering wheel, making it possible for a short person to move the seat up and reach the pedals while still sitting well behind the wheel. Moreover, many new cars are equipped with power adjustable driver seats [11]. Also currently available is a driver's seat that not only swivels, making it easier to enter and exit, but also turns perpendicular to the doorway and goes out and down toward the ground. A base with wheels can be put under it, and the driver has a wheelchair all set to go [12].

It is reported that some 2005 models will have headlights that swivel the way the steering wheel is turning, to provide earlier, better lighting through curves. One of these vehicles will also have rain-sensing windshield wipers that automatically adjust to the presence and amount of rain [13]. Both of these features are designed to improve visibility, and the latter will presumably eliminate the distraction of having to readjust the wiper speed as the rainstorm changes.

Some vehicles have rear-facing cameras to assist in backing up; they display what is behind the vehicle on a screen on the dashboard [11]. Some 2003 and 2004 cars are equipped with sonar to assist when parking. Sonar detects obstacles behind, in front, and at the corners of the car. According to one automobile dealer, when an obstacle, be it another car or a small child, is detected, a beeping sound begins inside the vehicle, and the closer the car gets to the object, the faster the beeping. In one car, the location of the object is displayed on the dashboard. The National Highway Traffic Safety Administration has estimated that, "an obstacle detection system could reduce rear collisions while backing up by 90 percent" [14]. Another high-tech device, an advanced cruise control, uses either radar or a laser beam to sense the distance to the car in front. This system maintains an appropriate distance between the two vehicles, given the speed being traveled. However, if necessary, it removes the slack from the safety belts in preparation for a crash and may slow the car to help avoid an accident [11, automobile dealer]. Similarly, a warning system to notify the driver that the car is leaving the lane, without activation of a directional signal, is planned for a 2006 luxury car [13].

Navigational systems now come standard in some models. With at least one system, the driver has the choice of reading step-by-step directions, looking at a diagram on the screen, or having a voice read the directions one-by-one. The driver can pick a specific destination and be directed throughout the entire trip. The safety benefit of this kind of navigational system, at least if the directions are audible, is that the driver need not have to reach for directions or try to read a map while driving. A voice-activated navigational system (which should help to keep the driver's eyes on the road) is reportedly coming out in the 2006 model year [13].

Allowing vehicles to determine which one will go first in various "conflict" situations may be another means of avoiding crashes. This futuristic thinking comes from Helen Greiner, Chairman and co-founder of iRobot Corporation [15].

To reduce injuries from accidents, some manufacturers are already adding more air bags to protect different parts of the body. For example, air bags for the knees, window curtain side air bags for the head, and larger front torso side air bags are available [11]. There are likely to be even more. Air bags have traditionally deployed depending on the location of the crash; for example, a frontal collision might deploy the front but not the side air bags. Now the industry is looking at air-bag deployment also being related to the size of the occupants, for instance, reducing the speed at which air bags deploy for smaller or frailer people so as not to harm them. A more futuristic idea is having the entire vehicle covered with foam, both outside and inside, upon impact [16].

While hand control substitutes for foot pedals have been available since the mid-20th century, General Motors has taken this idea a quantum step further. Its hydrogen-fuel celled concept car provides acceleration, braking, and steering through a pair of handles. Someone with limited lower body movement or strength could easily drive using its hand controls – there are no pedals. The driver with a short torso would not have a problem seeing over the steering wheel or hood of the car since there are none [17]. Suffice to say, there will be more spectacular vehicular and even highway innovations in the future.

At the 1939 World's Fair, General Motors had an eye-opening exhibit, a model of an automated highway system. Such a system is still being discussed and could even come to fruition this century. It might have cars traveling on a guideway close together, allowing for increased capacity, under automatic control so efficiency would be maximized and accidents would not occur. One could drive one's private car from home along normal feeder streets until reaching the guideway on a major artery or highway, or even underground. The driver would relinquish control of the vehicle for the time spent on the guideway.

Many of the high-tech systems mentioned above, and more, are expected to provide better protection for elders and all drivers by reducing distractions and stimulating appropriate reactions. However, there are at least two consequences that require study.

The first consequence is that instrument panels are becoming increasingly crowded with the controls necessary for all the new equipment. The instrument panel or high-tech systems may prove too complicated to learn or may overload the driver's attention. Whether such equipment and systems will increase safety remains to be seen. Volvo's 2004 YCC (Your Concept Car), designed by a team of women, includes a minimalist style interior including a bare instrument panel with only the essentials, the speedometer and the navigator, permanently on display. Other instruments are hidden away until wanted; the subtle gearshift controls are on the steering wheel [18]. It will be interesting to see if the minimalist (less is more) approach to dashboard design takes hold and whether drivers, especially older ones, prefer it.

A second consequence of utilizing high technology that requires study is the gradual reduction of human control over the vehicle. Although the research project's low-tech features described earlier in this chapter assist people with driving safely, the drivers using them are still in total control. The high-tech features go at least one step further. Some of the technology reminds the driver to act in certain situations; other technology takes over partial or full responsibility for certain tasks. A logical step down the road, the automated highway, would remove all human control for a period of time. At present, it is not known how loss of control over driving tasks will be received by drivers. Many enjoy driving and having the responsibility and control driving currently entails. This topic is bound to become a popular one for discussion as more and more innovations come into use.

Acknowledgements

The support provided by the Charles H. Farnsworth Trust to conduct this research project is gratefully acknowledged.

References

[1] U.S. Department of Transportation, Safe Mobility for a Maturing Society: Challenges and Opportunities, November 2003, Washington DC.

[2] National Center for Statistics and Analysis, National Highway Traffic Safety Administration, U.S. Department of Transportation, Traffic Safety Facts 2002: Older Population, Washington, DC.

[3] J.F. Coughlin, Beyond Health and Retirement: Placing Transportation on the Aging Policy Agenda, The Public Policy and Aging Report Vol. 11 No. 4, 2001.

[4] American Medical Association and U.S. Department of Transportation National Highway Traffic Safety Administration, Physician's Guide to Assessing and Counseling Older Drivers. American Medical Association, Chicago, 2003.

[5] J.F. Coughlin, Closing remarks at New Transportation Technology for Older People, an OECD/MIT International Symposium, September 24–25, 2003, MIT, Cambridge, MA.

[6] E.E. Johnson, Transportation Mobility and Older Drivers, Journal of Gerontological Nursing, Vol. 29 No. 4, 2003 34–41.

[7] State of Florida Department of Transportation, Florida Commission for the Transportation Disadvantaged, and National Center for Transit Research at the Center for Urban Transportation Research, University of South Florida, Senior Transportation Alternatives: Why Are They Important and What Makes Them Work? December 2003.

[8] N.M. Silverstein, J. Murtha, Driving in Massachusetts: When to Stop and Who Should Decide? University of Massachusetts Boston, Gerontology Institute Report, Boston, MA, April 2001.

[9] L.J. Molnar, D.W. Eby, L.L. Miller, Promising Approaches for Enhancing Elderly Mobility, Transportation Research Institute, University of Michigan, September 2003.

[10] A. Bandura, Social Foundations of Thought and Action, Prentice Hall, Englewood Cliffs, NJ, 1986.

[11] ConsumerGuide: Car Comparisons 2004, Vol. 711, Publications International, Ltd., July 2004.

[12] www.mobilityplus.net/seating.html, June 21, 2004.

[13] Car Buyer's Guide Presents, #49: Car Preview 2005, Harris Publications, Inc., New York.

[14] Grote Obstacle Detection System Aids Drivers Operating in Reverse, MSW Management: The Journal for Municipal Solid Waste Professionals, January 2004.

[15] R. Taylor, Lincoln automobile advertisement, special advertising supplement to the New York Times, June 22, 2004, p. ZL7.

[16] J. Pike, "Role of Technology in Protecting Older Vehicle Occupants," presented at New Transportation Technology for Older People, an OECD/MIT International Symposium, September 24–25, 2003, MIT, Cambridge, MA.

[17] J. O'Dell, GM Plans To Sell Hydrogen-Fuel Model in 2010, Los Angeles Times, March 4, 2003.

[18] S. Baruffaldi, When Women Design, Auto and Design, May/June 2004, 23–28.

[19] Channing L. Bete Co., Inc., Older Drivers – Making changes for the better, [a Scriptographic Product], 2000.

[20] Federal Highway Administration, U.S. Department of Transportation, Guidelines and Recommendations To Accommodate Older Drivers and Pedestrians, FHWA-RD-01-051, October 2001.

[21] Organisation for Economic Co-operation and Development, Ageing and Transport: Mobility Needs and Safety Issues. Paris, 2001.

[22] AAA Foundation for Traffic Safety, How to Help an Older Driver, A Guide for Planning Safe Transportation, Washington, DC, 2002.

[23] AAA Foundation for Traffic Safety, The Older and Wiser Driver, Washington, DC, 2003.

[24] P.R. LePore, When You Are Concerned – A Handbook for Families, Friends and Caregivers Worried about the Safety of an Aging Driver, State Office for the Aging, Albany, New York, 2000.

[25] S.D. Kaye, S.G. Thomas, S. Brink, Short Drivers and Air Bags, U.S. News & World Report. Washington: Nov. 11, 1996, Vol. 121, Iss. 19; p. 78, 1 p.

[26] Anonymous, Should You Get Pedal Extenders? Good Housekeeping. New York: Oct. 1998, Vol. 227, Iss. 4; p. 139, 1p.

[27] California Task Force on Older Adults and Traffic Safety, Traffic Safety among Older Adults: Recommendations for California, San Diego, CA, September 2002.

[28] K.W. Schaie and M. Pietrucha (eds.), Mobility and Transportation in the Elderly. Springer Series Societal Impact on Aging, Springer Publishing Company Inc., New York, 2000.

[29] National Highway Traffic Safety Administration, U.S. Department of Transportation and American Optometric Association, Driving When You Have Cataracts, DOT HS 805 594, June 2003.

[30] National Highway Traffic Safety Administration, U.S. Department of Transportation and American Optometric Association, Driving When You Have Glaucoma, DOT HS 809 595, June 2003.

[31] National Highway Traffic Safety Administration, U.S. Department of Transportation and American Optometric Association, Driving When You Have Macular Degeneration, DOT HS 809 596, June 2003.

[32] M. Jablow, On the Road: Driving and MS, Inside MS. New York: 2001, Vol. 19, Iss. 2, p. 14, 5 pgs.

Global Digital Healthcare Era – Enhancing Healthcare with Soft Technologies

Global Medicine Technology

Cindy MASON, Ph.D.
Visiting Research Scientist
Stanford Research Institute, Menlo Park CA, USA

Abstract. In little more than a decade, linkages between health care technologies of different cultures and continents have merged, resulting in global medicine technology. The next generation of young scientists and clinicians from both the research and clinical communities are merging established ancient technologies from outside the U.S. with modern medical technology and forging new ground in an increasingly challenging health care climate. Presently researchers, clinicians and communities are active in finding ways of using global medical technology to attack our most difficult and chronic (therefore expensive) health care problems. Using recent inventions, such as the fMRI, researchers and clinicians are understanding how and why they work. This chapter briefly discusses key ideas in the movement towards global medical technology: healthcare culture, mind-brain-body dialogue, and self-care including a self care exercise for the spine.

1. Introduction

American healthcare continues to evolve, sometimes painfully, inventing technologies that expand our ability to provide care [1–3]. Artificial Intelligence plays a significant role in future healthcare technology [4,5]. However, the fact of the matter is that the intelligence of future healthcare must come both from artificial and natural forms. Historically in healthcare, the west has had good fortune in developing science and technologies for healthcare, such as antibiotics and artificial intelligence, while the east has profited from *soft technologies* for healthcare based on mind[1] training that have evolved over thousands of years. For the first time in history, scientists can now shine a light on the mind, permitting investigation into how and why soft technologies work. The future of intelligence in our healthcare environments will include not just computational methods of intelligence as developed in the west but also from the natural intelligence that results from persistent mind training as developed in the east. This observation has profound implications for reducing healthcare costs while broadening accessibility and reducing dependence on healthcare providers. This view of health encompasses the notion that the source of health comes not only from without (the healthcare provider, healthcare system) but also from within (the individual, the self). "To be aware of a single shortcoming within oneself is more useful than to be aware of a thousand in somebody else…" [6].

A recent turn in the development of modern medicine is what is referred to as *global medicine*,[2] where ancient ways of health and healing still taught outside of western culture are being integrated with cutting-edge western medicine. Much like global telecommunica-

---

[1] The word mind, as used here, refers to mind and body. The brain and heart are also considered inseparable.

[2] A term coined by Dr. Mehmet Oz, heart surgeon at Columbia University.

tions and global markets, global medicine is medicine that benefits from the break down of cultural and physical boundaries. At Stanford University Hospital, stem cell transplant patients receiving daily Japanese acupressure sessions shaved up to 21 days of hospital time from what insurers typically expect to be a 40-day hospital stay [7]. Meditation training from India, China, Tibet and other cultures has become common as a means of working with medical complaints including pain, high blood pressure and stress [8–12,38]. Acupuncture, once viewed with skepticism, is now used in hospital surgery rooms to reduce the amount of anesthesia required and minimize side effects of surgical and other procedures [13]. At Columbia University, pioneering heart surgeons are investigating the impact of various alternative healing practices that can be combined with heart surgery to improve patient outcome [14].

At the same time that these unfamiliar healthcare philosophies and methods have found their way into our lives and medicine cabinets, unanswered questions must be answered regarding how, why, and when they work in order to preserve standards of care. Clinical trials using western scientific method are underway for some but not all of the techniques that constitute global medicine technology at the National Institute of Health [15]. Western scientists are attempting to uncover the effects of practices such as meditation and acupuncture on the mind and body at a number of governmental funded research institutions using detailed brain images with western technologies such as fMRI [16–19]. Mind training methods potentially fill a gap in our present healthcare system, addressing unmet needs of chronically ill, uninsured, and aging American public.

The practices also cultivate an attitude of self-care, reducing dependency on present healthcare providers, and potentially could be of service in the call for more broadly accessible care.

In this article we briefly discuss some key ideas in eastern mind training technologies and point to some of the ongoing activities in both clinical and research settings. Most of the ideas presented here embrace the notion that there is a relation, in fact a dialogue, between mind, brain and body. Concepts like self-awareness, mindfulness, forgiveness, and honesty, are also big players in the ancient technology of healing and the mind. Also included in this new health landscape are the ideas that mind, brain and heart are not separate organ systems, and that mind and body refer to the same concept. Mind training technologies were not developed in a laboratory nor do they rely on silicon chips or pharmaceuticals, rather, they were developed and passed down by "gurus" or teachers, sometimes religious leaders, who have developed deep insight into human nature and human behavior. Culture has preserved the teachings. Clinical success has kept them alive. They do not replace nor compete with western technology but are a marriage made in heaven for an ailing healthcare system, where patients feel alienated, hospitals are going broke, and doctors yearn for a system in which they, too, can slow down and provide compassion. In the article we discuss the role of healthcare culture in global medicine in the United States, examine mind-body-brain dialogue and its relation to health in practitioners and patients, and discuss directions and clinical work in self-care education. At the end of the chapter there is an example of global medical technology from Japan, an exercise in self-care for the interested reader.

2. The Culture of Healthcare

"It is probably true that, in general, the most fertile developments in the history of human thought are born at the intersection of two currents of ideas. The currents may originate in the midst of totally different cultural conditions, in diverse epochs and places."

Heisenberg, physicist

There is a significant cultural aspect to the integration of externally developed health-care and practices in both caregivers and patients. While Americans often wait until they are sick to think about health, most ancient technologies encourage daily practices and habits that encourage self-study, self-awareness and self-discipline as core ideas in preserving and maintaining health. The integration of these ideas into our healthcare system requires no less than a transformation in healthcare culture where self-care and health education become not only a priority but also a way of life. Behavioral changes resulting from self-knowledge and self-care play a major role in defining how we heal, how we age, and our quality of life. The integration of self-care practices like mindfulness meditation, yoga and qigong, into our own medicine cabinets carries the potential of real advances in our present system of care.

A revolution in western medicine, like in physics, will come from realizing that our method of questioning is limiting our solutions. The need to separate mind from body in order to describe and explain them fails to capture the interplay between mind and body. This interplay now appears to be fundamental in theories of healing and disease formation. Without realizing this interplay we will fail to utilize our full capacity to address not only clinical and financial healthcare issues but administrative ones as well. The fMRI diagnostic technique provides much needed evidence for western cultures to understand why and how some of these ancient medical teachings work – not only how they awaken, regulate, and influence the body's own healing mechanisms but how they work together with western medicine. Such evidence provides the key to our ability to integrate these methods successfully and transform an ailing healthcare system and restore the level of standards and scrutiny we have grown to expect from western medicine.

3. Mind-Brain-Body Dialogue

What we in the west are now referring to as the mind-brain-body dialogue is at the heart of traditional healing practices of Theravadan, Zen, and Tibetan Buddhist meditation. Other meditation practices involve repetitive slow body movements or repetitive thought exercises. These practices include yoga, tai chi, chi gong, chanting, prayer, and repetitive exercise. More than 35 years ago, researchers at Harvard were studying the origins and effects of stress and the cultivation of a relaxation response via meditation [20–22].

Clinical results of these practices, along with positive clinical results of acupuncture and acupressure, and studies of the mind during these practices, indicate there are a number of effects occurring in the mind/body as a result of these ancient technologies. Recent research in brain and cognitive sciences using fMRI, SQUID, and enhanced EEG show remarkable and highly positive changes occur in brain function as a result of prolonged meditation practice [27]. General information about fMRI and fMRI studies can be found at websites for a variety of places with on-going programs involving fMRI [23–26]. The invention of the fMRI provides details of the brain "in action" in a way previously imagined impossible. As shown in Fig. 1, the fMRI does not require an IV, thus it is less invasive than PET scans (for an introduction to fMRI, see [27,28]). It also requires fewer brain images to capture brain activity. We are now in a position never before experienced to understand how the mind creates changes in brain function over time, to watch the ways our mental and emotional lives affect our brain function, and to see the body's relationship to the brain. It is now possible to watch how persistent mind training produces enduring changes in the brain, beneficial for physical, emotional, cognitive and behavioral health.

Because many of the mind-body-brain technologies are relatively inexpensive, these studies have positive implications for a medical system pushed to its limits to find economical ways to help patients find solutions.

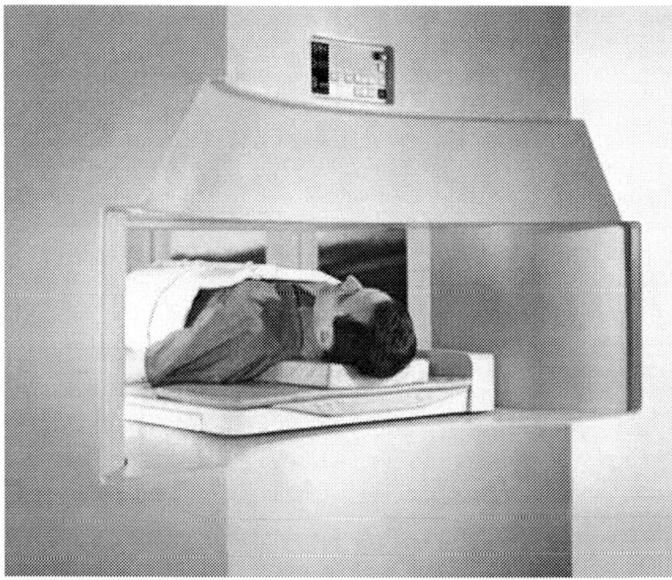

Figure 1. Functional MRI pictured below. The man is getting his head examined. Photo source: Radiology Info™ [25].

A core idea in many health cultures is that the link between mind, brain, and body is the breath, also known as prana, and qi.[3] Most if not all meditation instruction calls the student to develop practices involving the breath. Concentration practices and mindfulness practice are systems of mind training practices with core teachings relating to the breath, attention, and self-awareness. Figure 2 shows fMRI and EEG images that deomonstrate the influential relationship between meditation and brain activity. This study was performed at the Gollub Neuroimaging Lab at Harvard University [27]. The figure gives fMRI photos along with EEG records for regions of the brain including the brain stem (associated with cardiovascular control), hippocampus (associated with memory and learning), and anterior cingulated gurus, a region of the brain associated with concentration. While there are possibly more unanswered questions about mind-brain-body dialogue than there are questions about space exploration, these studies have profound implications for the use of natural intelligence and cognitive skills in our own healing. The study from which this image was taken demonstrated physiological effects of meditation including changes in activity of the brain involving emotion and breathing. For information on fMRI studies on mindfulness meditation the interested reader may wish to examine this and other Gollub Neuroimaging Lab projects [17], or the recent studies on Tibetan meditation practices at the University of Wisconsin [30].

The next set of fMRI images in Fig. 3, also from Gollub Neuroimaging Lab [27], shows the influence from body to brain, as an acupuncture needle insertion causes changes in the brain. The figure below illustrates the multiple effects of using acupuncture to needle an area of the body known as the Hoku point, Hegu point, or Large Intestine-4 (LI-4), located on the top side of the hand, in the highest place on the mound of tissue between thumb and index finger (think about the area where children draw faces on their hands and animate them, the inside corner of the mouth on that face points to LI-4). The area is one of the

---

[3] Qi (also called CHI, or KI) and prana are concepts that occur in most medical systems outside the west but appear to be difficult concepts in translation due to the differences between eastern and western thinking.

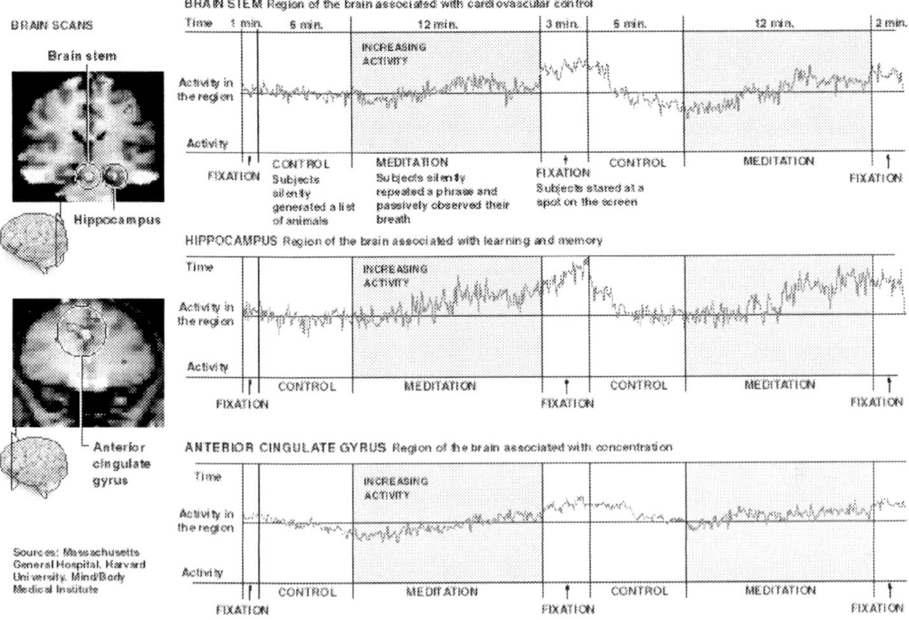

Figure 2. Physiological effects of meditation. Functional MRI images on the left, EEG on the right. Source: Gollub Neuroimaging Lab, Harvard University [27].

more well known acupuncture/acupressure locations and is commonly associated with pain relief but has multiple uses. The preliminary results of the study suggest that acupuncture needle manipulation on either hand relates to activity in the limbic system and subcortical structures. For more details on this project see [37].

To become a practitioner who works with prana, or qi, one of the more important aspects of training is to develop your own meditation practice. The strength of your practice and the quality of the teachers you encounter are central to the quality of care you will ultimately provide as a practitioner who works with qi or prana. Knowledge about meditation practices is passed down through oral teachings. As a result, the lineage of the teacher as well as access to the teacher is important. The path to health prescribed by lineage teachings includes systemic mind training such as meditation and spiritual practices as well as certain types of body meditation including yoga, qigong, tai qi, which work with the mind-brain-body dialogue using movement and breath together. Body meditation practices release tension in the body, freeing the breath, and uses postures and movements that open the spine, joints, and limbs, encouraging body fluids to move, at the same time relax the mind.

What type of meditation practices work for an individual is not a one-size-fits-all prescription. Generally, styles of meditation are a result of recommendations by friends or a result of personal inquiry. Often more than one type of meditation is explored before finding something satisfying, as there are many aspects to showing up for such teachings on a regular basis including location, availability of a teacher we feel comfortable with, the surroundings and social support offered in meditation community, family support in allowing time and space to develop the practice. Often there are weekend retreats and cost is still

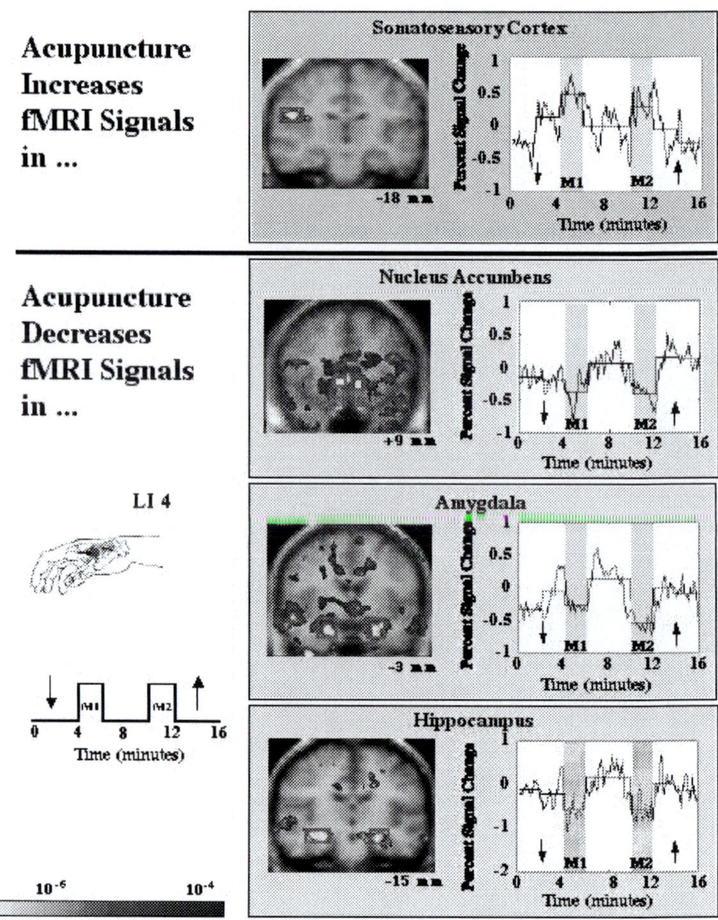

Figure 3. Physiological effects in brain from needle manipulation of the hand area known as Hoku or Large Intestine 4 (LI-4) point. Source: Gollub Neuroimaging Lab, Harvard University [27].

sometimes a factor when housing or travel is involved. Many hospital facilities and HMOs are beginning to offer education and support for these activities as a means of addressing patient needs. Stanford University, like many other hospitals, has recently begun a series of programs launching a new era in healthcare encompassing not only mind training but an emphasis on diet, exercise, social support and compassion [31].

The idea that meditation and mind training can influence health is not new. As long ago as 1975, Dr. Herbert Benson studied meditation and the development of a practice for cultivating the "relaxation response" as a means for combating hypertension [10]. What is new is the invention of technologies that allow us to see changes in brain activity as a result of such mind training practices. Recently Tibetan meditation has drawn the attention of neuroscientists and is the focus of studies at the University of Wisconsin [30]. Tibetan practices in meditation and healing are of considerable interest to American scientists for at least two reasons 1) the possibility that non-violent behavior and mediation may be linked – Tibetan culture, rich with meditation practitioners and a way of life conducive to meditation, enjoyed the status of a non-violence society for more than 2,000 years, and 2) the lineage of Tibetan mediation instructors has been rigorously preserved for as many years.

4. Self Care

An important aspect of the soft technologies is that of self-care. Many lineages encourage individuals not to become dependent upon a healthcare practitioner but to learn self-care methods. While these techniques are not in fact a substitute for seeing a practitioner, they are useful until that can be arranged, and help extend the benefits of other medical treatments. It is interesting to note that many individuals report being naturally drawn to taking better care of themselves as a result of their meditation practices, gaining the courage to make changes in habitual behaviors, increasing personal happiness that seems to spill over into every aspect of their life including their health.

Destructive behavior is at the root of many health problems, ranging from obesity and diabetes to domestic violence. The relation between emotional and physical health is most obvious among patients with heart problems [32], which are rated as the leading cause of death in this country. Although it is common sense to many of us reading this paper, there is now considerable scientific evidence that letting go of anger and resentment can reduce the severity of heart disease. In some cases, the release of anger has been shown to prolong the lives of cancer patients. Considering the relation between stress and the immune system, or stress and the adrenal response, the results of such studies are not surprising. Technological advances in surgical instruments, anesthesia, artificial hearts and heart valve materials may help patients manage symptoms of heart disease, but without fundamental changes in habitual responses, including emotional health, in a manner of speaking, we are pissing in the wind.

Destructive emotional lives have a price not only on health, but also on social structures. Families, workplaces, and schools all feel the price of violence, suicides and bullying that accompany emotional disharmony. Public institutions and school systems that cope with these problems are pressed to their limits to understand and prevent them (e.g. Columbine High School, International House at U.C. Berkeley). Meditation practices, mental or physical, increase awareness of feelings that may underlie such behaviors. Watching patterns of feelings in this way gives rise to self-awareness, and the opportunity to interrupt destructive habitual responses before they occur.

In an unusual example of global medicine, patients at Stanford University Hospital, Lucille Salter Packard Children's Hospital, Kaiser Permanente of Redwood City, Mills Peninsula, California Cancer Center of Marin, and other hospitals in the San Francisco Bay Area, are using the Japanese art of self-care known as Jin Shin Jyutsu physio-philosphy, to help manage side effects and emotional upheavals that adversely affect patients during major health projects, such as chemo, heart surgery, or transplants, and the treatments they involve [33–36]. Used in support of whatever treatment regime the patient is undergoing, patients subjectively report less fear, worry, and depression. During sessions with practitioners, individuals learn to monitor feelings and use simple recipes on themselves involving gentle touch to harmonize difficult moods, attitudes, or symptoms. These self-care methods can be used by even the sickest patients throughout the day and evening or when other treatments are unavailable to help with nausea, sleeplessness, pain, and anxiety, and other signs and symptoms. Practitioners quietly inspire a philosophical focus on reducing dependence on care providers by self-care training/instruction that guides individuals to use self-care exercises based on how they are feeling – physically, emotionally, mentally, and spiritually [36]. Interested readers are encouraged to try the Japanese exercises in self-care found at the end of the chapter. There is also an exercise that supports harmony of the spine and related functions. Jin Shin Jyutsu self-care is taught around the world by self-care instructors [36] and can be found on CD-ROM [33].

University of Wisconsin's Health Emotions Research Institute is using fMRI and other means to scientifically determine how positive emotions influence our health. Self- awareness, self-study, and self-care methods that work with emotions potentially can provide an economic and effective resource for the prevention of problems relating to individual health in schools, workplaces, and homes.

5. Conclusions

Future progress in solving some of the most pressing issues in healthcare will come by innovation and adaptation of ideas and methods that work. Healthcare access (especially preventative care) for a large number of uninsured, shortage of nurses, and the rising cost of healthcare in an aging population explosion are among just a few of the reasons to consider using global medical technology along side high-technology. Self-care education and meditation training are comparatively cheap ways of reducing the current pressures on our medical systems in the United States. By appropriate and thorough examination of the ways ancient soft technology works, we can maintain levels of standards in care in a cost-conscious healthcare environment. The addition of practices such as mindfulness meditation and self-care acupressure to our medicine cabinets is working to reduce numbers of hospital days, side effects and improve quality of life. Awareness of healthcare culture, confidence in the methods through scientific scrutiny and an openness to what works may not only work to save our healthcare system but the same methods for self-awareness for health also promise to reduce violence in schools, homes, workplaces, and public spaces.

Appendix A

JIN SHIN JYUTSU SELF-CARE EXERCISE

Figure 4 illustrates a self-care exercise called the "Main Central" for harmonizing spine functions as perceived in the Japanese healing art known as Jin Shin Jyutsu physio philosophy [36]. As prevention or maintenance, this exercise may be done upon waking, and/or before retiring at night. Use pillows as necessary for comfort. It may also be used as needed when working with health projects. It usually takes about 20 minutes when done properly, but may be interrupted and resumed without difficulty or loss of benefit. As this exercise proceeds, it is useful to visualize the breath coming up the back as you inhale, and down the front as you exhale. Figure 4a shows the physical locations for hands. Figure 4b gives directions for six hand positions referenced in Fig. 4a. Fingertips are often used, but palms, back of hands, or entire hand can also be used. It is important to be comfortable during the application of the exercise, avoiding noise, drafts, etc. Quiet music may be useful if you have trouble relaxing.

> **Step 1:** Place the fingers of the right hand on the top of the head (where they will remain until step 6). Place the fingers of the left hand on your forehead between your eyebrows. Hold for 2 to 5 minutes or until the pulses you feel at your fingertips synchronize with each other.

> **Step 2:** Now move the left fingertips to the tip of the nose. Hold them there for 2 to 5 minutes, or until the pulses synchronize.

> **Step 3:** Move the left fingertips to your sternum (center of your chest between your breasts). Stay there for 2 to 5 minutes, or until the pulses synchronize.

> **Step 4:** Move your fingers to the base of your sternum (center of where your ribs start, above the stomach). Hold them there for 2 to 5 minutes, or until the pulses synchronize.

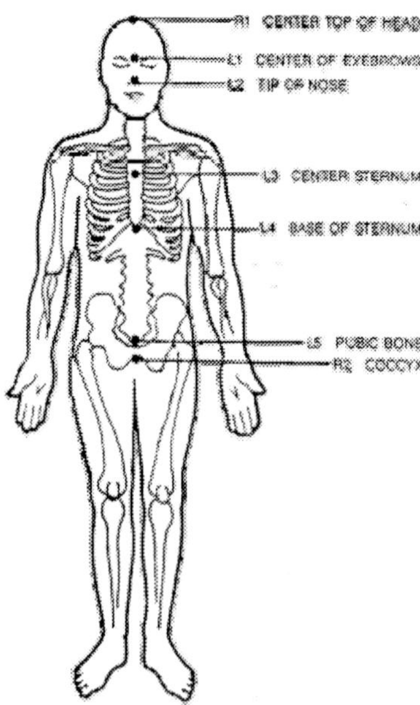

Figure 4a. Diagram shows hand positions used to administer self-care described in Fig. 4b. R1 refers to Right Hand position in Step 1. L1 is the Left Hand position in Step 1, L2 is the Left Hand position in Step 2, and so on. Source: Jin Shin Jyutsu Insitute [36].

Step 5: Move your fingers to the top of your pubic bone (above the genitals, center). Stay there for 2 to 5 minutes, or until the pulses synchronize.

Step 6: Keep your left fingertips in place and move your right fingertips to cover your coccyx (tailbone). Hold for 2 to 5 minutes or until the pulses you feel at your fingertips synchronize with each other.

Notes: The right hand remains on the top of the head while the left hand moves down the body until the final step. The practice is typically performed while lying flat, using pillows as necessary to maintain comfort. General instruction regarding the breath during the self-care practice is to envision the breath inhaling up the back of the spine/body and exhaling down the front of the spine/body.

Figure 4b. Gives the directions for a self care "recipe". There are six steps that move the hands according to descriptions below and follow the illustration in Figure 4a.

References

[1] Future of Health Technology Summits 1996–2002, www.fhti.org.
[2] National Institute of Health, www.nih.gov.
[3] The National Academies Institute of Medicine, www.iom.edu.
[4] Bushko, R., Defining Future of Health Technology: Biomechatronics, in *Future of Health Technology*, Renata Bushko, ed., IOS Press, Amsterdam, 2002.
[5] Mason, C. and Lieberman, H., Intelligent Agent Software for Medicine, in *Future of Health Technology*, Renata Bushko, ed., IOS Press, Amsterdam, 2002.
[6] Piburne, S. and Pell, C., The Dalai Lama a Policy of Kindness: An Anthology of Writings by and About the Dalai Lama/Winner of the Nobel Peace Prize Snow Lion Publications, Ithaca, New York, 1993.

[7] Mason, C., "Reduction in Recovery Time and Side Effects of Stem Cell Transplant Patients Using Physio-philosophy," in Psychoneuroimmunology Research Society Conference, 2003, www.pnirs.org.

[8] V.A. Barnes et al., *Proceedings of the 11th International Interdisciplinary Conference on Hypertension in Blacks,* New Orleans, LA, 1996.

[9] Norris, K., Stress Reduction in the Prevention and Treatment of Cardiovascular Disease in High Risk Minority Populations, presentation at The Congressional Prevention Coalition on Health Care for Minority Populations: Prevention of Hypertension and Heart Disease, on June 3, 1999.

[10] Herbert Benson, http://www.mbmi.org/.

[11] Center for Mindfulness, University of Massachusetts Medical School, www.umassmed.edu/cfm/.

[12] International Tibetan Qigong Association, www.tibetanqigong.org.

[13] http://www.stanfordhospital.com/clinicsmedServices/clinics/complementaryMedicine/index.html, Stanford Center for Integrative Medicine.

[14] www.columbiasurgery.org/divisions/cardiac/staff_oz.html,Columbia University Surgery Center.

[15] http://nccam.nih.gov/clinicaltrials/, National Institute of Health, National Center for Complimentary and Alternative Medicine.

[16] Gollub R.L., Hui K.K.S., Stefano G.B. Acupuncture pain management coupled to immune stimulation. Acta Pharmacologica Sinica. 20(9):769–777, 1999.

[17] Harvard Medical School Neuroimaging Lab, www.mgh.harvard.edu/depts/neuroimaging/gollublab.

[18] Lazar, S., http://www.mgh.harvard.edu/depts/neuroimaging/gollublab/meditation.html.

[19] Lazar, S.W., Bush, G., Gollub R.L., Fricchione, G.L., Khalsa, G., Benson, H. (2000) Functional Brain Mapping of the Relaxation Response and Meditation. NeuroReport. 11:1581–1585.

[20] Benson H., Beary J., Carol M. The relaxation response. *Psychiatry.* 1974; 37:37–46.

[21] Benson H., Greenwood M.M., Klemchuk H. The relaxation response: Psychophysiologic aspects and clinical applications. *International Journal of Psychiatry in Medicine.* 1975; 6:87–98.

[22] Benson H. Your innate asset for combating stress. *Harvard Business Review.* 1974; 52:49–60.

[23] A Public Repository of Peer Reviewed fMRI studies and their underlying data, National Science Foundation, W.M. Keck Foundation, National Institute of Mental Health, Sun Center for Excellance for Neuroscience, www.fmridc.org.

[24] www.fmri.org Columbia University Functional MRI Research Center.

[25] www.functionalmri.org.

[26] www.brainmapping.org, UCLA Brain Mapping Center.

[27] http://www.mgh.harvard.edu/depts/neuroimaging/gollublab/meditation.html.

[28] http://tezpur.keck.waisman.wisc.edu/ W.M. Keck Laboratory for Functional Brain Imaging and Behavior.

[29] http://www.fmrib.ox.ac.uk/fmri_intro/ Oxford University's Introduction to fMRI.

[30] Health Emotions Research Institute, Scientifically Determining How Emotions Influence Health, University of Wisconsin, www.healthemotions.org.

[31] Complimentary and Alternative Medicine Program at Stanford, http://camps.stanford.edu.

[32] Allison T.G., Williams D.E., Miller T.D., Patten C.A., Bailey K.R., Squires R.W., Gau G.T. Medical and Economic Costs of Psychologic Distress in Patients With Coronary Artery Disease. *Mayo Clinic Procedures.* 1995; 70:734–742.

[33] Mason, C., Integrating Self-Care Into Your Own Recovery, www.21stcenturymed.org.

[34] Sempell, P., Integrating The Healing Art of Jin Shin Jyutsu Into Western and Surgical Practice, San Francisco Medicine, June/July, 2000.

[35] http://www.marin-oncology.com/.

[36] Jin Shin Jyutsu Institute, www.jinshinjyutsu.com.

[37] http://www.mgh.harvard.edu/depts/neuroimaging/gollublab/acupuncture.html.

[38] Newton, V., Healing Energy, Master Zi Sheng Wang and Tibetan Buddist Qigong, China Books and Periodicals, Inc., San Francisco, California, 2000.

Shaping a Healthy Future:
Megabyte, Not Mega Bite!

Teresita B. HERNÁNDEZ, Ph.D.
President, Health Technomics, Inc, Annandale, VA, USA

Abstract. The globalization of obesity is not a myth. Scientific and technologic advances have increased food production and availability while decreasing demand for physical activity. These developments, in turn, have contributed to peoples' cognitive and behavioral relationship with food selection and consumption. The more you see, the more you want. Although disparities in food distribution and personal economics still exist, the problem of over consumption is becoming widespread among low income groups in developed countries and among the high income in developing countries. The development of innovative technologies such as described in this chapter may help ebb the tide of obesity and improve the global future of health.

1. The Obesity Problem—a Global Concern

The 21st century ushered in a public health concern that had had a low profile until the popular media gained insight into the increasing prevalence of overweight and obesity among the US population. The adage "big is beautiful" has lost its attraction; instead the term "obesity epidemic"[1] has been added to the public health vocabulary.

The 2003 report of World Health Organization (WHO) on Diet, Nutrition and the Prevention of Chronic Diseases[2] provides the global statistics that show changes over the past four decades in food supply and consumption, lifestyle, and the prevalence of chronic diseases that could be associated with obesity. Worldwide food availability expressed as kilocalories per capita per day increased from 2358 in the mid 1960's to 2803 in the late 1990's. Among developing countries, the increase was from 2054 to 2681 over the same period; the increase was specially pronounced in East Asia where the food energy supply increased by almost 1000 kilocalories per capita per day. There is no question that with food availability and rising income, obesity has now become a major concern in both developing and highly developed countries.

2. Part of the Problem—Technology

Technology has increased food production and has made packaging and transportation faster and easier. Indeed, there is an economic research report that concludes that 40% of the weight gain of the U.S. population in the past two decades may be explained by lower food prices due to agricultural innovations, and 60% may be due to a decline in physical activity because of technological innovations in the home and in the workplace.[3] An immediate consequence of technological innovations in agriculture and the food industry is the "super-sizing" of foods and beverages served in restaurants, fast food stores and food courts. Sizes of containers of ready-to-eat snacks and sweetened drinks have also been enlarged.[4,5]

If consumers were conscious of how technology has affected their lifestyle, if they knew what to do about it, and if they recognized that weight gain has a large behavioral component, then the obesity epidemic might have been prevented. Research on the increase in portion sizes of food and beverage consumed by the U.S. population over the past two decades supports the economic research findings. This is especially true for energy-dense but nutrient-deficient foods and beverages such as salty snacks, beer, and sweetened carbonated drinks.[6,7] Between 1989 and 1996, data from two independent national surveys (NHANES and CSFII) show mean portion intake of cola-type soft drink (excluding sugar-free, or low-calorie) increased from 11.6 to 14.78 fluid ounces for all users; at the 95th percentile, the change is from 18 fluid ounces in 1989–91 to 35 fluid ounces in 1994–1996.[8]

3. Providing a Solution with Technology

With creative, science-based instructional and behavioral modification tools, and the willingness of health professionals to maximize the use of such tools, technology can empower individuals in fighting obesity. As the title of this Chapter implies, the focus is on using computer technology for portion size definition and control. Within the limits of this chapter, there is no intent to address the problem of obesity in its entirety. The aim is to emphasize the need for recognizing the difference between food exposure (serving) and personal behavior or choice (portion), and further illustrate the difference between a health-based serving size and a market-based serving size. These concepts—serving versus portion, and health-based versus market-based—are not always explicit, even in many of our health and nutrition messages and have therefore become a source of confusion for the public.

There was a time when parents admonished their children at mealtime "Take only what you can eat" followed by "Eat everything on your plate." In this scenario, serving equaled portion. However, especially in this country, the abundance of the food supply and the busy lifestyle that has led to the growth of the "grab and go" food industry have made traditional meal preparation and serving almost obsolete. USDA reports that the frequency of dining out rose from sixteen percent of all meals and snacks in 1977–78 to twenty seven percent in 1995.[9] In 1970, the food-away-from-home sector captured about a quarter of total food spending and in 1995, about forty percent of the food budget was spent on food away from home.[10] These developments have also changed the meaning of "small", "medium" and "large" in relation to serving sizes.

A small informal survey that we conducted recently indicated that most (about ninety percent) dietitians and nutrition students use the terms serving and portion synonymously. This is highly influenced by a serving size defined in reference to the Diabetic Exchange, the Food Guide Pyramid, and sometimes the Nutrition Facts Label. On the other hand, consumers are continually exposed to serving sizes in the marketplace. These sizes get bigger and bigger in response to consumers' concept of "value", meaning "more for your money". The food industry uses this concept when introducing a new product or promoting sales. The opening of a new "burrito" restaurant in a college town in Maryland advertised its main attraction as huge (four-inch diameter) rolls! A famous cookie maker sends mail advertisement for its nine-inch cookie!

4. What This Chapter Is All About

This Chapter offers a new framework for defining serving size from two perspectives—one health-based, and the other, market-based. Health-based refers to serving sizes as defined

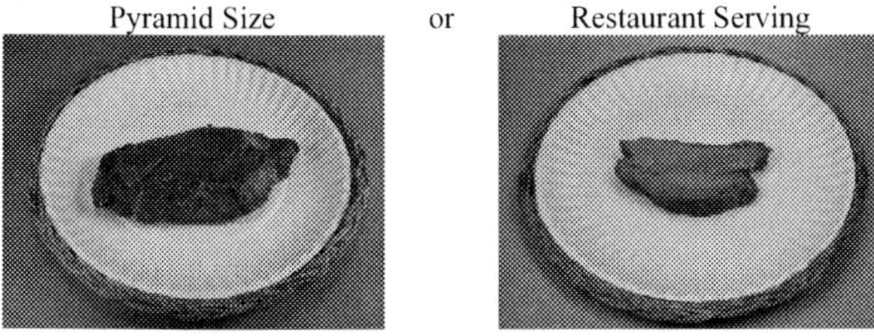

Figure 1. *Portion Basics:* Your Choice.

according to the Diabetic Exchange, the Food Guide Pyramid, and the Nutrition Facts Label guidelines. Market-based refers to single serving sizes encountered at grocery and convenience stores, at fast food counters, and in diners and full-service restaurants. It is important to note that serving size for a given food item varies even among the health-based references. For example, a serving size for orange juice is 4 fluid ounces in the American Diabetes Association's (ADA) Exchange List for Meal Planning, 6 fluid ounces in the US Department of Agriculture's (USDA) Food Guide Pyramid, and 8 fluid ounces in the Food and Drug Administration's (FDA) Nutrition Facts Label guidelines. However, it is even more important to note the large difference between the health-based and the market-based serving sizes. For example, the food guide pyramid size for steak is 2 to 3 ounces cooked (100g raw), whereas a restaurant serving size could be 3 to 4 times as large (see Fig. 1). The pyramid size for muffin is 1 ounce while muffins served at airports or sold in bakeries weigh about 5 ounces. And among foods for which pyramid servings are not clearly defined, for example, soft drinks, "super-sizing" of containers is the growing trend. As part of our project to develop an interactive desktop reference for serving sizes, we made many trips to fast food places, kiosks, food courts, and other convenience stores. This is a sampling of what we found among containers for soft drinks: the old 8 ounce "Dixie" cup is now called "kiddies"; a 16 ounce cup is "regular" or "medium"; 22–24 is "large", "Big Gulp" is 32, "Magnum" is 44, and "Double Gulp" is 64 fluid ounces. And if the container is filled to the brim, these volumes can increase by another 2–4 fluid ounces. Unfortunately, there is no requirement to label the capacity of containers. If shown, it usually appears encoded at the bottom of the cup. So if you want to know how much you had, you either have to finish the contents or spill it!

Keeping track of how much one eats and drinks is a difficult task. Even among professionals who are trained in food science and nutrition, few, if any, can accurately slice a 3 oz piece of meat or pour 8 fluid oz of juice without measurement tools. In the real world of food consumption, we must first acknowledge that the cognitive skills used in estimating sizes and amounts are not simple skills. They are brain functions—perceptual, mathematical, memory storage and retrieval—that differ from individual to individual. The degree to which these skills contribute to the accuracy of quantitative estimates is an area of research that we have only begun to address systematically. No professional group to date has defined an acceptable error rate in food measurement. Previous studies suggest that using visual portioning anchors tended to result in overestimation more frequently than underestimation for all types of food—solid, amorphous, or liquid—when estimation is done in real time or short-term recall.[11,12,13] In an attempt to establish a basis for a rational expectation of accuracy in portion estimation, our recently completed research suggests that cognitive adaptation to food exposure is a dominant influence in how consumers perceive portion sizes.[14,15]

Beyond these cognitive issues of measurement, scientists are beginning to document the effect of food exposure on personal consumption starting in early childhood.[16,17] To ebb the tide of obesity, it is important to explore the extent to which technology can assist as early in the formative years as possible. Our approach is to get both health professionals and the public to think visually, recognize the difference between health-based and market-based serving sizes, and make a distinction between serving (what you SEE, in other words, exposure) and portion (what you PARTAKE, in other words, personal behavior or choice). We have developed visual tools to promote this common reference for communication. The Health Technomics Computer-based Portion Anchors (HTCPA) is one of these tools.

5. The Health Technomics Computer-Based Portion Anchors (HTCPA)[18]

The Health Technomics Computer-based Portion Anchors (HTCPA) is a suite of programs that displays photographs of about 300 typical foods and 100 food and beverage containers commonly used in the U.S. Employing digital photography and a programming language that has both computational and pictorial database management capabilities, a pictorial database of at least two sizes for each food or container was created. Food was weighed and measured immediately before photographing. Foods with inedible parts, such as peel or bone, were again weighed and measured after photographing to obtain the edible portion weight. Capacity of containers was measured to the top and to about two centimeters from the top.

To communicate a health-based serving, a photograph of the USDA pyramid serving size for selected foods in each of the five food groups is available for display in the program. A universally recognized secondary anchor, a nine-inch paper plate serves to reinforce size perception without having to use a ruler. Weights, dimensions, and volume, where applicable, are available for each photograph in both English and Metric systems.

Photographs were taken under standardized studio settings. To maintain constant camera position for a specific view, several measurements were made for: a) the camera angle, b) position of the contextual anchor, and c) the tripod position. The product is: *testable, portable, upgradeable*, and *adaptable for multiple uses*.

HTCPA can be used for education and counseling, as measurement aids for dietary assessment, and for conducting cognitive research. *Portion Basics,* is the primary program for use in educational settings, or as a stand-alone visual aid during dietary assessment. For purposes of education or nutritional counseling, the teacher/student/client can browse the list of foods or containers and choose an item to view in two or more sizes. For foods, weights and measures can be displayed on demand. For container, dimensions and volume capacity can be displayed on demand. For some foods, there is also a picture of pyramid size serving for comparison with market servings as illustrated for steak below.

The second program, *Portion Counts,* is the clinical version for use in weight management, diet management in diabetes, or meal planning for heart healthy meals. *Portion Counts* allows the user to view the calories, carbohydrates, protein, fat, cholesterol and fiber content of each food displayed. It serves not only as a counseling tool, but can also provide reinforcement when installed on the client's computer. Figure 2 shows a computer screen from this program.

The third and most comprehensive program, *Portion Plus*, has all the functions of Portion Basics and Portion Counts, plus additional functions for data collection, storage, and retrieval. Thus, beyond educational and clinical uses, the program can serve as a tool for cognitive research in portion size estimation. For cognitive research, the user compares the size or amount of an actual serving of food placed beside the computer with what is displayed on the screen. For research on the effect of memory on portion size estimation, or for use as a measurement aid in dietary assessment, the user compares the size or amount of food eaten at an earlier time with what is displayed on the screen. Amount in every case can be expressed as a fraction or multiple of the amount shown on the screen. A portion estimation screen in Portion Plus is shown in Fig. 3.

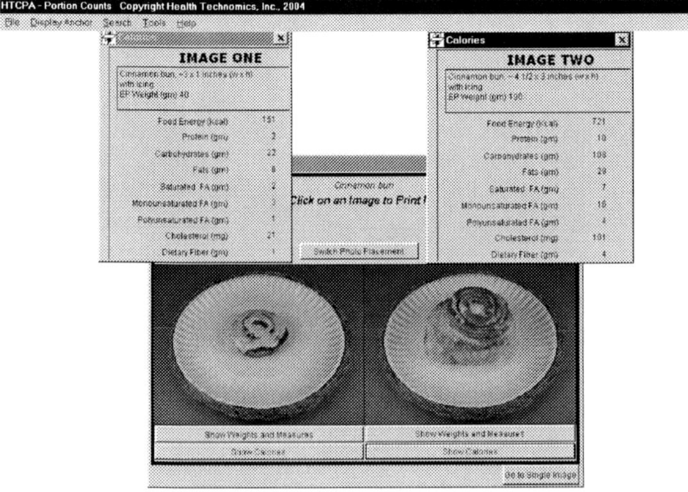

Figure 2. *Portion Counts*: When Calories Matter.

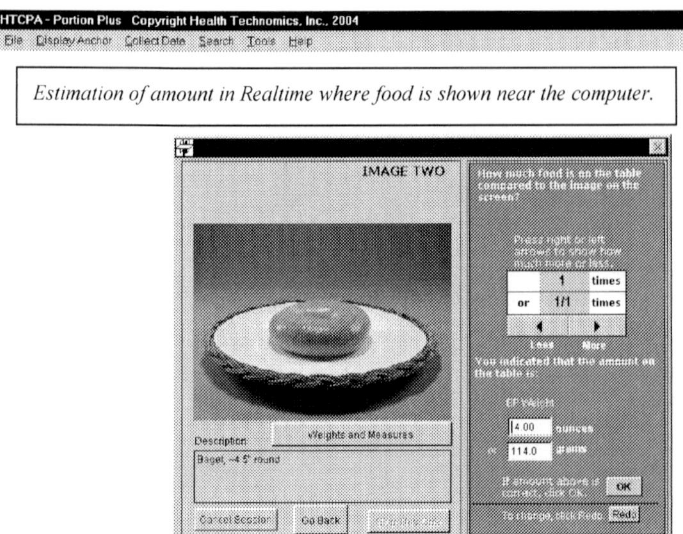

Figure 3. *Portion Plus:* Size Estimation.

6. Conclusion

While the problem of obesity and the phenomenon of "super-sizing" have become political as well as legal pursuits, and have created media frenzy, it is important for scientists to continue basic and applied research on this topic. There is still a long way to go in improving the quantitative aspects of portion size estimation and dietary assessment methods. But with a multidisciplinary approach and the use of appropriate technology to address the cognitive and behavioral issues in quantifying food intake, I am confident that we are on the right track in shaping a healthy future, megabyte by megabyte, not mega bite!

Acknowledgments

Small Business Innovation Research grants from the USDA made HTCPA development and testing possible. Co-developers are D. Kuehn for photography, K. Rubotzky, programming, and L. Wilder for content development and alpha test. Consumer testing at the University of Maryland was coordinated by P. Moser-Veillon and C. Wang, and at Tennessee State University by S. Godwin and C. Thompson. Dietitians in the Washington DC metropolitan area conducted the beta testing for operability and usability.

References

[1] Obesity in Science, Special Issue, February 7, 2003.

[2] Diet, Nutrition and the Prevention of Chronic Diseases, Technical Report Series 916, WHO, Geneva, 2003.

[3] Lakdawalla, D. and Philipson, T., The Growth of Obesity and Technological Change: A Theoretical and Empirical Examination, National Bureau of Economic Research Working Paper No. W8946, May, 2002.

[4] Hernández T., Kim K., Wilder L., and Sebrechts M., Serving versus Portion: Is there a difference? Does it matter? Fourth International Conference on Dietary Assessment, Tucson, AZ, September, 2000.

[5] Young, L., and Nestle, M. The Contribution of Expanding Portion Sizes to the US Obesity Epidemic, Am J Public Health. 2002; 92:246–249.

[6] Neilsen, S. and Popkin, B. Patterns and Trends in Food Portion Sizes, JAMA. 2003; 289:450–453.

[7] Smicklas-Wright, H. et al., Foods Commonly Eaten in the United States, 1989–1991 and 1994–1996: Are portion sizes changing? J. Am. Diet. Assoc. 2003; 103:41–47.

[8] Hernández, T. "Tracking intake of Core Food- cola carbonated beverage, 1989–1996", in Use of the Core Food Model to Estimate Mineral Intakes, J. Food Composition and Analysis. 2001, 14:305–307.

[9] Lin, Biing-Hwan, Frazĩo, Elizabeth and Guthrie, Joanne, Away-From-Home Foods Increasingly Important to Quality of American Diet. Food and Rural Economics Division, Economic Research Service, U.S. Department of Agriculture, Food and Drug Administration, U.S. Department of Health and Human Services. Agriculture Information Bulletin No. 749.

[10] Putnam J., and J. Allshouse, Food Consumption, Prices, and Expenditures, U.S.D.A., Econ. Res. Serv., SB-928, April 1996.

[11] Chambers E., McGuire B., Godwin S., Edwards E. Cognitive Methods, CDC, DHHS Working Paper Series No. 27, 1999.

[12] Hernández T., Kim K., Wilder L., Godwin S., and Sebrechts M. Computer based anchors and portion size estimation, Fourth International Conference on Dietary Assessment, Tucson, AZ, September 2000.

[13] Knous, B. et al., Grain-based foods portion size recall compared to portion photo selection, FASEB, San Diego, CA, April, 2003.

[14] Hernández T., Wilder L., Moser-Veillon P., Godwin S., Thompson C., and Wang C. Cognitive Adaptation and Portion Size Estimation: Is there a connection? Experimental Biology 2004, Washington, DC. April 18, 2004.

[15] Hernández T., Wilder L., Kuehn D., and Rubotsky K., Moser-Veillon P., Godwin S., Thompson C., and Wang C. Portion Size Estimation and Expectation of Accuracy, 28th National Nutrient Data Conference, Iowa City, IA, June 24, 2004; Submitted for publication, J. Food Composition and Analysis, July, 2004.

[16] Fisher, J.O., Rolls, B. and Birch, L. Children's bite size and intake of an entrée are greater with large portions than with age-appropriate or self-selected portions. Am J Clin Nutr 2003; 77:1164–70.

[17] Rolls B., Engell D., Birch L., Serving portion size influences 5-year old but not 3-year old children's food intakes. J Am Diet Assoc 2000; 100:232–4.

[18] Hernández T., Wilder L., Kuehn D., and Rubotsky K., Portion Perception: The Missing Link. Fifth International Food Data Conference/National Nutrient Databank Conference, Washington, DC, July 1, 2003.

Future of Intelligent and Extelligent Health Environment
R.G. Bushko (Ed.)
IOS Press, 2005

Digital Literacy in a Landscape of Data:
A Plea for a Broader Definition for
Citizens and Patients

Jean A. WOOLDRIDGE, M.P.H.
Principal, St. Cloud Communications, Bellevue, WA, &
Research Affiliate, Fred Hutchinson Cancer Research Center, Seattle, WA, USA

Abstract. The term 'digital literacy' is taking on a broader definition and greater urgency, as ubiquitous computing becomes a reality, and individuals and communities find their bodies and actions creating an exuberant wellspring of rich, complex data. These biological and sociological data can be ignored, used alone or shared with others for various reasons – for personal or social good or ill. Although strategies to protect our data from commercial, criminal, and governmental access are already being debated daily in the media, this paper is a brief plea for why we need to expand our concerns beyond the current financial and medical record security issues.

1. Introduction

There is a profoundly new conversation going on. Or, perhaps it is an ancient one, which we are now just joining. The language of that conversation is intimate, complex, and critical for the future of our individual bodies, our communities, and our planet.

This is a brief reflection on digital literacy – the language of the new conversation – and a plea to expand its current definition to the very broadest possible, as new roles emerge for citizens and for patients.

We are all citizens. We are all patients. We all seek the health of our families, our communities, our regions, nations, and our world. Because of technology, those two roles are converging and gaining more importance. We are increasingly aware of how connected we are all to each other through our technology – for peril, and for promise.

Technology (airplanes) spread SARS into an epidemic and showed us how quickly we affect each other's health across the globe. Technology (cell phones, DNA analysis, email) also showed us how quickly we worked together to contain the epidemic.

Citizens and patients rely on their government and healthcare systems to keep them safe and healthy, and to enable them to prosper and contribute to society. The more informed the citizen and the patient, the better the choices each can make. But many current ideas about digital literacy are already dangerously outmoded.

Most digital literacy discussions still focus on desktop standards and professional competence certifications driving workforce development for economic parity on the global stage. This is important but falls far short. Digital literacy needs to blend with many other kinds of literacy, including security literacy, in ways we haven't imagined before. Researchers and thought leaders, such as Michael D. McDonald of Georgetown University in the U.S., and Yoram Eshet of Tel Hai Academic College in Israel, are boldly illuminating these new landscapes.

2. Transparency and Boundaries

What would it mean to be literate, not in the conventional ways, but literate and aware about all the ways in which data "live" and in how we access, contain, and use it? What binoculars do we need for looking beyond the obvious Internet data-tracking of our current activities? Who or what are our border guards? How do they ensure that our data is being accessed and used with our knowledge, and to uses we approve of?

Think upon this:

- Our lives, privately and collectively, are being lived in a landscape of increasingly transparent data fountains. The data has always been there, we simply haven't had access to it before in such quantitative and qualitative ways. The data constantly being produced by our bodies, our communal actions, and the geography of our planet, is being broadcast and even amplified in ways never experienced before. Our bodies are talking to us through devices like smart shirts, wearables, smart homes, and monitoring sensors. Our communities are talking to us through online polls, GIS mapping of urban effects, and simulations. Our planet is talking to us through time-layered satellite photos of environmental degradation or redemption. (And, of course, our devices are all talking to each other.... particularly cellphones emboldened with photos, video, and GPS.)
- Natural boundaries are collapsing. In response, we need to continually redraw them – for other people and for things. RFID tags in consumer goods need killer switches so that our activities won't be tracked. Fabrics that can deliver vitamin C, antifungal agents, or nutrients for the endurance runner need to be clearly labeled for the right consumer. Medical monitoring data remotely sent to doctors from the homes of heart disease patients need to be protected. The federal medical data that use HIPPA law, need double guarding – protecting the privacy of individuals while avoiding unnecessarily delays of life-saving information in emergencies. In April, 2003, the state of Hawai'i in the U.S. passed a resolution protecting the individual liberties of its citizens and calling for the repeal of the most egregious provision of the USA Patriot Act, rushed through Congress in the aftermath of the 9/11 attacks. And data warehousing operations of marketers and governments need to have secure aggregation and privacy tools. As we've seen in 2004 and 2005, those tools are far from being in widespread use.
- Technological capability to monitor citizen actions and physiology for marketing or government purposes is clearly a two-edged sword with great potential for unintended consequences. Neuroimaging revealing the lives of our brains – already used in neuromarketing by firms that claim functional MRIs and other technologies can track direct physiological responses to new products and bypass the gender and SES biases in traditional focus group market research – is migrating from the lab to the marketplace and to the clinic. This is our most private data. This is not our credit card purchase log or our social security number, alarming as that is. This is the increasingly sophisticated record of how our *brains* work. Our most intimate data. Diagnostic, predictive, and possibly discriminating, data.

3. From "Dumb Environment" to "Intelligent and Aware"

Think upon this:

- As laypersons and scientists gain new ways to understand the consequences of individual health choices, the spread of epidemics, the correlations of economics and social violence, and changing weather patterns and their effects on economic conditions, technology is flattening the asymmetries in power and access to information.

- Individuals will manage their own health and chronic diseases, as they are managing their finances and retirement planning, as individuals are managing their legal affairs, and as private pilots are managing their flights. People will understand their genetic profiles, access their bodies' data, interpret risks, and plan actions, by using technologies in home lab kits, biosensors, simulations, cognitive style filters, and online information sources.

- Streams of technologies from chronic disease, sports medicine, the military, video-games, and genomics, are poised to add great value to the river of consumer health in the next three to ten years. Intel's Proactive Health Research and the Center for Future Health at the University of Rochester, are exploring the "smart medical home." VivoMetrics is developing "smart shirts" on 20+ physiological indicators. BodyMedia's wearable body monitoring products and technologies track many values beyond just the routine athletic ones and its SenseWear Patch is on display at the Cooper-Hewett Museum's "technical textile" exhibit in the fall of 2005. Prostate cancer patients at *CancerFacts.com,* are running "what if" simulations with various lab values to see if their treatments – and survival rates – can change. Patient we-blogs are bringing instant feedback to clinical trials and hospitals. Just as Smart Money's "Map of the Market" shows almost realtime U.S. stock market data changes, and ManyOne's new search engine and The Brain's lateral knowledge management show data relationships for planetary and corporate information, knowledge management graphic and haptic interfaces, many drawn from the video-game industry and the military, will allow us to absorb complex data and produce decision scenarios in synergy with our natural individual learning styles.

- Individuals, communities and global groups are sharing data from sensor mote networks embedded in sensitive ecologies for tracking changes. As the environment becomes alive and aware, generating its own data and interacting with other "things" as well as people, this "aware landscape" will be populated by various products: biosensors to collect data on weather, physiology, or the presence of chemicals, RFID chips that can track the position of every runner in the Boston marathon, or the journey of a fleece vest through distribution to point of sale, visualization graphic interfaces to display realtime data in meaningful ways to different audiences, from laymen to professionals, smart shirts and smart homes that can deliver nutrients and monitor activities of Alzheimer patients, robots that can assist elder people living alone or search through earthquake rubble for victims, wireless technologies that work in large "conscious clouds" with RFID chips embedded in everyday objects, groupware which fosters collaboration across nations and professions, affective and persuasive computing which creates machines that can recognize and respond to human emotions, and simulations for training and solving complex global challenges, or with insilico biology for more efficient clinical trials. The Semantic web will ensure that every piece of data has embedded metatags of information which can efficiently gather, analyze and present information to humans or machines or intelligent agents in ways we can only dream of now.

Mark Anderson vividly describes this future in his April, 2003, Strategic News Service letter:

> *"...I think it is difficult for people to conceive of an environment which is, of itself, intelligent and aware. We are quite used to the opposite: a "dumb" environment, in which we are safe and secure, where it takes almost superhuman effort and lots of money to get information in and out from wherever we might be.*

> *Who can imagine the opposite: an environment in which getting information in and out is almost omnipresent, and almost free? Even more shocking: one in which cameras and sensors are also ubiquitous, and in which embedded Radio Frequency IDs are, like their sensors, everywhere? ...*
>
> *The space around you is no longer a buffer, but is a conductor. For the first time in the history of the planet, you will not be hidden by your environment, but connected by it."* [1]

4. Voices for Broader Definitions

Fortunately there are voices already calling for a broader definition of digital literacy:

- Rima Rudd at the Harvard Health Literacy Studies project often invokes citizenship and rights as the basis for her health literacy work.
- The "21st Century Literacy Summit" held in March of 2002 in Berlin, Germany, sponsored by The Bertelsmann Foundation and the AOL Time Warner Foundation erected a new and broader tent for discussions – one closer to what is needed. It sought "to promote a transatlantic dialogue of decision-makers from government, business and academia" to address issues of technologies as catalysts for society as it shifts from industrial models to knowledge-based ones. The white paper presented on the global development of digital literacy skills defined four key literacies:
  - Technology Literacy: The ability to use new media such as the Internet to access and communicate information effectively.
  - Information Literacy: The ability to gather, organize and evaluate information, and to form valid opinions based on the results.
  - Media Creativity: The growing capacity of citizens everywhere to produce and distribute content to audiences of all sizes.
  - Global Literacy: Understanding the interdependence among people and nations and having the ability to interact and collaborate successfully across cultures.
  - Literacy with Responsibility: The competence to consider the social consequences of media from the standpoint of safety, privacy and other issues." (21st Century Literacy Summit, 2002.)
- Researcher Yoram Eshet at Tel Hai Academic College in Israel, who has proposed a "lateral literacy" that enables learners to build knowledge from non-linear hypertextual navigation through knowledge domains. Eshet asks us to consider that:

  > *"Digital literacy involves more than the mere ability to use software or operate a digital device; it includes a large variety of complex cognitive, motor, sociological, and emotional skills, which users need in order to function effectively in digital environments. The tasks required in this context include, for example, "reading" instructions from graphical displays in user interfaces; utilizing digital reproduction to create new, meaningful materials from existing ones; constructing knowledge from a nonlinear, hypertextual navigation; evaluating the quality and validity of information; and have a mature and realistic understanding of the "rules" that prevail in the cyberspace."* [2]

Just coming into the conversation, as more clinical and home-based uses of neuroimaging emerge, will be the ability to use technology to enhance and modify an individual's genetically- and environmentally-determined, thinking patterns and brain physiology.

The "aware environment" being constructed by the spread of sensor and wireless technologies, and transcranial electromagnetic stimulation, will demand the kind of richly associative thinking which Eshet proposes. With neurobiology mapping circadian rhythms and fMRIs and other imaging technologies giving unprecedented insight into how our brain works, developing technologies to capture how our thinking changes with technology, is an important area for thinking about how digital literacy will evolve.

5. Putting the Public in "Public Policy" and "Public Health"

Think upon this:

- As data becomes transparent to all stakeholders and all learning styles, and dialogue becomes "democratized", the word "public" takes up new residence in the terms "public policy" and "public health".
- Mike McDonald, of Global Health Initiatives and Georgetown University, envisions, in his still prescient 1995 dissertation, a layer to the national health information infrastructure, which would provide bridges to information resources for everyone from the schoolchild to the government policymaker:

  "Where datasets are available and understood, decision-makers – now including the engaged public – are beginning to utilize community health assessment algorithms within interdisciplinary community knowledge bases…that draw upon powerful simulation (models) and heuristic (rules for judgment) capabilities in order to participate and guide the evolution of their community."

  He continues, *"This new aspect of community governance through citizen participation, based upon an intimate knowledge of the socio-ecological factors, provides much greater understanding and participation by the people most affected by the problems at hand. There are a multiplicity of tools that aid the public in participating more fully in the process of governance, starting with their ability to visualize the nature and functioning of their community as well as mechanisms for identifying problems."* [3]

- In 2000, early steps to this vision were already being addressed in metric goals for the United States. Cynthia Bauer, at the U.S. Department of Health and Human Services' Office of Disease Prevention and Health Promotion, coordinates teams that monitor the progress of the nation in information technology for "Healthy People 2010". Part of their stated opportunities are in support of helping people to not only use existing information, but also to create tailored resources to manage personal health and to influence the health of their communities, as national and global health information infrastructures become integrated.

As technology illuminates social challenges, it helps us to make better choices, as patients and as citizens. It also holds us more accountable because the consequences of our choices are clearer.

So, how can we best participate in this "new" and ancient conversation in the land of data fountains?

Digital literacy. But a digital literacy that is broadly defined and inspires us to ask of ourselves – and our machines: How can we most wisely use the symbiotic stewardships we are forging with the machines we have created, for the good of the planet and our children's children?

References

[1] Anderson, M. (2003), April 30th Newsletter, Friday Harbor, WA, Strategic News Service, (www.tapsns. com).

[2] Eshet, Y. "Digital Literacy: A Conceptual Framework for Survival Skills in the Digital Era". Journal of Educational Multimedia and Hypermedia. 13 (1), pp. 93–106.

[3] McDonald, M., (1995), The Guiding Principle from "The Public Health Communications Toolbox: The role of the intelligent network and the sciences of complexity in advancing health and human prosperity", D.P.H. dissertation, University of California, Berkeley, 1995.

General References

Denning, P. and Metcalfe, R., Eds. (1997), "Beyond Calculation: the Next Fifty Years of Computing", Copernicus, Springer-Verlag, NY, Association for Computing Machinery.

Enriquez, J., (2001), "As the Future Catches You: How Genomics & Other Forces Are Changing Your Life, Work, Health & Wealth", NY, Crown Publishing.

Friere, P. (2003), "World Summit on the Information Society", February 2003 (http://main.edc.org/tours/literacy.asp).

Joy, B. (2000), "Why the Future Doesn't Need Us". In WIRED, Issue 8.04, April 2000, http://www.wired.com/wired/archive/8.04/joy.html.

MIT Media Lab, Health Special Interest Group, (2000), Cambridge, MA, http://www.mit.media.edu.

Wooldridge, J. (2002), "Our Wealth, Our Health – Bellwether Industries for Decision Support and Symbiotic Stewardships" in R. Bushko, *Future of Health Technology: Volume 80, Studies in Health Technology and Informatics*, (pp. 245–264), Amsterdam, The Netherlands, IOS Press (http://www.st-cloud.com).

"2003 World Telecommunication/ICT Indicators Meeting," (2003) the International Telecommunication Union, Geneva, Switzerland, January (www.intu.int/visions).

"21st Century Literacy Summit," (2002), The Bertelsmann Foundation and the AOL Time Warner Foundation, Berlin, Germany, March (www.21stcenturyliteracy.org/white/index.htm).

Other Resources

1) TED/MED3 Conference May 2003, www.tedmed.com. (Technology, Entertainment and Design/Medical) of Richard Saul Wurman, Information Architect. Detailed press reviews on emerging technology in public and private health; personal health dashboards.

2) Vivometric's SmartShirt, www.vivometrics.com, Continuous ambulatory monitoring products for physiologic data providing a "movie" of a patient's health, rather than a snapshot.

3) Intel's Proactive Health Research and Eric Dishman, www.intel.com.research. Use of sensor technology and the Semantic web to assist "aging-in-place". Multidisciplinary team led by ethnographic technologist from Paul Allen's Interval Lab.

4) NexCura's CancerProfiler technologies, www.nexcura.com. Decision support software featuring custom tailoring questionnaire linking patient preferences for quality of life to cancer disease stage and treatment recommendations, based upon peer-reviewed literature database.

5) Smart Money's Map of the Market, www.smartmoney.com. Unique graphic web interface of market data.

6) ManyOne, www.manyone.net. "… an intuitively organized, multimedia Web that will inform, educate, engage and involve people worldwide." Used by "a growing global alliance of researchers, scholars and experts…"

7) Strategic News Service by Mark Anderson, www.tapsns.com. Free one month newsletter subscription; May 2003 letter of Bill Pickard on "Ultimate Wi-Fi".

8) IHealthBeat by the California Health Care Foundation, www.ihealthbeat.org. Subscribers tailor e-newsletter to personal interests.

9) Conferenza Premium Reports, www.conferenza.com. Technology industry insider reports. $199/year for full; free for brief.

10) The Benton Foundation's Communications-Related Headlines, http://www.benton.org. Policy issues, many related to the digital divide. Free.

11) Harvard School of Public Health's Health Literacy Studies. www.hsph.harvard.edu/healthliteracy/links.html.

12) U.S. National Cancer Institute: www.cancer.gov. Usability research, treatment databases, and program planning for diffusion.
13) U.S. Department of Health and Human Services' "Healthy People 2010", www.healthypeople.gov. National prevention agenda to identify significant health threats and goals to reduce them.
14) National Resource Defense Council's BioGems, www.savebiogems.org. Citizen alert for endangered wilderness.
15) AACE (American Association for Computers in Education), www.aace.org. An "international, educational and professional not-for profit organization dedicated to the advancement of the knowledge, theory, and quality of learning and teaching at all levels with information technology."
16) FHTI (Future Health Technology Institute), www.fhti.org. "… focuses on key technologies and key challenges to the future of global healthcare to enhance health and lives."

Adaptive and Errorless Era – Adaptive Healthcare Process Management

Situated, Strategic, and AI-Enhanced Technology Introduction to Healthcare[1]

Renata G. BUSHKO, M.S.
Director, Future of Health Technology Institute, Hopkinton MA, USA

Abstract. We work hard on creating AI-wings for physicians to let them fly higher and faster in diagnosing patients – a task that physicians do not want to automate. What we do not work hard on is determining the ENVIRONMENT in which physicians' AI wings are supposed to function. It seems to be a job for social/business analysts that have their own separate kingdom. For the sake of all of us (potential patients!) social/business consultants and their methodologies should not be treated as a separate kingdom. The most urgent task is to achieve synergy between (1) AI/Fuzzy/Neural research, (2) Applied medical AI, (3) Social/Business research on medical institutions. We need this synergy in order to assure humanistic medical technology; technology flexible and sensitive enough to facilitate healthcare work while leaving space for human pride and creativity. In order to achieve humanistic technology, designers should consider the impact of technological breakthroughs on the organizations in which this technology will function and the nature of work of humans destined to use this technology. Situated (different for each organization), Strategic (based on an in-depth knowledge of Healthcare business), and AI-Enhanced (ended with a dynamic model) method for introducing technology to Healthcare allows identifying areas where technology can make medical work easier. Using this method before automating human work will get us closer to the ideal where there is no discontinuity between design and use of programs; where the technology matches users' needs perfectly – the world with humanistic technology and healthcare workers with AI-wings.

1. Is There a Cure for Diagnomania?

Diagnomania is an obsession with automating medical diagnosis while ignoring a real-world environment where diagnosis takes place. Medical AI research community suffers from diagnomania: it has been concentrating on the medical diagnosis for more than a decade despite of the fact that physicians do not want to automate it. Diagnomaniacs do not want to hear what an experienced neurosurgeon says: " I will never decide to operate on a patient based on a diagnosis of a machine." They ignore social setting of medical practice. Diagnomania, not physician's resistance to technology, is the reason that "the field of AI, which has attracted commercial attention recently as expert systems have been successfully implemented in industry has produced only a handful of narrowly focused commercial biomedical products [1]."

---

[1] Originally prepared for the Proceedings of the Workshop on the Medical Knowledge Representation, International Joint Conference of Artificial Intelligence, 8/1991, Sydney, Australia.

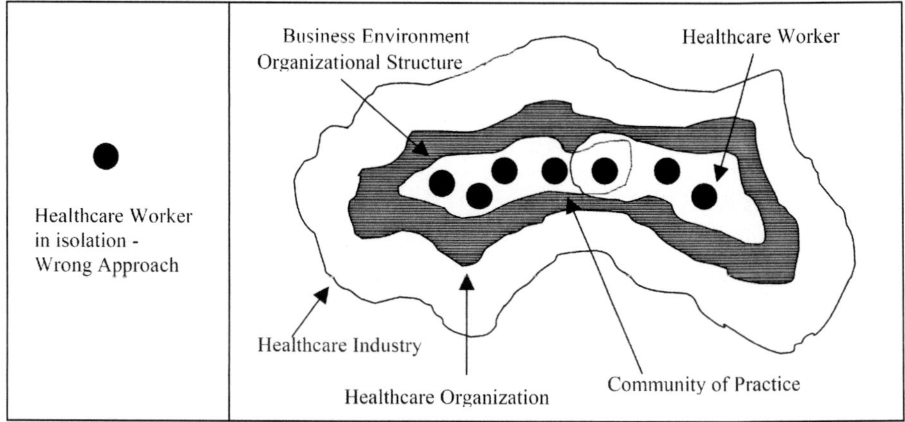

Figure 1. Healthcare worker in isolation and in a social context.

Because of Diagnomania healthcare workers do not have AI-wings yet and patients do not get a full advantage of achievements of modern computer science. It is time to change that! Diagnomania is not terminal. The cure involves internalizing that physicians and nurses do not deliver patient care in isolation but they function in communities of practice and in economically driven business organizations; that the way they solve problems and make decisions is effected by organizational structures (e.g., standard operating procedures) as much as their cognitive powers. These structures should not be ignored in defining AI projects aimed at creating new tools for healthcare!

On the contrary, the nature of medical workplace should drive the type and extent of research/application projects in healthcare. In addition, a unique organizational environment of healthcare institutions is what makes medical knowledge elicitation different from knowledge acquisition for other non-medical expert systems. Thus, we can increase both a rate of success of AI projects and accuracy/speed of medical knowledge acquisition by building models reflecting the nature of medical workplaces.

2. What Is the Nature of the Medical Workplace?

The nature of clinical work in medical communities of practice is highly nonroutine [2] and emergency-driven. It requires constantly inventing new ways to cope with unforeseen contingencies under time pressure and with limited resources. Patient care environment forces workers to "carry out their routine tasks and – often simultaneously – respond to unforeseen combinations of events [2]".

Medical work is based on dynamic, cross-functional, inter-departmental, and inter-organizational collaboration that requires constant communication and effective sharing of professional knowledge. It takes place in healthcare institutions that are constantly restructuring themselves in order to survive in a turbulent, competitive environment. Especially now healthcare executives must actively work on strategic repositioning of their organizations and their work is much like that of clinicians but their goal is a healthy organization in addition to healthy patients. CEOs and CIOs define social/business setting for medical practice, thus indirectly affect medical communities of practice.

3. What Kind of Tools Can Informate[2] Medical Work?

The irregular and ad-hoc nature of medical work (clinical and administrative) can be addressed by AI in three ways: (1) achieving high adaptability of programs (reasoning by analogy, approximate reasoning, machine learning, incorporation of neuro-fuzzy work validation methods), (2) getting automatic programming to work (healthcare workers create their own decision-support systems); (3) using social techniques and AI business modeling to precisely identify real need for medical decision-support systems within the reach of current technology.

(1) It is imperative that medical decision-support systems are flexible, non-brittle, and able to do "guessing" given incomplete knowledge. Research on analogical reasoning in large knowledge bases strives to create such adaptive applications but more work is still needed [3–5]. Neural and fuzzy solutions provide flexibility but we do not have good ways to validate them, thus we cannot rely on them in "main stream" patient care. (2) Automatic programming that could eliminate time/space discontinuity between design and use of programs is not mature enough to handle medical applications. (3) Social/business modeling (e.g., Situated, Strategic, and AI-Enhanced method) of the medical workplace, can and should be used NOW to define application areas where today's AI can really help by being incorporated into an enterprise-wide Integrated Healthcare Information System (IHIS).

4. Why Do We Need Situated, Strategic, and AI-Enhanced Method?

4.1. Why Situated?

Representing knowledge about technology in medical workplace is difficult because technology has a dual nature: it is easily manipulated by humans, but also molds behavior and organizational practice. "This reciprocal causation of dialectical relationships implies that a general predictive model of the interaction of technology with organizations is not meaningful [6]."

The specific institutional context (situation) has to be understood and this is the essence of the situated approach. We cannot count on preexisting, general knowledge relevant to a specific workplace. The only way to represent knowledge about a workplace is to do the "field work"; experience it – immerse in it and then represent it.

Thus, in order to understand a real medical community of practice a researcher/developer must have skills of a social scientist who is sensitive to the subtleties of motivational factors, power struggles, and frustrations within organizations.

4.2. Why Strategic?

We need to include knowledge about strategic positioning of a medical institution in an economic environment as a part of the workplace analysis because it affects the way communities of practice function and evolve (e.g., by the year 2000, nearly 80% [today 45%] of community hospitals will belong to hospital systems [7] which will change communication patterns within medical communities of practice).

A structurational model of technology derived from Gidden's theory of structuration can provide a framework for building a guidance system for situated and strategic organiza-

---

[2] Automating means introducing technology without paying attention to its effect on people; Informating goes beyond automating and prepares people and business process for technological change [9].

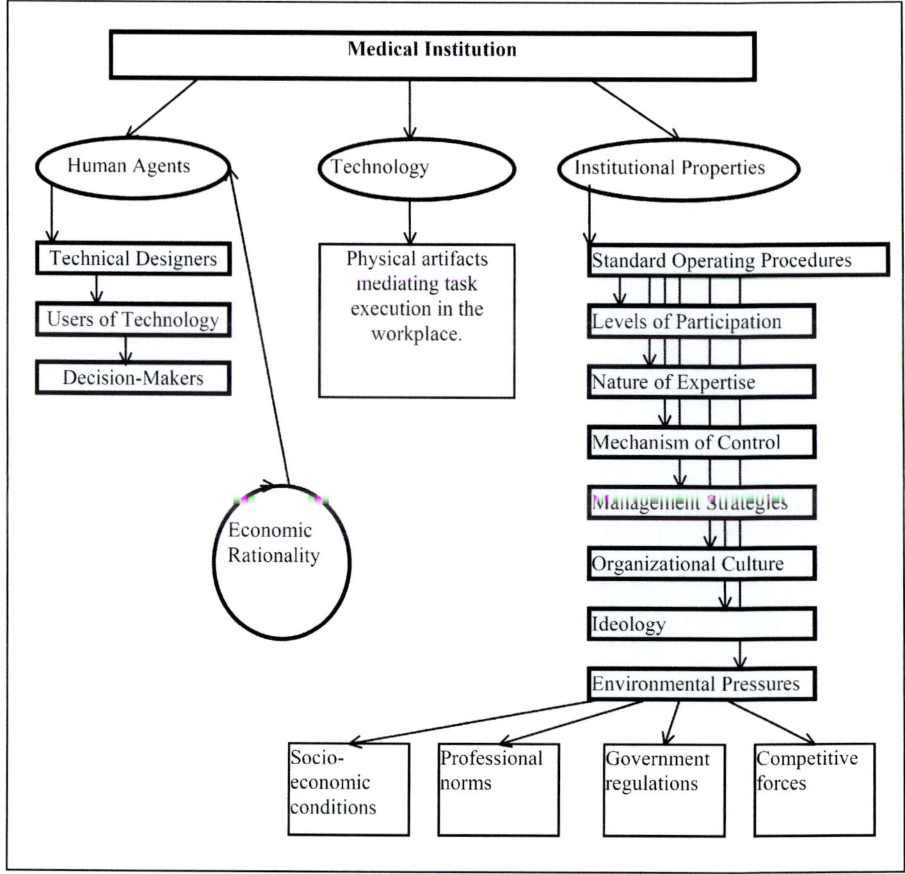

Figure 2. A Framework for Strategic Knowledge Representation.

tional knowledge representation. Giddens' theory describes reciprocal interaction of social actors and institutionalized social practices [Fig. 2].

4.3. Why AI-Enhanced?

Capturing real-time dynamics of a distributed business/medical process in a model allows for the discovery of bottlenecks in information flows and enhances the quality and speed of knowledge acquisition. A knowledge engineer communicates better with healthcare workers if model is used as a focal point; automatic knowledge acquisition tools can reuse "modeling knowledge". In addition, AI modeling enables technology designers to create a model of a future workflow (e.g., mediated by AI applications) before investing in implementation. This prepares users for the change, facilitates discovery of possible difficulties, and helps planning new applications' integration with Healthcare Information Systems. For example, modeling healthcare work with SYMMOD[3] allowed to encode, hard to otherwise

---

[3] SYMMOD is a symbolic modeling environment developed at a Digital Equipment Corp. that combines techniques of business analysis and discrete modeling with knowledge-based methods.

capture, knowledge about handling delays in radiology report distribution and made emergency-driven nature of physician-radiology communication process explicit.

Because medical knowledge "happens" in reaction to events (it is not static), an AI modeling tool able to represent this kind of knowledge has to easily support the following: (1) Multiple levels of abstraction, (2) Multiple logical views of the same process – different workers talk about the same process differently, (3) Emulation of dynamic interdependencies among activities and data over time; (4) Self-documentation; (5) Dynamic tracking of incomplete information – model assumptions [8].

5. Expectations

Using Situated, Strategic, and AI-Enhanced analysis of the workplace before automating human work assures that new technology makes this work easier and thus users fully accept it. Once researchers/designers get to use this method there will be more medical decision-support systems that are actually accepted and used in many areas of practicing medicine (e.g., patient referral, data analysis, policy monitoring, lab data analysis, health-education); there will be more enterprise-wide, scaleable AI applications integrated with Healthcare Information Systems. It is imperative that research on new ways to enhance medical work starts from the workplace analysis. AI modeling makes this analysis easier – a dynamic model helps to capture knowledge about the environment in which physicians and nurses work. Environment awareness enhances the quality and speed of knowledge acquisition. Situated, Strategic, and AI-Enhanced method of technology introduction will simply give healthcare workers AI-wings that let them fly where they want not there AI-designers think they should.

References

[1] Shortliffe, E.H., and Perrault, L.E., Medical Informatics, Computer Applications in Healthcare, Addison-Wesley, 1990.
[2] Kukla, C. and Cash, D., "I Like My Job because There's Nothing Repetitious About It": On the non-routine nature of workplaces, to be published in 1991.
[3] Bushko, R.G., KRA – Knowledge-Rich Analogy: Adaptive Estimation with Common Sense, MS Thesis, EECS Department, Massachusetts Institute of Technology, 1990.
[4] Lenat, D., and Guha, R.V., Building Large Knowledge-Based Systems, Adison-Wesley Publishing Company Inc., 1989.
[5] Minsky, M., Logical vs. Analogical or Symbolic vs. Connectionist or Neat vs. Scruffy, In Winston, P., Expanding Frontiers: Artificial Intelligence at MIT, MIT Press, 1990.
[6] Orlikowski, W., The Duality of Technology: Rethinking the Concept of Technology in Organizations, CCSTR#105, SSWP#3141, Sloan School of Management, 1990.
[7] Shortell, S.M., Morrison E.M., and Friedman, B., Strategic Choices for America's Hospitals, Jossey-Bass Inc. Publishers, 1990.
[8] Chaney, T., Symbolic Modeling, Digital Equipment Corp., internal white paper, 1990.
[9] Zuboff, S., In the Age of the Smart Machine, Basic Books, Inc., Publishers, New York, 1988. [3] Greenbaum, J. and King, M., Design at Work, Lawrence Erlbaum Ass., 1990.
[10] McDermott, J., The World Would be a Better Place if Non-Programmers Could Program, Machine Learning, April, 1989.
[11] Minsky, M., Why People Think that Computers Can't, Technology Review, November, 1983.

Future of Intelligent and Extelligent Health Environment
R.G. Bushko (Ed.)
IOS Press, 2005

Towards an Intelligent Hospital Environment: OR of the Future

Jeffrey V. SUTHERLAND, Ph.D.[a], Willem-Jan VAN DEN HEUVEL, Ph.D.[b],
Tim GANOUS[c], Matthew M. BURTON, M.D.[d] and Animesh KUMAR[e]
[a]*Chief Technology Officer, Patientkeeper, Inc., Brighton, MA, US*
[b]*Assistant Professor, Tilburg University, The Netherlands*
[c]*Grants and Programs, University of Maryland Medical System, Baltimore, MD, US*
[d]*Clinical Product Manager, PatientKeeper, Inc., Brighton, MA, US*
[e]*Systems Engineer, Inkriti, L.L.C., Watertown, MA, US*

Abstract. Patients, providers, payers, and government demand more effective and efficient healthcare services, and the healthcare industry needs innovative ways to re-invent core processes. Business process reengineering (BPR) [29] showed adopting new hospital information systems can leverage this transformation and workflow management technologies can automate process management. Our research indicates workflow technologies in healthcare require real time patient monitoring, detection of adverse events, and adaptive responses to breakdown in normal processes [22]. Adaptive workflow systems are rarely implemented making current workflow implementations inappropriate for healthcare.

The advent of evidence based medicine, guideline based practice, and better understanding of cognitive workflow combined with novel technologies including Radio Frequency Identification (RFID), mobile/wireless technologies, internet workflow, intelligent agents, and Service Oriented Architectures (SOA) opens up new and exciting ways of automating business processes. Total situational awareness of events, timing, and location of healthcare activities can generate self-organizing change in behaviors of humans and machines.

A test bed of a novel approach towards continuous process management was designed for the new Weinburg Surgery Building at the University of Maryland Medical [41,57]. Early results based on clinical process mapping and analysis of patient flow bottlenecks demonstrated 100% improvement in delivery of supplies and instruments at surgery start time. This work has been directly applied to the design of the DARPA Trauma Pod research program where robotic surgery will be performed on wounded soldiers on the battlefield [16].

1. New Strategies Needed for Healthcare Automation

New strategies are needed for intelligent automation in healthcare organizations to save time and resources, accelerate throughput, enhance patient safety, and improve outcomes. The complexity of modern healthcare has outrun the capabilities of manual and paper based operations. There are too many isolated silos of information and too many handoffs to deliver quality care. Resulting symptoms are obvious to a casual observer–the only thing that kills more people every year than inpatient medical error is heart disease and cancer [42]. In addition, institutional behaviors, conflicting incentives, and cultural issues make healthcare enterprises highly resistant to adoption of new technologies.

"Even though U.S. medical care is the world's most costly, its outcomes are mediocre compared with other industrialized nations. A recent World Health Organization (WHO) report ranking the world's health systems placed the United States 37th. The 2001 Institute of Medicine Report, "Crossing the Quality Chasm," characterized the U.S. system as fundamentally broken and called for major federal investment in information technology as crucial to achieving necessary changes, such as "elimination of most handwritten clinical data by the end of the decade." Better use of information technology is essential to providing better care at lower cost." [7]

Complex manual processes for patient care are often impervious to automation, particularly when change to established procedures is required. Cultural resistance to innovation is strongest where workflows are most inefficient and new process is perceived as disruptive. Change may be most effectively introduced in stealth mode by transparently saving physicians' time and improving their ability to treat patients. Disruptive, but invisible, innovation is required to cure dysfunctional healthcare systems [12].

1.1. Creating an Automated Safety Net for Patients

The pace of events that need monitoring in a high velocity surgery facility make manual analysis and control of daily operations high risk, painful, and ineffective. Methods are needed to automate standard protocols, to monitor execution of processes, to alert staff about required interventions, and to identify and predict adverse events. A useful metaphor for solving these problems is the introduction of the autopilot in the aircraft industry.

Initially, autopilots were simple devices that kept the aircraft on course while the crew could pay attention to higher level tasks. These systems have now evolved to full control of takeoff and landing of commercial airliners. Beginning with the Boeing 777, full fly-by-wire controls became available on commercial aircraft [11] and Boeing test flights of new aircraft are done on autopilot to avoid risking the lives of crew members.

An autopilot acts as a safety net to keep the aircraft on course at the right altitude while the pilot's attention is occupied elsewhere. If the aircraft starts to veer off course, all systems interoperate to gently steer the aircraft back on course.

1.2. Early Automated Feedback Prevents Process Breakdown

Autopilots operate by feedback mechanisms that cause small corrections back to course, so that large corrections are never needed. Interventions that are too late and require large corrections can be damaging and fatal.

An autopilot is needed to guide process execution for routine healthcare events and warning lights and alarms need to be available just as they are for an aircraft pilot when an engine is overheating or a collision is immanent. Healthcare needs an air traffic control system that assures operating rooms are ready, staff and equipment are in place, the patient is properly staged and prepped through the process, and beds and follow-up treatment are available when the patient clears the operating room.

"As concerns about patient safety have grown, the health care sector has looked to other industries that have confronted similar challenges, in particular the airline industry. This industry learned long ago that information and clear communication are critical to the safe navigation of an airplane. To perform their jobs well and guide their planes safely to their destinations, pilots must communicate with the air traffic controller concerning their destinations and current circumstances (e.g., mechanical or other problems), their flight plans, and environmental factors (e.g., weather conditions) that could necessitate a change in course. Information must also pass seamlessly from one controller to another to ensure a safe and smooth journey for planes flying long distances; provide notification of airport

delays or closures due to weather conditions; and enable rapid alert and response to an extenuating circumstance, such as a terrorist attack." [28]

1.3. Current Automation Often Does Not Fit Physician Workflow

In a perioperative setting, hundreds of patients and staff may be flowing through dozens of operating rooms on a daily basis in a single facility. One third of the patients are unscheduled and identified only on the day of surgery. The resulting chaos can be overwhelming, even with some form of electronic health record (currently available in 12% of hospital systems [58]). Orchestration of behavior between information systems is ad-hoc, and paper based. Computer systems are dedicated to isolated operations or departments with no computational means to communicate with one other.

A deeper problem is the majority of clinical decision support systems are failures or underutilized because of an impedance mismatch between the analytical, linear process forced on clinicians by automation, and the way they work which is quite different.

"Technical artifacts (such as computer systems) can be viewed as embodying the implicit theories of their creators about how work is done, what characterizes workers and their environment, what problems they face, and how they will use the artifact... However, there is quite a large mismatch between the implicit theories embedded in these computer systems and the real world of clinical work. Clinical work, especially in hospitals, is fundamentally interpretative, interruptive, multitasking, collaborative, distributed, opportunistic, and reactive... The result of this mismatch is that many of the failed attempts at computer-based clinical systems were bound to fail because the model of health care work inscribed in these tools clashed too much with the actual nature of clinical work." [59]

1.4. Six Sigma Quality in Healthcare Requires Workflow Process Management

The autopilot metaphor facilitates more creative thinking about innovation in clinical automation because an autopilot does not force a linear, artificial workflow on the pilot. Along with other systems on an airplane, it works collaboratively with the crew and the flight control team (air and ground) to provide a safety net for operations.

Industry best practice is known as Six Sigma Quality. Companies like Motorola and General Electric have committed themselves to reducing the frequency of defects in their business processes to fewer than 3.4 per million, the Six Sigma goal. As a contributor to Six Sigma Quality an autopilot incorporates characteristic features important to healthcare quality improvement:

- An autopilot operates in stealth mode;
- Removes work from the pilot without interrupting normal workflow;
- Alerts the pilot in the case of unforeseen events it cannot handle and returns control to the pilot.

Limitations of current healthcare systems provide great opportunities for workflow collaboration and process improvement efforts. It is rare for any activity in healthcare to reach Six Sigma Quality. Inpatient medication accuracy is more error prone than airline baggage handling. Post heart-attack medications and mammography screening results are even worse. The only area of medicine that has used industry best practices to systematically reduce error is anesthesiology where in the last decade error rates have been reduced to 3.4 per million events [13].

Because of the general lack of industrial quality practices in healthcare 100% improvements are possible as noted in the supplies and equipment example later in this paper.

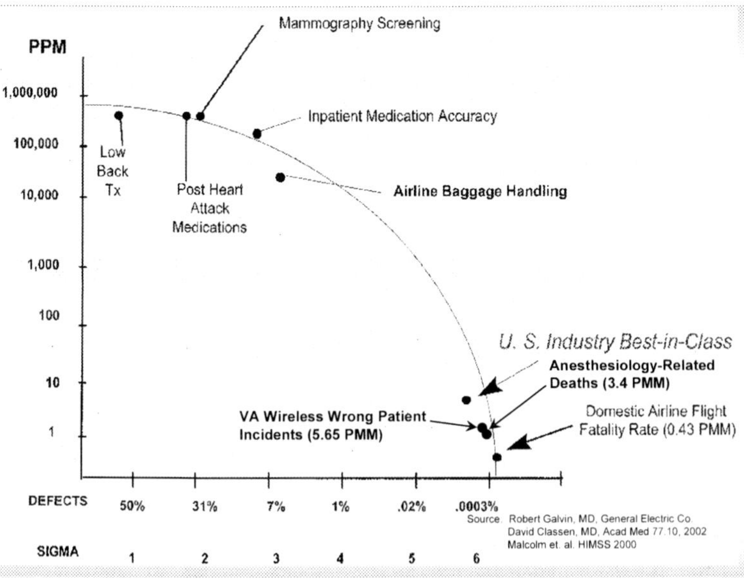

Figure 1. Number of errors per million events for some healthcare practices compared to airline safety [50].

1.5. Radical Improvement in Quality of Patient Care Is Possible

Enhanced automation and integration to avoid oversights, mistakes, and medical errors are only the tip of the iceberg in improvement possibilities for healthcare. Radical improvement in the overall quality of care is possible by reducing the incidence of medical errors through deeply reinventing existing healthcare processes around cognitive workflow of clinicians, evidence based medicine, and clinical guidelines.

Important areas for continuous business process redesign related to the success of current medical practices entails statistical analysis of new clinical protocols and design of disease management systems. Business process integration offers a promising solution for rapid adoption of new treatments in practice by promoting new techniques through automated alerts and recommendations, while reducing negative side effects by displaying warnings and recent analyses of outcomes.

It currently takes an average of 17 years for evidence based medicine to be integrated into clinical practice [5] and research shows that physicians incorporate the latest medical evidence into treatment only about 50% of the time.

"Our results indicate that, on average, Americans receive about half of recommended medical care processes. Although this point estimate of the size of the quality problem may continue to be debated, the gap between what we know works and what is done is substantial enough to warrant attention. These deficits, which pose serious threats to the health and well-being of the U.S. public, persist despite initiatives by both the federal government and private health care delivery systems to improve care." [34]

Opportunities for unobtrusively automating the introduction, suggestion, or recommendation of the latest evidence based medical practice into clinical processes could generate a revolutionary improvement in patient outcomes. The impact of monitoring and managing small increments of clinical behavior can have enormous consequences.

A recent study showed that inpatient medication error is the fourth leading cause of death in the U.S. (113,000 deaths) with nosocomial infections not far behind (90,000 deaths) [42]. Inpatient surgery and postoperative care appear to significantly con-

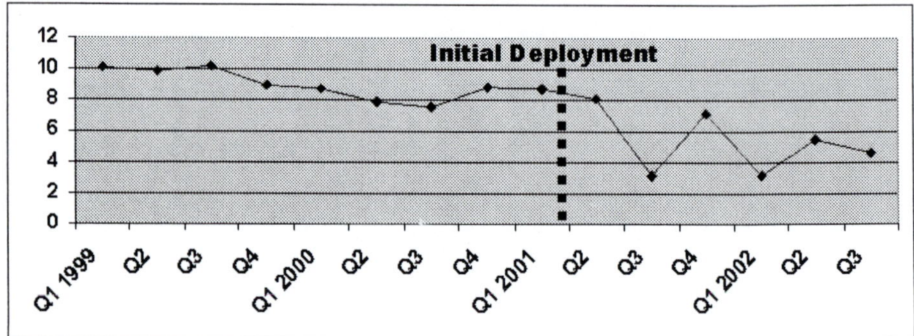

Figure 2. Postoperative deep wound and organ space infection rates per 1,000 elective surgical cases [28].

tribute to adverse events. An analysis of 15,000 nonpsychiatric hospital discharges revealed that 66% of adverse events were found to be related to surgery [8].

An example of a surgery related medication error is failure to give antibiotics within two hours before surgery. This doubles the postoperative deep wound and organ space infection rate, compounding medical error with nosocomial infection. Automated monitoring and alerting on this relatively simple event generates a significant improvement in care [30].

Automated monitoring of order entry and medication administration is easily implemented with new information systems coming on line and even with older systems. For example, it is currently possible with systems in place at the University of Maryland Medical Center to monitor order status of a medication and to generate an automated query to a care provider prior to patient surgery to confirm proper antibiotic delivery.

2. Towards a Solution – Adaptive Process Control

Healthcare processes require coordinating clinical events and patient scenarios that can span many departments and extended periods of time. Healthcare workflows are dynamic due to regular upgrade of treatment protocols and unexpected changes in patient status [3]. Wireless communication devices, context-aware applications, and adaptive workflow engines can help overcome these problems.

Workflow systems implemented in most industrial settings are not appropriate for healthcare. For example, widely deployed Enterprise Resource Planning (ERP) systems are adopting standards-based workflow engines to control process flow. These systems are designed to control "predictive processes," i.e. the steps of the process are highly predictable in advance.

Healthcare workflows can be highly *unpredictable* due to organizational or medical complexity. The problem in healthcare is how fast a system can adapt to unexpected events [14]. In the University of Maryland Medical System (UMMS), for example, 1/3 of the surgeries are unanticipated and enter the process at unpredictable times during the day. Then there are the inevitable and unexpected complications during surgery.

A highly adaptive system is needed to control this "empirical process". In the chemical industry where process research is a core competency, it is well known that trying to apply a "predictive process" control system to an "empirical process" has caused many plants to explode [36]. In healthcare, this same mistake increases morbidity and mortality.

Conversely, applying an "empirical process" to control unpredictable events in chemical plants is commonplace. For example, the same chemicals can be used to make vanilla to bake a cake or nerve gas for chemical weapons. The difference in the result is primarily due to the temperature of one of the vats where the chemicals are heated. An "empirical process" watches the temperature of the vat. When it gets too high, the system executes a rule dependent strategy to bring the vat into the right temperature band, or failing that, shuts the process down. This same strategy is appropriate for healthcare settings and is analogous to the operation of an autopilot.

Complex adaptive system theory (*cas*) has been applied to analysis of information systems in healthcare and other industries [49]. The healthcare enterprise is a complex adaptive system and the field of adaptive system theory provides fertile ground for research on healthcare process improvement strategies [33,60]. Advanced empirical process controls strategies in this paper are rooted in *cas*.

2.1. Context-Aware Workflow as Autopilot

An effective use of adaptive workflow engines in the healthcare enterprise is as an autopilot. An autopilot does not fly the plane and it does not perform the tasks of aircraft subsystems. It monitors and observes that the plane is veering off an established course and makes minor adjustments by gently tweaking subsystems to push the aircraft towards level flight on a predetermined heading. In this way, the autopilot prevents major errors by handling multiple small errors and correcting them. Advanced autopilots use terrain following radar and other subsystems to automatically fly the plane. Even then, they rely on a hierarchy of subsystems to actually execute flight.

For example, work described in this paper has been used in design of the DARPA Trauma Pod [16], an autonomous vehicle planned to perform robotic surgery on the battlefield. In that system the workflow engine will not do the surgery. It will check that the Trauma Pod is ready for surgery, handle the logistic aspects of assuring supplies and instruments are available, cleanup after robotic surgery is complete, restock, sanitize, and prepare for the next surgery. In addition, it will assure no sponges are left inside the patient using RFID technology. When it sees exceptions, it will alert hierarchical subsystems or external systems to take appropriate action.

MIT Professor Rodney Brooks calls this approach a "subsumption" architecture, the best way to take a large collection of dumb subsystems and orchestrate them to exhibit intelligent behavior in robotic design [9]. The same approach can be taken to monitor distributed systems in a healthcare enterprise, which are "dumb" in the sense they cannot communicate with one another or adjust well to one another. A higher-level workflow engine can alert subsystems or clinicians to perform adjustments to patient processes before major problems occur. In this manner, a large collection of "dumb" subsystems can be made to appear "smart."

An adaptive workflow engine can be used to orchestrate behavior of disparate systems in a surgery center through direct integration via web services, HL7 standards-based messaging, a hybrid solution, or proprietary adaptors [48]. The ability to "capture" the function of legacy components in an enterprise is a standard complex adaptive systems strategy and the basis for introduction of intelligent agents into advanced software systems [4].

Another important aspect of an autopilot is *total situational awareness* of what is happening and using that awareness to unobtrusively alter aircraft behavior. The pilot of an aircraft wants an autopilot to do its task so well that its operations are transparent. In order to promote user adoption of new clinical processes in a healthcare enterprise, the workflow engine must be transparent to routine operations and only become visible when a critical event occurs. The introduction of RFID technology for capture of critical data on patients, staff, instruments, and supplies helps to make this possible.

2.2. Stealth Mode of Automated Data Collection

A stealth mode of data collection is needed to introduce new technology without disrupting current manual processes. By stealth mode, we mean automated collection of data that is normally observed; yet irregularly captured because of lack of time and tedious manual data entry procedures. It is essential data for managing operations in a high stress environment, where erroneous perceptions generate suboptimal organizational response.

RFID technology can automatically monitor flow of patients, staff, supplies, and equipment. Baseline data can be captured for critical process points, bottlenecks identified, and process improvement plans developed. Monitoring critical events and evoking selective orchestration of behavior is required across multiple healthcare information systems and care providers that move a patient through the perioperative system with dozens of points of clinical and administrative interaction.

Passively monitoring operations with RFID technology provides real time data useful in constraint theory analyses [21]; an approach that can identify bottlenecks and target selected initiatives that cause radical improvement in throughput in an enterprise in a short period of time. In addition, sensing systems combined with workflow engines and inferencing applications can anticipate future events, and trigger interventions that alter the course of action, potentially saving patients' lives, and certainly improving efficiency.

RFID capabilities are now being integrated into 802.11 access points so that location data can be seamlessly delivered to a central network or database, with transaction specific accuracy for the location of patients, staff, equipment, and supplies [18]. Future refinements allow real time determination of procedures performed by analysis of proximity of clinicians, patient, and instruments for an appropriate period of time. Intelligent video can identify the nature of processes underway in an operating room.

Baseline data can be gathered for targeting high yield process interventions. In the initial phases, process improvements programs should be implemented manually. When the manual solution demonstrates success and the return on investment (ROI) is positive, real time process monitoring can be implemented to expand initial gains, widely deploy the implementation within the organization, and support an ongoing process improvement methodology.

Data mining of historical information can generate new insights for process intervention. Real time adaptation, combined with post-process automated reflection generating new strategies for future adaptation is a powerful feedback process that can progress a system from strength to strength through continuous process improvement.

3. RECIPE for Incremental Evolution and Process Improvement

Research results from the Operating Room of the Future project at UMMS led to a technology introduction strategy that maximizes probability of adoption by minimizing disruption of ongoing surgery operations. We call this process a RECIPE for REal-Time proCess ImProvement in hEalthcare.

RECIPE focuses on identifying bottlenecks in current processes that leads to development of small incremental improvements. Most opportunities for intervention generate 30% improvement and 100% improvements are often achieved [53]. Strategically introducing small incremental changes into current processes can evolve over time into major institutional transformation.

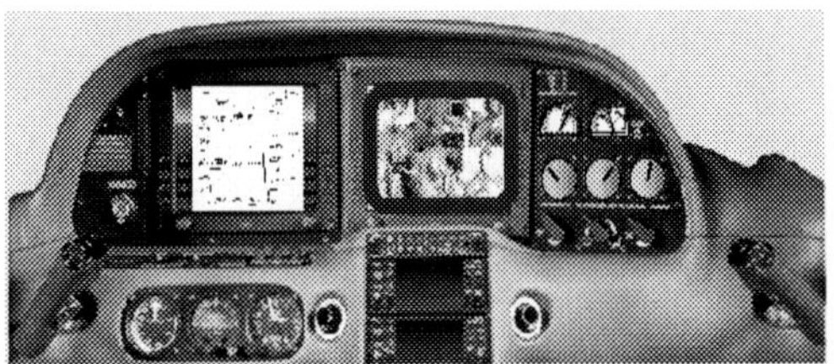

Figure 3. The RECIPE Cockpit.

3.1. The RECIPE Approach

The RECIPE research project adopts a hybrid research methodology, blending empirical (positivist) with non-empirical techniques. During the course of a project, we first scrutinize manual execution of processes, and then incrementally inject more intelligent workflow technology to improve the process. This way of working is chosen based on the hypothesis that redesign and automation of manual processes may significantly improve processes.

Manually reengineering business processes often yields dramatic improvements by itself. Automating business process change requires standards-based workflow management techniques, particularly when change requires orchestrating behavior between humans, new information systems, and legacy applications.

Production workflow systems today are largely implementations of predictable and repetitive document processing [40]. These systems are not well suited to healthcare where standard workflows may not exist, exceptions are routine, and breakdown of workflows is a daily reality. In addition, healthcare workflows are patient centric rather than document centric, and patient identification and location are often indeterminate in a fluid hospital setting [14].

At each stage of automation, medical workflows are designed using the following abstract process pattern:

1. Analysis state of the art processes
2. Develop a business case
3. Redesign business process
4. Evaluate

During analysis (Step-1), the analyst concentrates on "break-downs" in the material, financial, information or process flow. The aim is to chart nodes and related business rules in the workflow that may heavily influence other nodes; e.g., improvements of these nodes have a ripple effect all through the workflow. Some initial findings about this new approach to workflow modeling have been reported [54].

To justify any changes in the workflow, the methodology defines a business case, stipulating expected costs, revenues, risks etc. of the proposed adaptation (Step-2). Once business considerations are assessed, problems in processes may be ranked (e.g., processes with the highest costs are considered first). Top-priority issues for healthcare processes can be further analyzed by modeling the workflow.

Redesigning processes aims at optimizing medical workflows so that they are better equipped to meet the organization's goals. RECIPE allows processes to be manually tested in the healthcare domain to assess feasibility and return on investment. Acceptable improvements are automated and introduced gradually to manage disruption of production work patterns. Real-time process improvement implies that processes may be evaluated and calibrated with virtually no delay between the operation being executed, and monitored. In many cases, manual testing may not be needed.

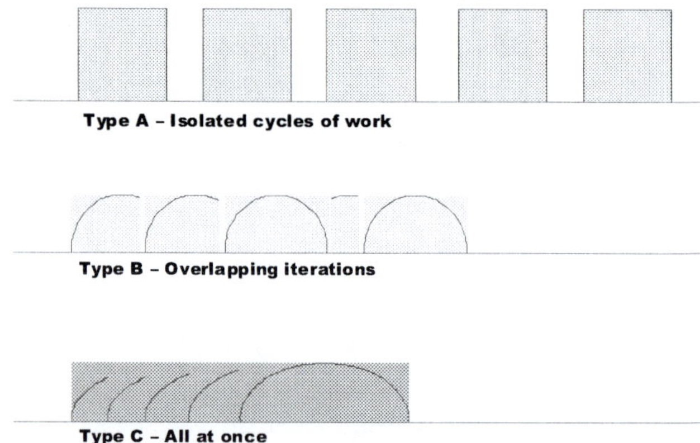

Figure 4. Type A, B, and C strategies for delivering product [55].

Evaluation of process improvements (Step 4) takes place by carefully comparing metrics measured after introduction of a process improvement with that of the original process. Several metrics may be analyzed in stealth mode, including quality of service, revenues, costs, improvement in patient care, and level of adoption of the process improvement.

Repeatedly performing these steps will evolve clinical processes to new levels of automation improving efficiency and safety. Injecting the workflows with more intelligence causes them to morph from rather dumb, manual processes to autonomous, intelligent workflow systems that are capable of surviving break-downs, intrusions and new execution contexts.

3.2. RECIPE Supports Agile Process Improvement

RECIPE has a highly iterative character. The iterative approach has been shown to produce good results in the U.S. and Japan as demonstrated by Takeuchi and Nonaka [56] in their analysis of best business practices. They noted that the U.S. National Aeronautics and Space Administrations phased program planning (PPP) severely compromised speed and flexibility because it separated phases of the project like a relay race with multiple handoffs (Type A). They observed Type B overlap of phases which eliminates handoffs at Fuji-Xerox and Type C multiple phases at once at Honda and Canon (see Fig. 4). It has been observed on software development projects that Type B and Type C overlapping approaches radically increase throughput [44,45,47].

Ideally, a Type C project would implement manual process mapping concurrently with RFID tagging and tracking of patients, staff instruments and supplies. Automated analysis of RFID data would clarify and validate process maps. In addition, real-time RFID data on patient, staff, and logistics flow would identify bottlenecks in patient flow allowing application of constraint theory analysis to increase throughput [21].

It is important to note that process improvement strategies require an iterative approach. When a process bottle is eliminated, new bottlenecks appear in unexpected places. RFID data will clearly reflect that. The need to first make minor change, then watch the system to see where the next change should be made is not intuitive to the naive observer. It is central to the RECIPE approach. Minor incremental change evolves over time to transformative change.

This paper describes the method of the RECIPE real time process improvement methodology and an example introduction of the methodology into a high velocity surgical environment at the University of Maryland Medical System [52]. The approach is suitable for all types of healthcare processes and for evolution of next generation systems, including the DARPA Trauma Pod [16], an autonomous robotic vehicle for performing fully automated diagnosis, treatment, and surgery on wounded soldiers on the battlefield. See Appendix I for more detail on application of RECIPE to perioperative system design.

3.3. Step-1: Process Analysis at the University of Maryland Medical System (UMMS)

Introduction of process improvements into an organization requires understanding current processes, mapping out desired future processes, and developing an intervention plan to revamp current operations. The natural tendency for a traditional organization is to make this a linear process, extending time to deployment in the hope that slowness of movement with minimize disruption and maximize throughput.

Divergent views of project goals, an extended need to educate staff on best business practices in workflow, and the early stage of RFID technology forced the UMMS project into a Type A scenario. Research objectives to get a prototype running were compromised by operational needs to immediately improve processes manually. Manual process mapping was accomplished first before anything else could be done.

Manual assessment of start times and equipment readiness at first surgery of the day in all operating rooms was accomplished concurrently and senior staff members worked on operating room shifts to directly experience problems, identify bottlenecks, and establish priorities. One of the goals was to minimize analysis lag time by doing high level process mapping across the perioperative process and deep analysis only on top priorities for process improvement. This, combined with an awareness of best business practices in workflow, allowed substantial initial gains to be made in a priority area using manual techniques.

At the beginning of the project, an external consulting team was hired to review all internal perioperative processes and make recommendations. After review and analysis, many manual changes were made to current processes. The area identified as highest priority was case cart readiness of supplies and instruments at start of surgery.

The two changes that had the most impact on supplies and instruments availability in the operating room were raising the qualifications and pay rate of supply personnel and increasing the inventory of supplies and instruments. The design of the new building created an unanticipated requirement for a higher number of instruments to be on hand. It was only through process analysis on the front line that sufficient management data was available to justify the considerable investment in increases salaries and instrument inventories.

Concurrently, the authors undertook a deeper analysis of inventory problems and determined there were three disparate information systems currently supported supplies and instruments management operations:

System 1. Equipment and Supplies Management System. The Pathway Material Management System (HBOC Star) is the primary inventory system for UMMS. The system provides a minimal set of information to an ESI Surgery Scheduling System (product name, item number, hospital number, other identifying number, number in inventory, change number, cost, date, location, and whether chargeable to the patient).

System 2. Scheduling System. The ESI Surgery Scheduling System was used for managing surgery operations. The responsibility updating surgical preference lists was not clearly defined. Updates and changes to the inventory system were forwarded by email to individuals working on the ESI system. This created a large backlog of unresolved changes and updates to inventory needed for surgery schedules. Any updates had to be manually entered into the surgery scheduling system. In addition, specialty carts for different surgery types were not in the surgery scheduling system. These supplies were kept in the hallways and new nurses often had difficulty finding equipment needed for surgery.

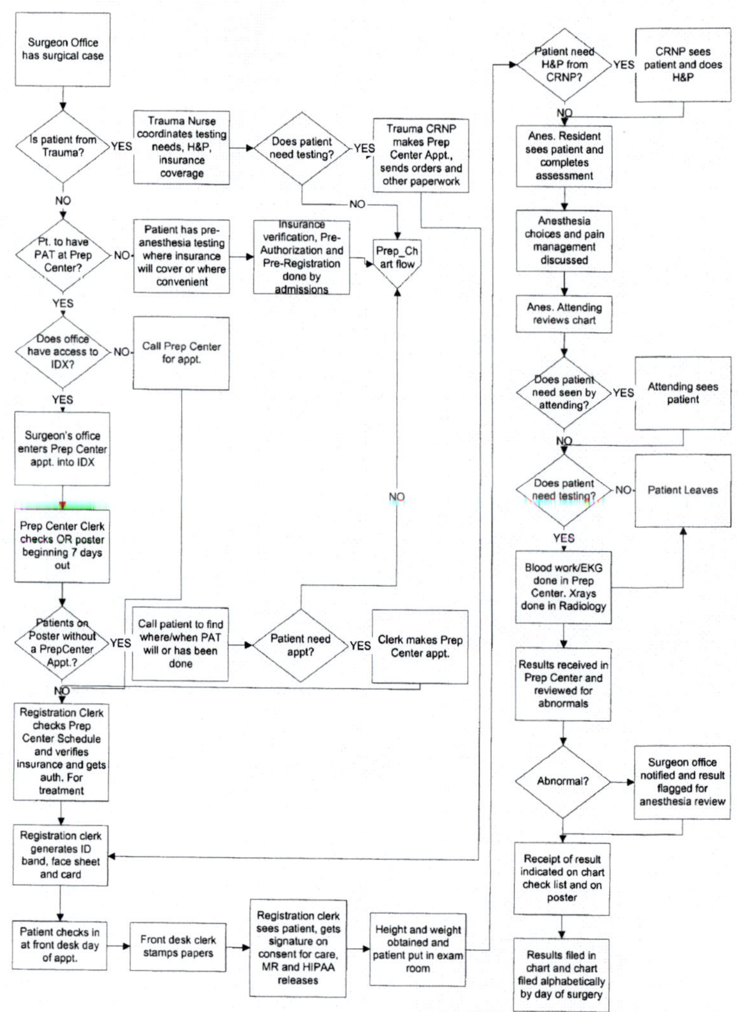

Figure 5. Perioperative process map of patient preparation visit prior to surgery at the University of Maryland Medical Center. Data prepared under contract with Perioptimum on 24 May 2004.

System 3. Instrument Tracking System. The third critical system was the SPM Instrument Tracking System in the basement of the surgery center where supplies and instruments were handled. Information was entered into this system via barcodes that were swiped for instruments received, decontaminated, prepped and stacked, then sterilized. People often did not swipe the instrument barcode, making information inaccurate.

The lack of automated interfaces between these systems generated extensive manual intervention and error-prone rework. Analysis of each system with the technical owner showed that in most cases, there was an easy way to automate an interface.

There was no easy way for an end-user (a surgical nurse missing a piece of equipment) to update any of these systems or alert anyone that supplies were missing. On daily rounds it was common to see a frustrated nurse trying to call the supply area with an angry surgeon standing by. Often, the line was busy. If the line was not busy, there was no way to easily determine why a missing supply or instrument still had not appeared in the operating room 45 minutes later.

Lack of automated interfaces between systems caused discrepancies between the inventory system and the surgery scheduling system. An attempt was made to reconcile these problems by manually reviewing monthly reports from each system. Discrepancies and complaints were handled by email and volume of email was unmanageable.

3.4. Step 2: Business Case Analysis

Workflow implementation is based on detailed analysis of current clinical process and development of a desired new process. The implementation must initially support legacy processes without disrupting operations and gather baseline data to support later analysis of research results. Process improvements are identified, manually tested, introduced through automation, and the effect on the system is tracked, evaluated, and compared against baseline. Considerable preliminary work was completed to (1) evaluate clinical processes, (2) prioritize targets of opportunity, (3) and analyze the top priority target of opportunity.

A high level design of a workflow system was developed as a reference model for analysis of solutions in the perioperative environment. The Perioperative System Acceleration Tool (PSPAT) was designed to monitor existing disparate systems as well as RFID data on patient, equipment, and staff location, and to intervene by communicating between systems and people. The goal was to provide a system that would observe impeding process failure and alert staff so that crises could be averted. See Appendix II for a detailed description of PSPAT.

Based on work with members of the surgical teams at the University of Maryland Medical Center, a list of top priorities for automation was developed. Strategies for solving these problems were identified.

1. **Posting process** – A surgery case needs to be understood and placed in the schedule appropriately. PSPAT will monitor patients the day before scheduling for surgery to assess completeness of documentation and preparation. When the patient gets placed in the schedule, the surgery information system sends PSPAT an update.
2. **Preference lists** – Supplies, instruments, and equipment for operating room along with case carts are prepared the day before surgery. If the cart is not set up right or not in the right location at the right time, the surgery schedule is compromised. PSPAT will be monitoring the location of the carts, its relationship to a patient and surgeon, and payload. It will notify the right people if the carts are not in the right place at the right time. To do this, PSPAT receives the updated schedule from the surgery information systems and alerts the surgery information system of events that will compromise the schedule.
3. **Add-in cases** – Unanticipated surgery cases disrupt the surgery schedule and case cart requirements. This causes a scramble and unplanned work for nursing, anesthesia, and scheduling. PSPAT assumes the surgery information system will manage the schedule. If it changes, PSPAT is alerted in real time.
4. **Anesthesia staffing** – Staff shortages cause major problems with anesthesia staffing. PSPAT will know where the anesthesiologists are and whether they can meet scheduling commitments. Problems will cause PSPAT to alert the appropriate individuals. If the schedule is going to be compromised it will alert the surgery information system. Surgery schedules will be updated in response.
5. **Efficiency of patient transport** – PSPAT monitors location of patients and analyzes traffic flow. It will predict schedule changes that need to be made and make recommendations. Alerts will be sent to the surgery information system which must respond appropriately.

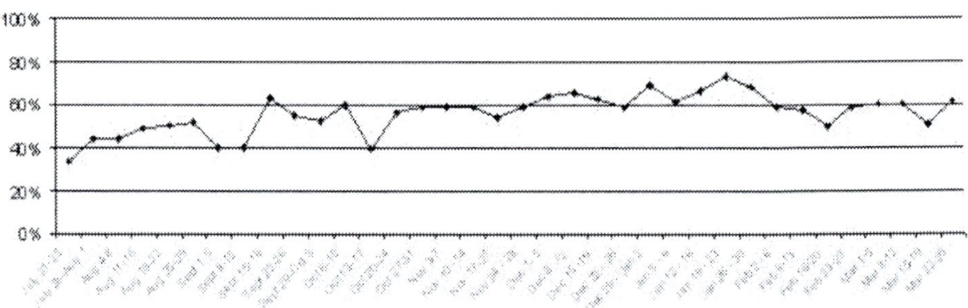

Figure 6. Case Cart Readiness.

6. **Patient consent forms and labs** – A major problem is assuring lab tests are completed and consent forms are signed. PSPAT will monitor and detect conditions where the surgery schedule will be compromised. Alerts will be sent to the surgery information system which must respond appropriately.

7. **Outflow from the OR** – Post-Anesthesia Care Unit (PACU) and the Intensive Care Unit (ICU) bed bottlenecks are a problem. PSPAT assumes that another system does bed management. That system must provide appropriate information to PSPAT.

Based on data collected on the first surgery of the day for each operating room, the items generating the most frustration and delay in the operating rooms schedule was availability of supplies, instruments, and equipment at the start time of each surgery. On daily rounds, the head nurse in each operating room was asked what problems occurred that impeded the smooth execution of the surgery schedule. During early weeks of surgery in the new Weinberg building, many processes established over many years in the old surgery facility no longer worked. In particular, completeness of case carts with respect to instruments and supplies availability was averaging 40–60%.

3.5. Step-3: Real Process Improvement Evaluated

During the initial phase of this project, the most interesting change in operations in the surgery center was the rise of case cart readiness from 40% to 80%, a 100% improvement before the introduction of any automation. This was the result of clinical staff doing process analysis for the workflow project and discovering management changes that could be made to improve throughput. It was difficult to implement and maintain this improvement manually. Follow-up with improved systems and automated support was essential to sustain 80% readiness and drive it higher.

3.6. Step-4: Automated Process Enhancement of Supplies and Instruments Delivered to Operating Rooms

At the beginning of the project, construction of the operating rooms had just been completed and all the latest technology had been installed along with easily accessible computer screens. Yet there was no visible surgery schedule, no visible patient list, and no automated access to surgical preference sheets to help resolve equipment and supply discrepancies. The environment was ripe for simple, easy, and efficient automation.

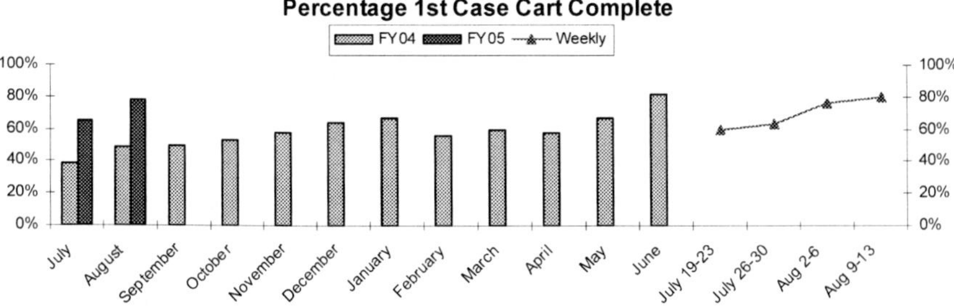

Figure 7. 100% process improvement in case cart readiness observed in surgery center during design phase of project.

The University of Maryland Medical System had installed the PatientKeeper application platform for physician mobile devices, tablets, and desktops. Each physician has a patient list or lists for all appropriate clinics or services. All clinical information on patients in displayed on these devices. Providing a schedule of patients for all operating rooms each day would be an improved configuration for the operating room. Demographic data, residents, attending physicians, and surgeons are linked to patients. The surgery scheduling system could be accessed to provide surgeon preference sheets for each patient/surgery combination so a surgery staff could quickly view this information on a mobile device, a tablet, or operating room workstations.

During the first surgery of each day for each operating room, the surgical nurse is queried on staff readiness and surgery start time. If there are any missing supplies or equipment items, the first step is to review the surgery preference list. If the item is on the list, but not on the case cart, a phone call is made to the supply area. Often the phone line is busy. When the call gets through and expedited service is requested, there is no way to easily determine what happened when the requested item is still missing 30 minutes later.

With a mobile device, the clinician could select a missing item and have it automatically transmitted to the supply area with time of request and priority automatically highlighted on screen in the supply area. A workflow engine could monitor the fulfillment of this request, alert all staff when delays were encountered, and provide recommendations for actions to solve the problem.

If the missing item were not on the surgery preference sheet, the practice was to request a change by email sent to multiple parties. When this was approved, the change was manually entered into the surgery scheduling system. It often took weeks to get a preference list updated and there were so many emails involved that items often missed getting updated.

The solution is to have clinical staff use a mobile device to request addition of an item to the surgeon's preference sheet and have that automatically communicated to the mobile devices or desktops of those individuals who need to provide approval. The workflow engine can monitor the protocol for updating these items and check the surgery scheduling system on a daily basis to assure that preference lists have been properly updated. If there are errors, the workflow engine triggers a series of actions that resolved the problem automatically.

There are many other critical scenarios for resolving equipment and supply problems that are beyond the scope of this paper. The problem resolution protocol for any one of them can be maintained and supported by a properly configured workflow system.

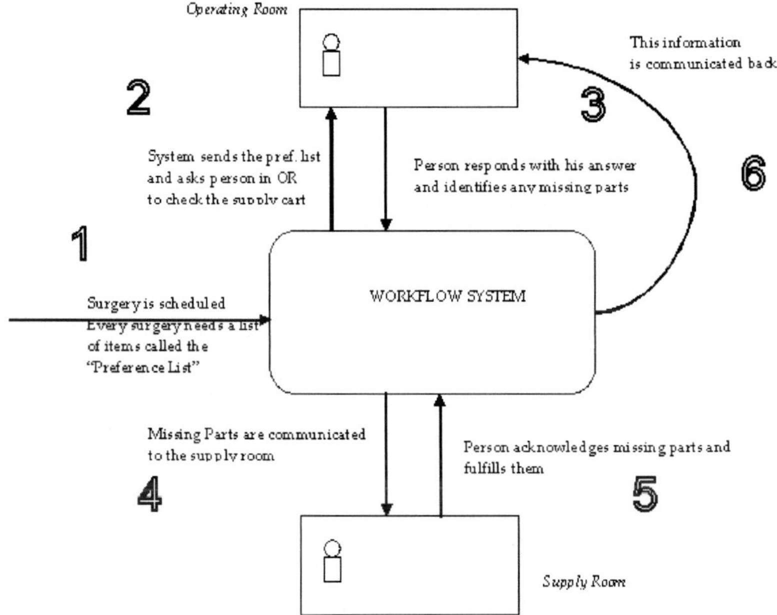

Figure 8. Supplies/Instruments Workflow.

4. Example: Workflow System Prototype

A workflow system for managing supplies/instruments needs to be robust, scalable, and highly configurable and provide support for pluggable components and subsystems. Such a workflow system will interact with several external systems for providing its functionality.

A prototype workflow for supplies and instruments was implemented using OSWorkflow – an open source workflow engine from OpenSymphony (http://www.opensymphony. com/). OSWorkflow is a flexible workflow engine based on finite state machine concept. OSWorkflow supports an XML based workflow definition descriptor. This allows a simple XML file to be translated into a business workflow.

Workflow Descriptor XML fragment

```
<workflow>
  <step id="1" name="Schedule Surgery">
   <actions>
     <action id="1" name="Schedule Surgery">
       <pre-functions>
        <function type="class">
          <arg name="class.name">workflow.function.ScheduleSurgery</arg>
       </function>
      </pre-functions>
        <results>
        <unconditional-result old-status="Finished" status="Underway" step="2" />
      </results>
     </action>
    </actions>
   </step>
```

```
<step id="2" name="Email OR Attendant">
<step id="3" name="Submit Preference List">
<step id="4" name="Email Supply Personnel Missing List">
<step id="5" name="Submit Missing Parts">
<step id="6" name="Email OR Attendant Missing List Fulfillment">
</workflow>
```

4.1. Workflow Steps

Step 1 – Schedule Surgery: A surgery is scheduled for a particular surgeon and surgery type and on a particular date. Clicking on the "Schedule" button triggers the workflow execution. Surgical preference list is obtained from the database and set in the workflow execution context object.

Surgeon	▽	
Surgery Type	▽	**Schedule**
Date		

Step 2 – Email OR Attendant: An email is sent to the email id configured in the DB for the OR attendant. The email contains link to a JSP page which displays the items to be verified in the supply cart.

Subject	Alert for checking surgical preference list in the supply cart
Description	Please click here to confirm whether all the items are available in the cart

Step 3 – Submit Preference List: The OR attendant configures the missing quantities of items and updates it in the database.

Item	Quantity	Description	Vendor	PO Number	Available in Full?	Quantity Missing	
A8	3	Swab	IM	123	○ Yes ○ No	☐	**Submit**
N1	2	Steth	GE	ABC	○ Yes ○ No	☐	

Step 4 – Email Supply Personnel Missing List: If one or more required items are missing, an email is sent to the email id configured in the database for supply personnel.

Subject	Alert for Missing Parts in the Preference List
Description	Please click here to confirm that the items have been requested for supply

Step 5 – Submit Missing Parts: The email sent in step 4 above contains link to a JSP page that displays the missing parts in the preference list. Supply personnel can then configure the items which have been reordered.

Item	Quantity	Description	Vendor	PO Number	Quantity Needed	Reordered?	
A8	3	Swab	IM	123	1	○ Yes	**Submit**
N1	2	Steth	GE	ABC	2	○ Yes	

Step 6 – Email OR Attendant Missing List Fulfillment: An email is then sent out by the workflow system to OR Attendant that the missing parts in the preference list have been fulfilled.

5. Research Directions

RECIPE will continue to be a proof of concept effort at heathcare institutions with focused research in the areas of interoperability of medical systems and development of open source Web services protocols. Work in this area has been promising although there is a need for a dedicated Surgical Extensible Markup Language, which will make brokering information between surgery based systems and technology easy and inexpensive.

5.1. Web Services

Some of the current interfaces in healthcare, particularly financial interfaces, are still batch oriented. The majority of clinical system interfaces are point-to-point using HL7 Version 2 formatted messages [25]. These are difficult to implement and maintain because the HL7 Version 2 standard specifies format, but not the semantics of the data put into formatted areas. As a result, every interface in unique and it is sometimes impossible to overcome semantic differences in the meaning of data items as they exist in disparate systems.

HL7 Version 3 [26] specifications are based on the HL7 RIM object model and specify structure, semantics, and constraints on data to improve system interoperability. The HL7 standard also specifies XML implementations useful for processing transactions on the web. The concept of HL7 Electronic Health Record (EHR) services that could be used generically for any EHR to access data in any other EHR is in the early stages of analysis and design. It is fundamental to true interoperability of clinical systems and medical devices and would facilitate tight coupling of systems via web transactions.

Full specification of HL7 Version 3 web services would streamline implementations of PSPAT by allowing the PSPAT workflow engine to more easily orchestrate behaviors across disparate healthcare systems and medical devices. Early work is underway jointly by HL7 and the Object Management Group [37], and a software factory implementation using the latest Visual Studio tooling has been specified by Microsoft [1].

The highest stage of interoperability (Phase 5 above) would allow agents to implement goal seeking behavior based on collaborative orchestration of higher level services provided by one or more workflow engines [31]. These will be essential to future military systems such as the DARPA Trauma Pod now being prototyped using autonomous robots as surgeons [16].

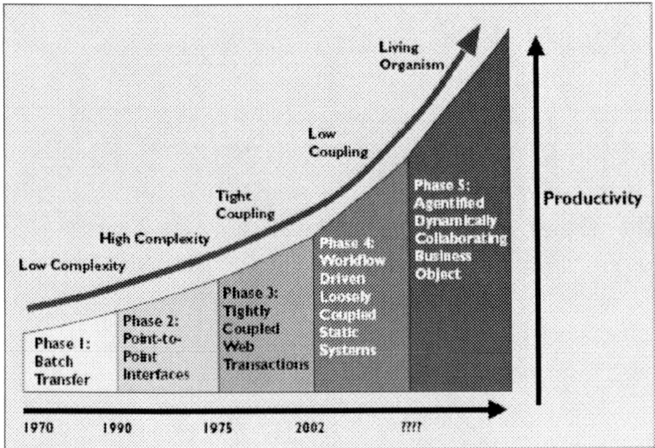

Figure 9. Improved enterprise integration leads to enhanced interoperability, more access to critical function-ality, lower implementation and maintenance costs, plug and play architectures, and more flexible and intelli-gent systems [31,49].

5.2. DARPA Trauma Pod

During the development of RECIPE and PSPAT, the Defense Advanced Research Projects Agency (DARPA) solicited a proposal for a Supply Chain Management Subsystem (SCMS) in a robotic vehicle that would perform surgery on the battlefield. This is part of a military strategic objective to be 30% robotic by the year 2025.

The goal of the DARPA Trauma Pod Phase I is to demonstrate feasibility of performing a surgical procedure without a human Surgeon, Circulating Nurse or Scrub Nurse in the Operating Room. The proposed Supply Chain Management Subsystem will support this goal by demonstrating the interaction between the surgical robotic client(s), an automated surgical item dispensing system and non-attached back-end legacy systems that include pe-rioperative distribution center activities such as restocking and reordering, as well as proce-dure coding.

The supply chain management system will be developed to manage information regard-ing the inventory in the automated dispensing system and to track the life cycle of all items used during the demonstration of the Trauma Pod. The technical challenge is, "how will the automated dispensing system maintain situational awareness during operations without costly and fragile interfaces with its robotic clients and other heterogeneous systems?"

To solve this problem SCMS will be developed in a Web Services technology environ-ment utilizing open source, standards based tools. A web services message bus will facili-tate supply chain information exchange with internal and external systems. In order to eliminate the costs of creating direct data feeds between the dispensing system and its ro-botic clients, SCMS will utilize a light weight medical encounter record to monitor and re-cord relevant activity during the surgical process. Data accumulation in the Medical En-counter Record will be synchronized with real time activity in the Trauma Pod via the proc-ess workflow engine, under development at the University of Maryland Medical System's Operating Room of the Future and PatientKeeper.

RFID technology will be utilized to uniquely identify and track the physical location of all supply items within twelve inch zones utilizing Class I RF tags. For Supply items such as lap sponges that may require additional information regarding their altered state while in use, Class III RF tags with imbedded sensors capable of measuring dampness and tempera-ture will be implemented. Finally, accumulated data in the Medical Encounter Record will

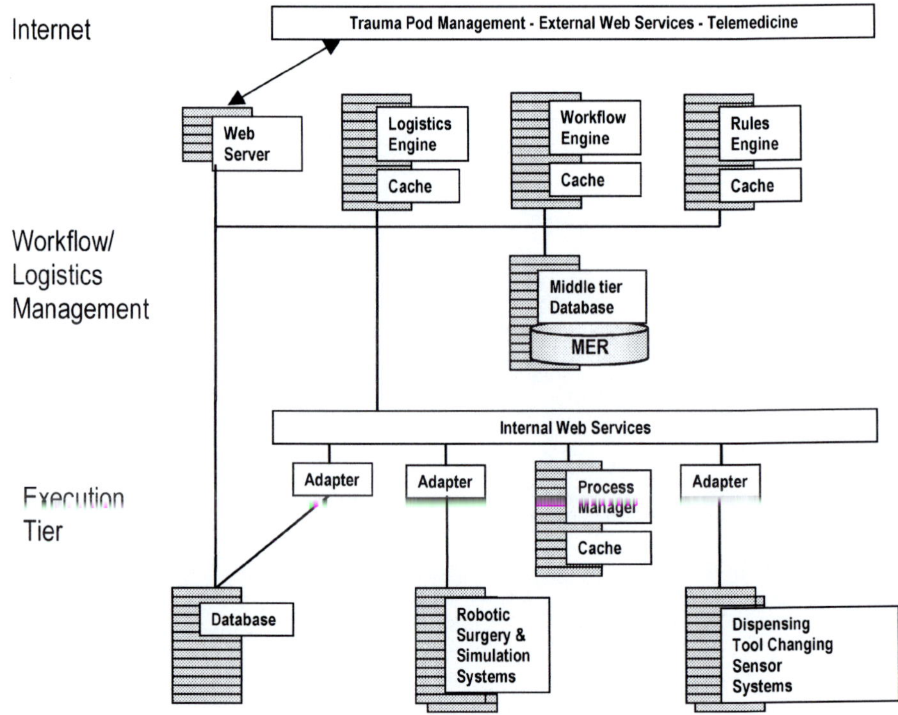

Figure 10. Web services architecture for SCMS.

be analyzed and translated into data elements required by military logistics systems (DMLSS) and electronic medical records (PIC, TMIP).

This work draws upon over a decade of research at the National Institute of Standards (NIST) in their "Intelligent Manufacturing Systems". Among other topics the NIST program addresses interoperability of manufacturing systems including robotics, supply chain and other legacy systems.

Off the shelf components will be used to accelerate development and lower cost:

- PatientKeeper Mobilizer middleware platform – provides web services bus and external interfaces.
- Apache web server
- Tomcat application server
- Oracle database
- OS Workflow – open source workflow engine

Development efforts will focus on building adapters to connect Trauma Pod subsystems to the web services bus, interfaces to input medical and logistics data, and Oracle database schema to store logistics information and the MER.

Base technology will use proven components with widespread deployment in production. The system will read inbound medical and logistics data, assure adequate supplies and instruments are available for surgery, reorder and re-provision as required, document procedures and association medical information, and provide visibility on each aspect of its functionality to an outside observer.

Sandberg and Ganous [41] described perioperative systems design and a comprehensive process involving dozens of activities embedded in nested timelines. The proposed approach can be extended to cover perioperative systems activities that will be essential in a production version of multiple Trauma Pods interoperating on the battlefield.

6. Conclusions

Work on the Operating Room of the Future at the University of Maryland Medical System is the first known prototype implementation of a standards based workflow engine in an operating room suite to monitor, manage, and improve throughput, while enhancing patient safety and patient care.

The advent of new technologies including Radio Frequency IDentification (RFID), mobile/wireless technologies, automated business process management (internet workflow systems and intelligent agents), Service Oriented Architectures (SOA) and Business Process Management (BPM) opens up new ways of automating business processes, overcoming barriers to technology adoption, and resolving problematic issues like patient, staff, and equipment location [35]. Total situational awareness of events, timing, and location of critical healthcare activities, makes possible real time process improvement by (1) anticipating future behaviors of complex systems, (2) displaying the probable futures of complex operations to all affected personnel, (3) generating self-organizing change in behaviors of humans and machines, (4) erasing a possible negative future outcome, and (5) replacing it with a modified future outcome that meets organizational goals.

The potential gains from this approach are enormous in terms of improved efficiency and patient safety. Workflow enhancement of clinical processes generated a 100% improvement in supply and instrument readiness in a large operating room suite. Full implementation of an automated workflow facility with integration into production clinical systems could induce a radical reinvention of clinical process integration resulting in improved patient outcomes, an enhanced staff working environment, significant cost reduction and enhancement of institutional revenue.

Implementation of the RECIPE approach automates feedback mechanisms for systematic enhancement of clinical processes. Implementation of intelligent automated systems in other domains with computerized feedback loops have led to emergent architectures with higher adaptability, capability, extensibility, and maintainability than could be initially conceived by the original designers of such systems [10,15]. This approach opens up ways to move away from medical production systems, and facilitate ad-hoc, autonomic workflows that are capable of adjusting themselves to new situations, monitor and recover from disruptions, and deal with attacks from anywhere.

References

[1] *A Software Factory Approach to HL7 Version 3 Solutions*. 2005, Microsoft and Blueprint Technologies.

[2] Allen, S., *Emergency Room Recovery*, in *The Boston Globe*. 2004: Boston. p. A1.

[3] Anyanwu, K., et al., *Healthcare enterprise process development and integration.* Journal of Research and Practice in Information Technology, 2003. **35**(2): p. 83–98.

[4] Arthur, W.B., *On the Evolution of Complexity*, in *Complexity: Metaphors, Models, and Reality. Proceedings Volume XIX, Sante Fe Institute Studies in the Science of Complexity.*, G.A. Cowan, D. Pines, and D. Meltzer, Editors. 1994, Addison-Wesley.

[5] Balas, E.A., et al., *Improving preventive care by prompting physicians.* Arch Intern Med, 2000. **160**(3): p. 301–8.

[6] Barkmeyer, E. and J. Lo, *Experience with IMDAS in the Automated Manufacturing Research Facility*, in *NISTIR 4132*. 1989, National Institute of Standards and Technology: Gaithersburg, MD.

[7] Bates, D.W., et al., *A Proposal for Electronic Medical Records in U.S. Primary Care.* J Am Med Inform Assoc, 2003. **10**(1): p. 1–10.

[8] Beyea, S.C. and P. Kilbridge, *Setting a research agenda on patient safety in surgical settings.* Semin Laparosc Surg, 2003. **10**(2): p. 79–83.

[9] Brooks, R.A., *How to build complete creatures rather than isolated cognitive simulators*, in *Architectures for Intelligence*, K. VanLehn, Editor. 1991, Lawrence Erlbaum Associates: Hillsdale, N.J. p. 225–239.

[10] Brooks, R.A., *Intelligence without representation.* Artificial Intelligence, 1991. **47**: p. 139–159.

[11] Buus, H., et al. *777 Flight Controls Validation Process.* in *14th Digital Avionics Systems Conference (DASC).* 1995. Cambridge, MA.

[12] Christensen, C.M., R. Bohmer, and J. Kenagy, *Will Disruptive Innovations Cure Health Care.* Harvard Business Review, 2000. **Reprint R00501**: p. 102–111.

[13] Classen, D.C. and P.M. Kilbridge, *The Roles and Responsibility of Physicians to Improve Patient Safety within Health Care Delivery Systems.* Acad Med, 2002. **77**(10): p. 963–972.

[14] Dadam, P., M. Reichert, and K. Kuhn. *Clinical Workflows – The Killer Application for Process-oriented Information Systems.* in *BIS 2000 – Proceedings of the 4th International Conference on Business Information Systems.* 2000. Poznan, Poland: Springer-Verlag.

[15] DARPA, *One Year Countdown to Grand Challenge 2005: DARPA Publishes Rules, Team Application Status Report*, in *Thomas Goodwin (contact), Arlington, VA.* 2004.

[16] DARPA, *Operating Room of the Future Workshop*, in *Executive Summary.* 2003. p. 1–2.

[17] Dhaliwal, J.S., et al., *Using Enterprise Modelling to Reengineer Healthcare Processes.* SIGGROUP Bulletin, 1997. **18**(1): p. 51–53.

[18] Exavera, *eShepard FAQ (Frequently Asked Questions).* 2004, Exavera Technologies: Portsmouth, NH.

[19] Ganek, A.G. and T.A. Corbi, *The Dawning of the Autonomic Computing Era.* IBM Systems Journal, 2003. **42**(1): p. 5–18.

[20] Gatersleben, M.R. and S.W. van der Weij. *Analysis and simulation of passenger flows in an airport terminal.* in *Proceedings of the 31st Conference on Winter Simulation: Simulation–a bridge to the future.* 1999. Phoenix, AZ: ACM Press.

[21] Goldratt, E.M. and J. Cox, *The goal: a process of ongoing improvement.* 2nd rev. ed. 1994, Great Barrington, MA: North River Press. 351 p.

[22] Han, Y., A. Sheth, and C. Bussler. *A Taxonomy of Adaptive Workflow Management.* in *1998 ACM Conference on Computer-Supported Collaborative Work.* 1998. Seattle.

[23] HDM, *PDAs Help Boost Hospital Revenue*, in *Health Data Management.* 2003.

[24] Henckels, C., *Wrong Site Surgery: A Study of Medical Misadventure Claims.* 2003, ACC Medical Misadventure Unit.

[25] Henderson, M., *HL7 Messaging.* 2003, Aubrey, TX: OTech.

[26] Hinchley, A., *Understanding Version 3: A primer on the HL7 Version 3 Communication Standard.* Understanding HL7 Series. 2003, Munich: Alexander Moench Publishing.

[27] Holland, J.H., *Hidden order: how adaptation builds complexity.* 1995, Reading, Mass.: Addison-Wesley. xxi, 185.

[28] Institute of Medicine (U.S.) Committee on Quality of Health Care in America, *Patient Safety: Achieving a New Standard for Care.* 2004, Washington, D.C.: The National Academies Press.

[29] Jacobson, I., M. Ericsson, and A. Jacobson, *The object advantage: business process reengineering with object technology.* 1995, Wokingham, England; Reading, Mass.: Addison-Wesley. 347.

[30] Larsen, R.A., et al., *Improved perioperative antibiotic use and reduced surgical wound infections through use of computer decision analysis.* Infect Control Hosp Epidemiol, 1989. **10**(7): p. 316–20.

[31] Maamar, Z. and J. Sutherland, *Toward Intelligent Business Objects: Focusing on techniques to enhance BPs that exhibit goal-oriented behaviors.* Communications of the ACM, 2000. **40**(10): p. 99–101.

[32] Manolescu, D.A. and S. Paul, *An Evaluation Framework for Workflow Engines.* Personal communication, 2003: p. 1–21.

[33] Marsland, S. and I. Buchan, *Clinical Quality Needs Complex Adaptive Systems and Machine Learning*, in *MEDINFO 2004*, M. Fieschi, Editor. 2004, IOS Press: Amsterdam.

[34] McGlynn, E.A., et al., *The quality of health care delivered to adults in the United States.* N Engl J Med, 2003. **348**(26): p. 2635–45.

[35] Minear, M.N. and J. Sutherland, *Medical informatics--a catalyst for operating room transformation.* Semin Laparosc Surg, 2003. **10**(2): p. 71–8.

[36] Ogunnaike, B.A. and W.H. Ray, *Process Dynamics, Modeling, and Control.* Topics in Chemical Engineering. 1994: Oxford University Press.

[37] OMG, *Health Level Seven, Object Management Group Begin Joint Healthcare Software Services Standardization Work: Combined Effort Leverages Strengths of Each Organization*, in *OMG Press Release 03–08–05.* 2005, OMG and HL7: Needham, MA.

[38] Paul, S., E. Park, and J. Chaar, *Essential Requirements for a Workflow Standard*, in *Business Object Design and Implementation II: OOPSLA '96, OOPSLA '97, and OOPSLA '98 Proceedings*, D. Patel, J. Sutherland, and J. Miller, Editors. 1998, Springer-Verlag: London. p. 100–108.

[39] Paul, S., E. Park, and J. Chaar, *RainMan: A Workflow System for the Internet.* 1997: IBM T.J. Watson Research Center.

[40] Reichert, M., C. Hensinger, and P. Dadam. *Supporting Adaptive Workflows in Advanced Application Environments.* in *EDBT Workshop on Workflow Management Systems.* 1998. Valencia.

[41] Sandberg, W.S., T.J. Ganous, and C. Steiner, *Setting a research agenda for perioperative systems design.* Semin Laparosc Surg, 2003. **10**(2): p. 57–70.

[42] Starfield, B., *Is US Health Really the Best in the World.* JAMA, 2000. **284**(4): p. 483–485.

[43] Steinert-Threlkeld, T., *Extreme Returns*, in *Baseline.* 2003. p. 26–28.

[44] Sutherland, J., *Agile Can Scale: Inventing and Reinventing SCRUM in Five Companies.* Cutter IT Journal, 2001. **14**(12): p. 5–11.

[45] Sutherland, J., *Agile Development: Lessons Learned from the First Scrum.* Cutter Agile Project Management Advisory Service: Executive Update, 2004. **5**(20): p. 1–4.

[46] Sutherland, J. *Future of Scrum: Pipelining of Sprints in Complex Projects.* in *AGILE 2005 Conference.* 2005. Denver, CO: IEEE.

[47] Sutherland, J., *Future of Scrum: Pipelining of Sprints in Complex Projects with Details on Scrum Type C Tools and Techniques.* 2005, PatientKeeper, Inc.: Brighton, MA. p. 1–27.

[48] Sutherland, J. and S. Alpert, *"Big Workflow" for Enterprise Applications.*, in *Business Object Design and Implementation III: OOPSLA '99 Workshop Proceedings*, D. Patel, J. Sutherland, and J. Miller, Editors. 1999, Springer-Verlag: London.

[49] Sutherland, J. and W.-J. van den Heuvel, *Enterprise Application Integration and Complex Adaptive Systems: Could System Integration and Cooperation be improved with Agentified Enterprise components?* Communications of the ACM, 2002. **45**(10): p. 59–64.

[50] Sutherland, J.V. *Advances in Mobile Computing: Disease Management.* in *TEPR Conference and Exhibition.* 2003. San Antonio, TX.

[51] Sutherland, J.V., *Architectural Vision for MANUFACTURING and 3CI Support.* 1989, Object Databases: Cambridge, MA.

[52] Sutherland, J.V. *Medical Informatics.* in *TATRC Advanced Medical Technology Principal Investigators' Review.* 2003.

[53] Sutherland, J.V. *RECIPE for REal time proCess ImProvement in hEalthcare.* in *13th Annual PHYSICIAN-COMPUTER CONNECTION Symposium.* 2004. Rancho Bernardo, CA: American Society for Medical Directors of Information Systems (AMDIS).

[54] Sutherland, J.V. and T.J. Ganous. *Back To The (OR) Future: The Perioperative Systems Performance Acceleration Tool.* in *Healthcare Information Management Systems Society Annual Conference and Exhibition.* 2004. Orlando, FL: HIMSS.

[55] Takeuchi, H. and I. Nonaka, *Hitotsubashi on Knowledge Management.* 2004, Singapore: John Wiley & Sons (Asia).

[56] Takeuchi, H. and I. Nonaka, *The New New Product Development Game.* Harvard Business Review, 1986(January-February).

[57] TATRC: Telemedicine and Advanced Technology Research Center, *Advanced Medical Technology Principal Investigators Review*, in *TATRC Operating Room of the Future, Medical Modeling and Simulation.* 2003.

[58] Thompson, T.G. and D.J. Brailer, *The Decade of Health Information Technology: Delivering Consumer-centric and Information-rich Health Care – Framework for Strategic Action.* 2004, U.S. Dept. of Health and Human Services: Washington, D.C.

[59] Wears, R.L. and M. Berg, *Computer Technology and Clinical Work: Still Waiting for Godot.* JAMA, 2005. **293**(10): p. 1261–1263.

[60] Zimmerman, B., P. Plsek, and C. Lindberg, *Edgeware: insights from complexity science for health care leader.* 1998: VHA, Inc.

Appendix I: Applying RECIPE

I.1. The Business Case for RECIPE

The healthcare goals of increasing revenue, reducing cost, enhancing patient care, and improving customer satisfaction are difficult to achieve due to high costs of integration of legacy systems, cultural barriers to adoption, and the intrinsically complex nature of healthcare processes. Healthcare processes typically require deep knowledge and expertise, are highly error prone, and demand a significant requirement for cross-functional workflow [17]. These issues present many barriers to adoption of new technologies.

Healthcare is the largest service industry in the United States and still largely paper based. The opportunity for improved efficiency and error reduction is huge ($70B). Inefficiencies from paper based processes in healthcare are similar to public sector operations where a single project providing automated management reporting on the web for fire, police, paramedic services, water, and other departments achieved a 1986% ROI annually, with an initial investment of $852,000. Overall expenses for the entire City of Albuquerque, NM, budget were cut by 6% with this single project [43]. This project demonstrates one important aspect of RECIPE, elimination of costly manual silos of information, and replacement with transparent and accurate reporting.

In healthcare there is there is an additional opportunity for revenue enhancement through real time process improvement. Brigham and Women's hospital in Boston introduced mobile capture of patient charges for procedures in the hospital and observed over 15% increase in revenue for PDA users in the first month of operation [23]. Charges are entered by the physician immediately at the point of care. Edit rules execute immediately to give the physician feedback in order to correct information or formulate it according to insurance processing requirements. Real time reporting allows identification of missing charges and automated follow-up assures that associated revenue is found and collected. This project demonstrates a second aspect of RECIPE where automated rules allow real time corrections and data mining after the event generates an adaptive, corrective response.

The focus of all these efforts is to bring knowledge gained in other industries into healthcare, such lessons learned from airport logistics [20] where deployment of these techniques has placed Amsterdam Airport Schiphol in the top three airports in the world with respect to the passenger experience. Throughput can typically be enhanced in virtually all operations: inventory can be reduced through just in time delivery, quality can be enhanced, and patient satisfaction of medical products can be optimized through innovation and fine tuning at the level of individual clients.

"...Boston Medical Center, the city's safety net hospital, is becoming a model of how to bring relief to the nation's beleaguered emergency rooms, reducing treatment delays and closures to ambulances when ERs are more crowded than ever. BMC emergency doctors are treating more patients than they did last year and have reduced average time in the waiting room from 60 minutes to 40 minutes. The secret lies in a radical idea for medicine, but one that has guided airport managers and restaurant hostesses for years: Keep the customers moving." [2]

I.2. RECIPE Components: Planning, Testing, and Technology

The RECIPE for incremental evolution of administrative and clinical processes consists of a planning component, a testing component, and a technology component.

The planning component is the responsibility of clinical domain experts and requires:

- High level maps of end-to-end healthcare processes.

- Prioritized opportunities for operational or clinical improvements.
- Detailed process maps of selected process improvement areas.
- Selection of precise mechanism for process improvements.
- Establishment of research objectives and collected of data for outcomes analysis.

The testing component requires:

- Communication and validation of planned improvements with all stakeholders.
- Manual introduction of the process change in a targeted area of the institution.
- Data collection to analyze and document the effect of the process change.
- Recommendations for automation of the process improvement.

The technology component requires domain knowledge and expertise in new technologies areas. Specifically:

- RFID technologies need to be evaluated, pilot projects initiated, and data collection and monitoring strategies need to be defined.
- Workflow engines are increasingly embedded in ERP and CRM systems for specifying, automating, and updating operational protocols. This technology needs to be evaluated, selected, and fine tuned for healthcare operations.
- Alerting and messaging systems need to be implemented to reach any member of the clinical or operational staff on any available device.
- Service Oriented Architectures (SOAs) need to be deployed to provide cost effective integration with enterprise and departmental systems.
- An operational database needs to be established to store protocol specifications, state of protocol executions, and essential data collected as part of a Medical Encounter Record (MER) that is used for workflow execution.
- Dynamic application generation of real-time workflow requests for action or information must be specified and implemented.
- Automated reporting is essential for real time operations information and data mining of historical workflow data.
- Monitoring and reporting on changes in baseline data affected by incremental process improvement needs to be automatically delivered to clinical and administrative staff on a routine basis to demonstrate and maintain process improvements.

I.3. RECIPE and PSPAT

PSPAT constitutes architecture, a backbone, and a tool for managing and monitoring the Pre-Operative Period, the Intra-Operative Period, and the Post-Operative Period. RECIPE is a research project that builds on top of PSPAT and explores real-time improvement of healthcare processes. In particular, the RECIPE project aims at capturing best practices and heuristics into a methodology that will include a "cookbook" and a supporting suite of tools for supporting real time process improvement, depending on a blend of SOA, workflow technology and Business Process Management techniques. The approach provides immediate value to an organization by first improving manual management of current tasks, then incremental addition of automation to eliminate manual overhead. Adoption is enhanced by demonstrating measurable improvement in small steps, while avoiding technology disruption of established workflows.

I.4. RECIPE and Continuous Process Improvement

RECIPE facilitates continual evolution of business processes. In contrast to continuous business process improvement, continual evolution methods allow us to *incrementally* improve business processes, commencing with rather straightforward automation of manual tasks, evolving towards more sophisticated levels of automation that are equipped with more intelligence. The higher the level of automation, the better it conforms to the medical processes and policies that are required by the organization.

In particular, several stages of workflow automation are distinguished, ranging from pure manual tasks to the level of full automation using autonomous agentified workflows that may adapt their own behavior, being equipped with reflective capabilities, and heal themselves without any involvement of humans. Currently, the following levels are identified including: basic level (0), managed level (1), predictive level, (2) adaptive level (3) and the autonomic level (4). This taxonomy is in line with the indexation of autonomous computing [19].

Firstly, the workflows residing at the basic level are characterized by rather a rather informal and very local process landscape. Typically, management has some knowledge about the time these processes take to finish, and coordinates them centrally. Next, the managed level workflows are usually designed according to best practices, and optimized using feed-back loops. Packaged software solutions, e.g., ERP packages, are prototypical examples that support medical processes fitting in this category. The predictive level revolves around the evaluation of medical workflows by considering their ROI, possibly at the level of individual transactions. While doing so, future projections are created that take into account potential risks, benefits and costs. At even a higher level of sophistication, workflows are provisioned automatically, and optimized so that they meet required levels of transaction performance. This performance may be described using several Key Performance Indicators (KPIs), each of which identifies a measurable, and business-strategy related process improvement area. The autonomic level entails the most refined level in the framework of Fig. 6. Workflows at this level are able to monitor and quickly tune themselves to new e-business process requirements (KPIs), and react to disruptions in medical processes. The latter characteristic implies that autonomic systems are self-healing.

RFID comes in the picture from level two, and aims at creating a comprehensive "cockpit" overview of a healthcare-related business process. In particular, the RFID is used to observe and graphically represent the situation in which the process is executing so that managers may quickly visualize anomalies.

The RECIPE approach makes it possible to unobtrusively introduce real time process improvement into an operational healthcare environment through:

- RFID tracking of patients, staff, supplies, instruments, equipment – accumulating baseline data
- Analysis of patient flow bottlenecks and development of process improvements targets

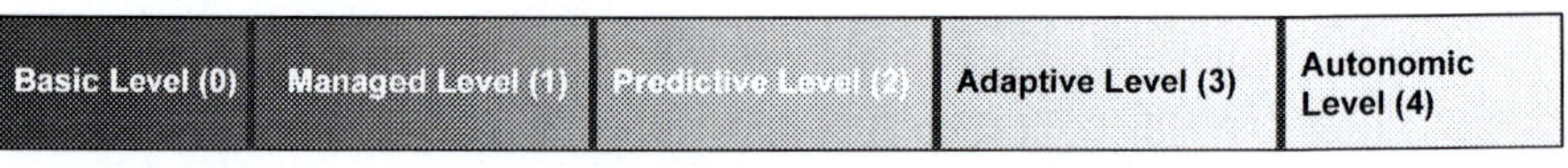

Figure 11. From Basic to Autonomic Computing.

- Manual testing of process improvements
- Integration of a standards-based workflow management system into the enterprise IT infrastructure
- Small incremental process improvements introduced through the workflow engine with rapid fine tuning
- Automatically deal with disruptions when possible – otherwise make them visible proactively
- Orchestrate human and machine behavior to anticipate and resolve problems
- Dynamic application generation: real time support for workflow engine to obtain information needed at any step of process

I.5. RECIPE and Agile Practices

RECIPE is based on Agile process theory [46] which, in turn, in based on complex adaptive system theory [27]. It is designed to unobtrusively and systematically transform an organization. It can be rapidly implemented with Agile teams using best business practices [55] for product development. Failure to implement Agile practices will generate excessive delay and ensure a long and painful transformation. It is highly recommended that institutions implementing RECIPE get ongoing training from Agile coaches experienced in team process and team development.

Appendix II: Perioperative Systems Process Acceleration Tool (PSPAT)

II.1. Perioperative Systems Design

Perioperative Systems Design describes a rational approach to managing the convergent flow of patients having procedures from disparate physical and temporal starting points, through the operating room and then to such a place where future events pertaining to the patient have no further impact on OR operations. The process for an individual patient can be envisioned as a nested set of timelines: a coarse-grained timeline beginning with the decision to perform an operation and ending when the patient definitively leaves the post-op occurrence, and a fine-grained timeline encompassing the immediate pre-op, intra-op and post-operative course. At each point, physical infrastructure and work processes impact the progress of patients along these timelines. Starting from this construct, Perioperative Systems Design can be conceptualized, studied and optimized like any industrial process in which many materials, actors and processes are brought together in a coordinated workflow to achieve a designed goal [41].

The Fig. 12 shows nested, interactive timelines around the Pre-Operative Period, the Intra-Operative Period, and the Post-Operative Period. Of interest, is that there are more activities before and after surgery than during surgery. Wrapping a workflow monitoring, management, and alerting system around the Inter-Operative Period tasks an appropriate separation of concerns. We call this "wrapper" around the surgery procedure the Perioperative Systems Process Acceleration Tool (PSPAT).

Perioperative Process Timeline

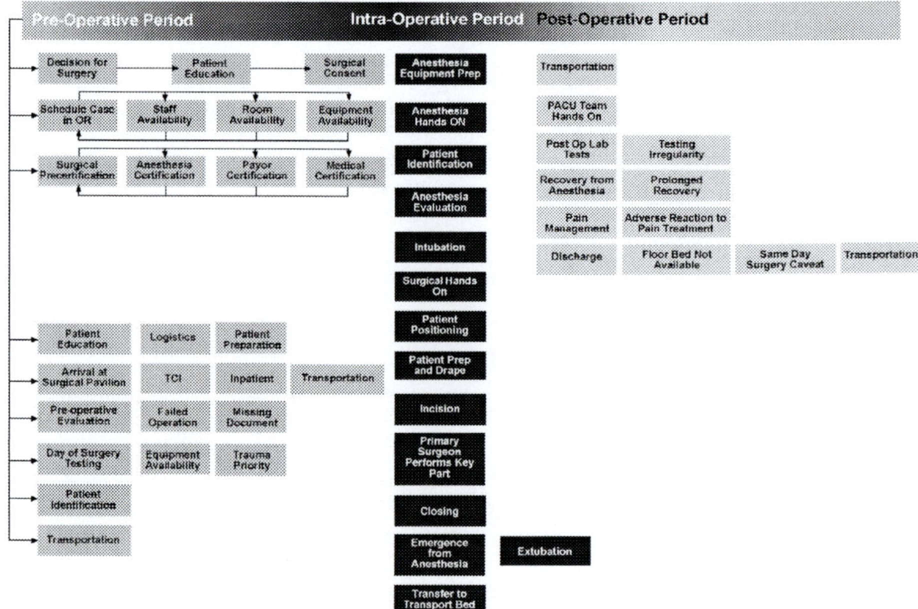

Figure 12. Perioperative Process Timeline [41].

II.2. PSPAT in Pre-Operative Period

In the Pre-Operative period PSPAT needs to orchestrate and monitor the following activities:

- Patient identification
- Diagnostic workup
- Incoming patient medications and allergies
- Surgery schedule
- Determine staff readiness
- Confirm operating room readiness
- Assure supplies and equipment availability
- Capture data on incoming medical record, capture vitals, I/Os, pre-operative medications, tests, and scans
- Monitor patient entry into operating room
- Monitor patient readiness

The first two tasks identify the patient and the corresponding diagnoses to avoid mistakes. For example, wrong site surgery makes up 2% of medical error [24]. A surgery scheduling system is used to schedule patient, staff, and operating room. At UMMC, one third of surgeries each day are unscheduled so the scheduling problem is extremely difficult in a surgical setting. There are many moving parts to be coordinated and many unanticipated events.

Supplies and equipment must be prepared before surgery and the case cart with all items needed must be in the operating room before surgery. Case cart readiness was a major problem at UMMC prior to beginning this study. A substantial amount of paperwork and lab tests must be gathered an interpreted before surgery. There are many points where delays can be induced in the system. As a result, surgery start times are often late which has major revenue and cost implications. Process mapping, monitoring of critical points, and implementing process improvements can significantly increase patient throughput.

Monitoring patient entry into the operating room and patient readiness for surgery are critical to successful outcomes, particularly with respect to patient safety. Automated monitoring of positioning and timing of the patient can reduce manual data entry, increase accuracy, and also provide analytical data essential to planning for process improvement.

II.3. PSPAT in Intra-Operative Period

Intra-Operative tasks include:

- Anesthesia equipment preparation
- Anesthesia
- Patient identification
- Anesthesia evaluation
- Intubation
- Surgical hands-on
- Patient positioning
- Patient prep and drape
- Incision
- Primary surgery
- Closing
- Emergence from anesthesia

- Extubation
- Patient transport

PSPAT assumes that the anesthesiologist intubates and monitors the patient, while the surgical team does the surgery. It monitors surgery start and stop time, manages schedule irregularities, assures proper inventory of supplies, instruments, and equipment, and communications externally when operating room needs arise. Patient safety is supported by patient identification and RFID technology used to check inventory and make sure no supplies are left inside the patient.

II.4. PSPAT in the Post-Operative Period

Post-operative issues include:

- Patient transportation
- Patient handoff to recovery area
- Post-op lab tests
- Assessing lab test irregularities
- Monitoring recovery from anesthesia
- Dealing with issues around prolonged recovery
- Pain management
- Adverse reaction to pain treatment
- Discharge

When surgery is complete, the patient is moved to a recovery area and monitored carefully. Appropriate laboratory tests are performed and any abnormalities are assessed for further treatment. Pain is carefully managed along with any adverse reactions to the surgery, allergic responses, and post-surgery medication or treatment.

All of these issues need to be deal with by a combination of human and automated systems. At a minimum, PSPAT maintains a Medical Encounter Record (MER). This consists of all relevant data on patient flow through the perioperative process. It is collected, processed, evaluated, and updated by a workflow engine. The MER provides data for the discharge summary, and updates the external medical record. In addition, PSPAT may be tasked with monitoring protocols around lab tests and pain management, as well interfacing with transportation subsystems and handoff of the patient to external systems.

II.5. Perioperative Event Flow in the DARPA Trauma Pod

In the context of a robotic OR of the Future project such as the DARPA Trauma Pod [16] it is essential to map the clinical processes required for surgery, develop protocols for management of critical process events, establish rules for decision making during PSPAT execution of clinical protocols, and orchestrate behavior between heterogeneous complex systems. In particular, it is essential to orchestrate the interaction between surgical robots, a surgical item management system (dispensing) and non-attached back-end systems including perioperative distribution center activities (restocking and reordering) and procedure coding, utilizing a workflow engine embedded with intelligent goal seeking agents.

The DARPA Trauma Pod provides a microenvironment that totally automates the surgery process. PSPAT is designed to provide operational support for both major surgery centers and the Trauma Pod. Thus lessons from one environment enhance research and development on the other environment.

In the Trauma Pod, PSPAT manages the environment surrounding diagnostic and surgical procedures which are the responsibility of robotic subsystems.

- Respond to incoming event alert
- Analyze current state of trauma pod for surgical readiness
- Register inbound patient
- Read medical record from soldier's dog tag
- Provide external telemedicine view of all data and events
- Monitor vital signs and I/Os
- Provide for external telemedicine input as required
- Support diagnostic workup
- Capture diagnostic data and treatment plan
- Maintain order sets relevant to treatment plans
- Initiate and monitor execution of order sets by surgical subsystems.
- Manage inventory of supplies, instruments, and equipment
- Monitor post-operative process and discharge of patient
- Update external systems
- Restock inventory
- Monitor sanitization of pod

PSPAT activities in the Trauma Pod are defined initially as a streamlined set of functions. Responsibilities start when the soldier enters the Pod and terminate when the soldier leaves the Pod. Initial assumptions are that robotic subsystems will manage most surgical activities leaving overall coordination to PSPAT. It is highly likely that PSPAT will absorb more activities as testing for deployment of the Trauma Pod proceeds and the robotic engineers are required to support the full scope of patient management.

The DARPA Trauma Pod provides a controlled microenvironment for developing optimal perioperative workflow without the distraction of institutional issues, cultural resistance, or re-education of humans trained in suboptimal workflow. It is a useful test bed for design of process improvements which then can be migrated into the human perioperative environment.

II.6. PSPAT at the University of Maryland Medical Center

The University of Maryland Medical System is developing a Perioperative Systems Acceleration Tool (PSPAT) that provides an integrated workflow engine, rules engine, logistics engine, Medical Encounter Record (MER) repository, and interface engine, coupled with extensive connectivity to all relevant external enterprise systems. PSPAT will passively monitor the location and availability of patients, staff, supplies, instruments, equipment, and operating facilities, watch the convergence of the surgery team, supplies, instruments, and equipment around the patient, and intervene to assure that critical personnel and physical requirements are met in real time, and initiate alternative protocols and actions when planned perioperative schedules cannot be met or patient safety is at risk.

The basic concepts in PSPAT are information uptake from a wide variety of clinical systems, calculation of current state of clinical processing, and generating a set of reactions to current state in order to move it towards organizational goals for efficiency, safety, and improvement of patient outcomes.

In the context of an automated OR of the Future, it is essential to wrap information technology around the surgery to support the entire perioperative process and orchestrate behavior between heterogeneous systems which exist outside, yet support the surgical pro-

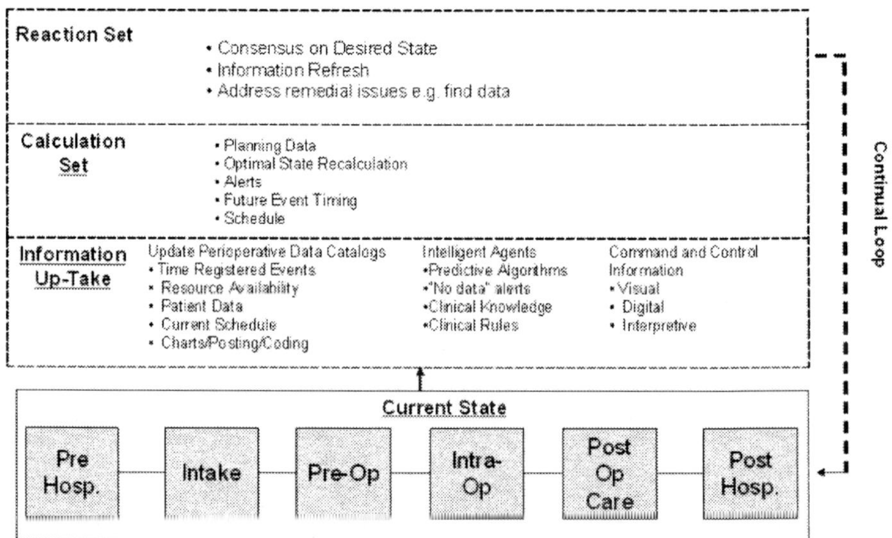

Figure 13. Perioperative Systems Process Acceleration Tool.

cedure, and are mandatory for patient safety and support of treatment before and after surgery. In particular, it is essential to provide a lightweight MER repository capable of managing the information input of a patient record, diagnostic and triage information, vitals and I/Os data collection, automated lab tests and patient scans, treatment plans, order sets and protocols, surgeon preference lists for supplies and equipment, web-based visual display of patient information for external telemedicine clinicians, reordering and restocking supplies management. For post-surgical care, discharge summaries, and externally posting of updates to the patient's medical record are of critical importance. The medical facility picking up the patient for post-surgical care must have up to date medical information that incorporates all procedures, medications, and diagnoses, along with discharge medications and recommendations for follow-up.

PSPAT in the University of Maryland Medical Center uses existing clinical and logistics systems to the maximum extent possible. For example, there is an enterprise wide clinical repository that supports computerized physician order entry. A new surgery scheduling system is currently being installed. Several equipment and supply information systems support perioperative activities. Integration with these systems allows PSPAT to use these systems as both data sources and implementation systems for adaptive process improvement.

For the DARPA Trauma Pod PSPAT implementation, there are no other clinical repositories in the Trauma Pod. The PSPAT MER must read the incoming patient record off a soldier's smart dog tag. It then will aggregate all relevant clinical and logistic data in the MER. Upon release from the Trauma Pod, the soldier's medical record on the dog tag will be updated with the latest clinical information.

II.7. PSPAT Components

This section provides a conceptual overview of PSPAT. Work on specific components is ongoing. In some cases technology is available and implemented. In others, selection activities are underway. Some components are in the prototype stage. Others are based on available commercial products.

II.7.1. A Workflow Engine

The workflow engine lies at "heart" of the PSPAT. It understands the steps of the perioperative system design and "beats" as it executes perioperative processes step by step. It "pumps" information and moves it through various "organ systems" of the PSPAT. The "organ systems" provide services to the workflow engine that help it execute its tasks. The key service components of the workflow engine are (1) adapters to extract information from any human or machine source of essential data, (2) a virtual information repository to store the Medical Encounter Record (MER), along with process definitions and key information elements required for process execution, (3) a rules engine to do intelligence processing of essential information to answer questions posed by the workflow engine as to current state, (4) an alerting and messaging system to inform or request other parts of the healthcare system to perform tasks, request information, or advise on completion of critical tasks, (5) a reporting system to monitor timely task completion and provide summary data for outcomes analysis, (6) a logistics subsystem to manage inventory and ordering of supplies, instruments, and equipment, and (6) a web-based telemedicine view of all data and process states for external human interaction and observation.

Workflow Engines designed to streamline, automate, and re-engineer business processes are rarely deployed in healthcare. Here we will assess the most prevalent initiatives in this domain. For this purpose it is important to make a distinction between Workflow Management Systems products of the 1990s which were monolithic in nature and current Workflow Engines designed to be embedded as a software tool in a Service Oriented Architecture [32]. The most advanced Workflow Engine prototype for healthcare designed specifically for web-based integration with legacy systems was "Big Workflow," developed at IDX Systems in the late 1990's in collaboration with computer scientists from IBM Watson Laboratories [39,38,48]. Several prototypes have been developed for clinical and administrative systems using the University of Georgia METEOR Workflow Management System [3]. Strategies for using workflow technology to "capture" legacy systems and repurpose them for use with more current technologies are critical for healthcare and have been well documented [49]. Enterprise modeling for business process transformation in healthcare, serving as a basis for configuring medical workflow engines, has been examined in Singapore [17].

II.7.2. Adapters to Gather Information from Any Human or Machine Source

The role of the interface engine and adapters is to transform all data into XML on a web information bus. This allows standards-based web technologies and open source tools to be applied to ongoing PSPAT enhancement.

PSPAT has an interface engine and adapters designed to support a wide variety of interface types:

- XML remote procedure calls used for system integration over IP networks
- HL7 transactions used to transport medical data between medical information systems.
- SQL interfaces designed to interact with any SQL database, e.g., Oracle or SQL Server.
- Custom interfaces of any type for specialized systems such as medical devices or robots.

The strategic goal of PSPAT is to reduce integration maintenance costs by at least an order of magnitude. This is critical as new process improvement targets may require acquisition of data from new systems on an ongoing basis. The software architecture for PSPAT

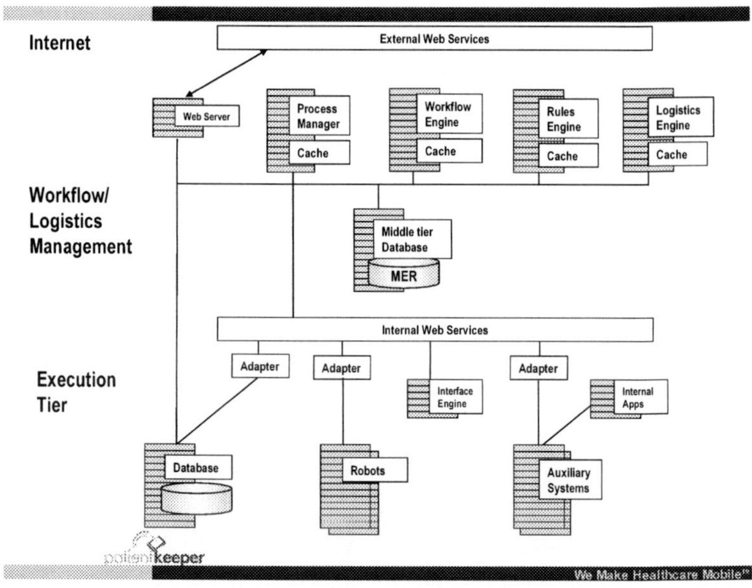

Figure 14. Software architecture for DARPA Trauma Pod [53].

in the University of Maryland Medical Center is envisioned to be similar to that in the DARPA autonomous robotic Trauma Pod show above.

II.7.3. MER: Virtual Information Repository for the Workflow Engine Access

A key concept for management of process workflows is a "package" of information that flows with the patient through every point in the perioperative process. Updating that "package" shows the real-time state of the patient in process sufficient for the workflow engine to determine what step of the process the patient is in, whether a step in the process is complete, if conditions are met that are necessary to move to the next step, or to ask a specialist to tell the system what the next step should be. This "package" or Medical Encounter Record (MER) captures essential real-time data necessary to efficiently and safely manage patient flow.

This "package" concept is an essential component of the architecture for Boeing Computer Systems and follows an airplane or missile through the entire assembly line process. It is stored in a virtual repository in that primary data resides in hundreds of heterogeneous financial, design, and factory automation systems throughout the Boeing Company. The concept was refined through work with the NIST Automated Manufacturing Research Facility (AMRF) [6] and Titan Systems Corp [51]. It is here extended to healthcare.

MER information is "fuel" for workflow engine processing. The workflow engine will seek out the required information from multiple data sources related to each step the patient goes through in the perioperative process. These sources include, but are not limited to the electronic medical record used house-wide, the perioperative software system, the pharmacy software system, the clinical laboratory software system, the picture archiving system (PACS) used for accessing digitized images, and others. Having users' interfaces for the workflow engine Web-based, PDA-based, and wireless, will provide for easy access to any data source from any location to obtain whatever information is needed for the current step of the workflow process.

II.7.4. A Rules Engine to Provide Intelligent Agent Support for the Workflow Engine

When a workflow engine executes a workflow process with a defined series of steps there are pre- and post-conditions, or constraints that must be met when moving from step to step. Often these constraints require sophisticated decision-making which is aided by a rules engine. There are robust rules engines available commercially and as open source, that can be used to augment the workflow engine when complex decisions need to be made. The core development of a workflow engine can then focus on quick execution of workflow protocols, dealing with error conditions, integrating with other systems, and so forth, without trying to reinvent a proven technology for automating complex decisions.

The rules engine evaluated for this project maintains a state network or a set of constraints representing medical policies, so that at any point in time (present or historical) the state of all patients for which data has been received is known. Therefore, upon receipt of new data, the network is updated to reflect any changes in patient, staff, operating room, equipment, or supplies state.

Additionally, actions are defined for rules that have become satisfied. The rules engine is designed to work in conjunction with a physician mobile application platform that will run clinician applications and display appropriate alerts, reminders, and requests for information. The rules incorporated in such applications push them to the level of intelligent agents.

In addition, since the rules engine can store the state network of information for all patients in the perioperative process, it can detect scheduling and other issues across all patients in real time. This is achieved by checking the state of patient data extracted from underlying databases that are accessed through adapters.

Rules may be modified, extended, or included to accommodate new medical insights, hospital or governmental policies. As a result the rules environment can evolve with human input to maximize patient throughput, efficiency, and safety of the perioperative process.

II.7.5. An Alerting System to Ensure Timely Completion of Clinical Events

The workflow engine will use as a service a comprehensive alerting system to send messages of any type to any device type, supported by the rules system. It has the additional capability of sending a dynamic query form to an external human interface for data the rules engine needs to process a clinical pathway. In essence, these are "smart alerts." The alerting system can incorporate remote telemedicine experts into the surgery process as required.

II.7.6. A Reporting System to Access Outcomes Data in Real Time

The MER stores the state of each patient in a comprehensive clinical data repository and keeps a record of important state transitions for future analysis. This allows the development of queries to determine improvement in outcomes over time with respect to patient care, efficiency of scheduling and utilization of resources, and the frequency of adverse events detected in the perioperative systems processes.

II.7.7. A Logistics Subsystem to Manage Inventory

The workflow engine orchestrates processes and manages communication of needs and requirements to external systems. It assures that required inventory is on hand to support scheduled surgery and manages reorder of consumable supplies.

II.7.8. Web-Based Telemedicine View

The PSPAT rules engine has the capability of dynamically generating web-based views of all clinical data, processes, and process states. It can also generate dynamic applications to request or transmit data to any human or machine participant in the perioperative process. This capability will allow external human observers or participants in the perioperative process to view process flow inside the operating room or Trauma Pod.

II.8. PSPAT Summary

PSPAT is designed to observe the clinical setting, notice when something is going wrong, and advise people and systems on corrective courses of action. As it evolves into more and more automation it provides an autopilot to coordinate actions between silos of activities. It watches the patient traverse the healthcare system and notes what has been done, what has not been done, and the patient status. In its ultimate incarnation, it will evolve into a personal nurse for the patient making sure every action is directed towards better outcomes for the patient. It is designed to be the safety net that catches the patient when they fall through the cracks in the healthcare system.

Future of Intelligent and Extelligent Health Environment
R.G. Bushko (Ed.)
IOS Press, 2005

Framework for Measuring Adaptive Knowledge-Rich Systems Performance

Renata G. BUSHKO, M.S.
Director, Future of Health Technology Institute, Hopkinton MA, USA

Abstract. The universe is non repeatable in nature – most of events cannot be prestated and do not repeat themselves. The only way to create systems that are truly useful is to make them adaptive (able to reason by analogy and learn) and rich in knowledge (including common sense knowledge). Adaptive and knowledge-rich health management could get us closer to errorless health care where small incremental adjustments happen all the time preventing occurrence of an error. In the era of adaptive systems we need to have a way to evaluate their performance. Are they truly adaptive? How adaptive are they? Are they accurate enough? Are they fast enough? Are they cost effective? This chapter presents general framework for measuring adaptive knowledge-rich systems' performance and includes among others definitions of adaptiveness factor, britt (a unit of brittleness) and uso-quant (unit of usefulness of a piece of knowledge). Measuring adaptive knowledge-rich systems performance is one of the most important research areas that can have a big pay-off in healthcare now and in the future.

Motto

"How do we ever understand anything? Almost always [...] by using one or another kind of analogy – that is, by representing each new thing as though it resembles something we already know. Whatever a new thing's internal workings are too strange or complicated to deal with directly, we represent whatever parts of it we can in terms of more familiar signs. This way, we make each novelty seem similar to some more ordinary thing. It really is a great discovery, the use of signals, symbols, words and names. They let our minds transform the strange into the commonplace." Marvin Minsky, The Society of Mind

1. Introduction

By providing Artificial Intelligence (AI) programs with a large amount of knowledge and a way to reason by analogy, such programs will be able to mimic human ability to solve hard problems—the ability to adaptively arrive at crude, vague, but close to correct solutions by guessing values of unknown and crucial details while omitting known but unimportant details.

By providing programs with metaknowledge in the form of problem-independent agents and a way to analogize, we could create programs that would assemble new methods for solving novel problems – exhibiting adaptive and smart behavior. Reasoning and task metaknowledge elicitation and its representation in the form of problem-independent agents needs more attention before a program adaptively assembling new problem solving methods can be built.

A combination of a knowledge-rich environment and an analogy engine will be called Knowledge Rich Analogy (KRA).

We assume that KRA is sufficient to solve a wide variety of hard real-world problems accurately enough, quickly, adaptively, cost-effectively, and in a non-brittle manner. The power of KRA grows with an increase in the amount of metaknowledge. Metaknowledge enables KRA to exhibit meta-adaptiveness: the ability to configure effective problem solving methods to novel problems.

We do not know how to imitate the commonsense-intensive nature of human thinking, we do not have a ready to represent pool of metaknowlege (knowledge of how and when to use what type of knowledge to solve problems), and in addition, we lack concepts enabling a systematic examination and evaluation of KRA systems and KRA applications. In order to investigate the power of various kinds of knowledge and their effect on KRA application performance, a new set of methodological tools has to be created. New measures for evaluating accuracy, timeliness, adaptiveness, cost-effectiveness, non-brittleness, and KB-preparedness of KRA applications are preconditions (means) to achieve a goal of true adaptiveness.

2. Need for Automation of Estimation Tasks

Estimation tasks usually appear at the very first stage of problem solving when all the information needed for the full analysis of the problem is not yet available because of the time and cost constraints. Humans, however, fill in the gaps by using approximate and analogical reasoning to arrive at crude estimates. Automating estimation tasks would substantially improve flexibility of expert systems, especially in engineering design and modeling, for it is in these activities that the estimation of the boundary conditions and numeric threshold values of parameters constitute a major difficulty.

In addition, more and more often, modern technology requires computer modeling of catastrophic phenomena (e.g., strength of composites). This is possible only if the problem of modeling discontinuous functions, that characterize catastrophic phenomena, is solved by commonsense estimation. The success of a KRA approach would open up doors for modeling discontinuous processes.

Automated estimation tasks are also potentially applicable to a wide variety of computational problems that rely on approximations and abstractions, including decision-making, planning, design, simulation, diagnosis and others. These problems are usually in NP, thus in order to automate them, a program has to do the guessing (estimation) itself.

3. Need for Research on Reasoning by Analogy

Current research on computational analogy uses mainly toy problems and reasoning about relatively simple physical objects and processes. Estimation tasks require representation of complex, real-world, dynamic events and analogizing between them. Moving from "toy analogies" to "real analogies" would give AI systems more adaptivenss (non-brittleness). "To make any real-world application program resourceful, we must supplement its formal reasoning facilities with matching facilities that are heuristically appropriate for the problem domain it is working in. ...Different types of problems and representations may require different concepts of similarity" [1]. "Intelligent" software should be able to do interdomain expertise transfer by looking for relevant analogies among far-flung, seemingly unrelated knowledge.

4. Need for Research on Common Sense

AI has managed to make programs that solve mathematical problems (e.g., hard integration problems) considered difficult even by mathematicians; AI has produced expert systems highly competent in narrow, highly specialized domains like glaucoma diagnosis; AI has gotten very good at playing checkers and chess. AI has not yet been able to create an agent that is able to stop solving a mathematical problem in order to help somebody who fainted in the same room. Solving a mathematical equation turns out to be easier than recognizing various aspects of the environment in which the equation is being solved. We need to build a "common sense engine" in order to create and agent able to deal with the complexity and diversity of everyday situations.

Marvin Minsky in "The Society of Mind" defines common sense as "an immense society of hard earned practical ideas—of multitudes of life-learned rules and exceptions, dispositions and tendencies, balances and checks." These balances and checks are especially useful in performing estimation tasks, where we deal with incomplete information. Programs with common sense or "do something sensible" programs [2] would be non-brittle, easy to use, not always perfect but always on target. They would have to "automatically infer for themselves a sufficiently wide class of immediate consequences of anything they are told and what they already know" – according to John McCarthy in "Programs with Common Sense".

The body of commonsense knowledge is enormously large; consists of things that almost everyone knows, but is too divers to characterize any other way. A KRA environment like CYC KB gives hope of providing AI programs with enough knowledge from various domains that would make them non-brittle and adaptable to the rich environment in which they have to function. Capturing common sense will bring big payoffs both in science and in business. "We can hardly expect to make machines to wonder before we find out how to make them do ordinary, sensible things." [2]

5. Need for Metaknowledge in Adaptive Systems – Metaadaptiveness

In order to achieve adaptiveness of problem solvers (metadaptiveness) we need to represent knowledge describing when, why, and how various types of knowledge are used (metaknowledge). Metaknowledge is used to plan or modify reasoning strategies to adapt them to achieve a predetermined goal from a given situation. It is reasoning about how to act to achieve that goal. And on a longer time scale, software should be able to reflect creatively on its past experience and use this experience to improve performance on new tasks. How can it be done?

Let's assume that an "agent" is a reusable component of the problem solving method (subject to certain informational requirements). If research on analogical meta-reasoning is successful, it will be possible to derive new problem-solving agents from known agents as follows: Agent M known to work for task T1 of type T, can probably be successfully applied to similar tasks T2, T3…Tn of type T. It can also be a potential source of similar agents N1, N2…Nm working for tasks from a different class C that is in some way similar to T. If an efficient way of matching problems analogically is devised, it can be used to analogize between agents for solving those problems. This may result in highly adaptive problem solvers.

But representation of metaknowledge is impractical in first order predicate logic because "Predicates [of FOP] expressions are prohibited from referring in certain ways to one another. This prevents the representation of metaknowledge, rendering those systems incapable of describing what the knowledge that they contain can be used for. In effect, it precludes the use of functional descriptions. We need to develop systems for logic that can reason about their own knowledge, and make heuristic adaptations and interpretations of it, by using knowledge about knowledge but these limitations of expressiveness make logic unsuitable for such purposes." [1]

6. Significance of the Methodology to Evaluate Adaptive Knowledge-Based Systems

Developing a set of concepts for evaluating and comparing KRA applications is a precondition of success. Because of the novelty of knowledge-based systems, we are far from having well defined performance objectives and measures. I believe that we should try to emulate older and better structured sciences and develop measures of performance that could be used to compare applications created by various researchers. Objective measures of the performance of progress or success can become as hard as the problem that we are trying to solve; I think that it is the right place to start.

7. Research on Analogy – History

Research on computational analogical reasoning gained momentum in the 1980's [1,3–12,83,15]. Two distinct trends appeared in the course of these works: pragmatic and syntactic. All pragmatic theories argue that the mapping process is critically under the control of the system's current goals while the syntactic school concentrates on 'the higher order constraining relations' in the mapping process. Holyoak in ACME showed some evidence for the pragmatic claims; Gentner represents the syntactic approach.

Still, despite all that effort, the study of analogy is still in its infancy. The study of purpose-directed analogy is a particularly important aspect of the analogy phenomenon.

"…we rarely use a representation in an intentional vacuum, but we always have goals—and two objects may seem similar for one purpose but different for another purpose. Consequently, we must take into account the functional aspects of what we know, and therefore we must classify things according to what they can be used for, or which goals they can help us achieve," [1] Pragmatic theories are now getting more and more attention and even Gentner incorporated goals as the front end of SME. This work supports pragmatic theory. Both the syntactic and pragmatic schools agree that analogy is the most powerful tool of human problem solving not well mimicked by AI programs yet.

8. Metaknowledge – Marvin Minsky's Agents and John McDermott's Mechanisms

Making a conceptual connection between a theory of human cognition [9] and research on the taxonomy of problem-solving methods [16,17] should be investigated. Perhaps there exists a meaningful mapping from the types of agencies described by Marvin Minsky and types of mechanisms postulated by John McDermott. This seems to be quite plausible if we imaging K-lines activating a set of specific agents after recognizing certain salient task features. The activities of those agents will constitute what McDermott perceives as mechanisms. I expect that looking for the agents-mechanisms mapping, even if the direct simple mapping is not found, will result in improvements to both Minsky's and McDermott's approaches, putting the agents' based SOM theory to practical use and enriching the criteria used for mechanism selection and description. Another result may be the discovery of clusters of mechanisms typical of certain agencies or societies; that would shed light on the granularity level used by humans then thinking about their tasks.

Agents-mechanisms mapping may be done by representing activities performed by agents in the CYC KB and looking for some convergence with mechanisms also represented in the same KB. Using the same ontology for the representation of agents' activities and mechanisms should create "a common denominator" phenomenon therefore simplifying mapping.

9. Hard Problem Definition

"For a hard problem, it may be almost as difficult to recognize 'progress' as to solve the problem itself." [9] The following definitions define when the progress has been made in investigating analogical problem solving in a Knowledge-rich Adaptive environment. As Marvin Minsky points out, the task of defining measures of progress or success can become as hard as a problem that we are trying to solve but this is the right place to start. The set of definitions listed below were developed in the real-world task of creating adaptive knowledge-rich system [18].

Definition 1: Knowledge
"We tend to think of knowledge as good in itself, but knowledge is useful only when we can exploit it to help us reach our goals". [9]
"Knowledge is generated by an observer, relative to his point of view, in the process of making sense (modeling)." [19]
"Knowledge can only be created dynamically in time." [20]
"Knowledge of the world cannot be captured in a finite structure." [20] (p. 107) as interpreted by Clancey. [19]

Definition 2: Hard problem
A problem is hard if it requires commonsense knowledge in addition to specialized knowledge and a set of non-obvious to the non-expert heuristics in order to be solved effectively and accurately. A body of knowledge required to solve a hard problem is not algorithmical but it is not totally intuitional either (neither algorithm not black box) leaving some space for symbolic reasoning. A hard problem manifest itself by the following facts:

- There exist experts that can solve the problem better (significantly faster, with greater accuracy) that an average human; these experts consider the problem easy!
- Providing solution involves some symbolic reasoning and some commonsense reasoning that is perceived as intuition
- Training humans to solve this kind of problem is a long-lasting, difficult, and not always successful process
- Even experts' accuracy leaves some space for improvement
- Hard problems always require some sort of guessing and verifying that guess. This makes them NP problems. We do not know the algorithm generating the solution but we can easily verify the positive solution once a guess is provided.

Definition 3: Real-world problem
A problem is called here a real-world problem if it is routinely performed by people and needed in some agents' (human, organization, society) existence.

10. Accuracy and Time-Effectiveness

Definition 4: Accurate results
   Results of the problem solution are accurate

- If they seem intuitively correct to a domain expert or
- If a similar case is found in the real world or
- If automatically obtained results agree with the results obtained by applying a complete, correct theory of a phenomenon to the problem at hand (if such theory exists)

Definition 5: Quick results
   A solution to a hard problem is quick

- For time-critical problems – if the solution is obtained by the system equally fast or faster than if obtained by unaided human
- For non-time-critical problems – if the solution is obtained in acceptable time; the definition of the term "acceptable" depends on the application type (no general definition possible)

If time of arriving at the solution is longer than that of a human expert then solution should improve accuracy or lower the cost as compared with the cost and accuracy of the solution derived by a human expert.

11. Variability

Definition 6: Variability
   A variability of knowledge of certain type is measured with variability factor.

Definition 7: Variability factor
   Variability factor is obtained by dividing the number of different kinds of cases represented in the KB by the approximate number of different kinds of cases occurring in the real world.
   E.g., There are approximately 100 different organizational functions, KB contains 10 of them. Variability factor = 10/100 = 0.1 (V-global).
   The same measure can be applied to the novel cases covered by the system.
   E.g., There are 2 novel cases covered by the system for 10 cases fully represented. Variability factor of novel cases = 2/10 = .02 (V-global)

12. Adaptiveness

Definition 8: Adaptiveness
   A KRA problem solver is adaptive if it produces accurate solutions to novel problems (cases) not fully represented and substantially, qualitatively different from cases fully represented in the KB. The set of novel cases to be tried is intuitive extension of full cases. Adaptiveness of the KRA application is measured with an adaptiveness factor.

Definition 9: Adaptiveness factor
   The ratio of the amount of different cases that can get solved successfully by the system to the number of cases fully represented in the KB. The total amount of cases is comprised of cases fully and partially represented.

FC = number of cases fully represented
SPC = number of partially represented cases solved acceptably
PC = number of novel partial cases as predicted by human given a list of fully represented cases

Adaptiveness factor for the entire system; Min (AS-global-i) = 1:
AD-global = (number of partial cases solved acceptably + number of full cases) / number of full cases
Adaptiveness factor for the system's Growth Stage-I; MAX (AD-local-i) = 1:
AD-local = number of partial cases solved acceptably / number of partial cases

13. Cost-Effectiveness

Definition 10: Cost-effectiveness
In general KRA, application is cost-effective when development cost is justified by the benefits coming form the working application.
Cost of development (C):
   A. cost of knowledge acquisition
   B. cost of representing knowledge
   C. cost of developing user interface
   D. cost of testing the application
   E. cost of using the application

Benefits from the application
   A. adaptiveness and/or
   B. increased accuracy and/or
   C. speed and/or
   D. ability to explain the solution

KRA environment should provide the possibility of minimizing the cost of knowledge representation. The analogy engine should provide the possibility of maximum adaptiveness. Thus two following aspects of cost/benefit analysis are most important when we deal with KRA applications: cost of knowledge representation and adaptiveness.

Definition 11: Total Additional knowledge (dK)
dK consists of a problem and method knowledge (PK + MK) that have to be added to the already large KB in order to build an application program that solves a particular kind of problem or in order to improve performance of this program. dK should be very small in comparison with the entire KB and BK to satisfy cost-effectiveness.

Definition 12: Background knowledge (BK)
BK is the knowledge from the KB that is obviously and directly relevant to the problem at hand. dK should be very small in comparison with the entire BK to satisfy cost-effectiveness. The ratio dK/BK must be reasonably small.
   * Let's measure the amount of knowledge in assertions of the form Unit-slot-value (U-s-V) r frames or slots
   * Let's assume that the cost of representing knowledge is proportional to its amount.

Definition 13: Cost-effectiveness – based on the cost of knowledge representation and adaptiveness
A KRA application is cost-effective when:
The cost of the representation of additional domain specific knowledge (dK=MK+PK) needed in order to cover a significant number of novel problems and ability to solve them adaptively is reasonably small.

Definition 14: Cost effectiveness (dK-factor = KB-reusability factor)
dK-factor is an indirect measure of the relative costs of representing knowledge in KRA applications; it is a ratio of the amount of dK to the amount of BK; dK / BK.

Definition 15: Cost-effectiveness (savings approach)
Another possible measure of cost-effectiveness could be the number of problem solving sessions (N) that have to be performed in order to return the development cost of an application (break-even point).
- $dS = dS1 + dS2 + dS3$ = average savings per one run of the application
- $dS1$ = average savings from improvements in accuracy in $
- $dS2$ = average savings from improvements of adaptiveness in $
- $dS3$ = average savings from improvements in speed in $
- C = development costs
- $N = C / dS$

14. Non-Brittleness – the Key to Adaptiveness

Definition 16: Britt (a unit of non-brittleness)
The non-brittleness claim of KRA can be expanded into a following claim:
KRA eliminates a positive reinforcement between specificity, brittleness, and power (the more specific, the more brittle, the more powerful). A large KB of human commonsense knowledge allows methods to be highly specialized, powerful, but at the same time nonbrittle and degrading gently.

One Britt is the amount of knowledge that needs to be added to a heuristic with degradation level x in order to increase its power (Lenat's appropriateness) by a unit without changing the degradation level (steepness to the heuristic's slope).

Or alternative approach:

One Britt is the amount of knowledge that needs to be added to a heuristic with power P and degradation level y so that its peak power remains the same, while the degradation level decreases by 0.5 (50%).

15. Power, Amount and Growth of Knowledge

Definition 17: Power of knowledge in the system when applied to problem P
"Can we give, say, an equation for how to measure the effective power of the knowledge in a system, when it is applied to a problem P? It is premature to even attempt to do so – it may never be possible to do so. [] First approximation of the power of the knowledge in the system, we might simply superpose all the power curves of the heuris-

tics that comprise the knowledge. That would give us an overall idea of the power of the system as a function of what problem it was applied to. If we're interested in applying the system to a particular problem P, we could then read off the value of this curve of point P [21]". Power here refers to Appropriateness.

Definition 18: Horizontal knowledge increase – Accumulation

Horizontal increase in the amount of knowledge means adding new assertions of the type that already exists. It is equivalent to accumulation. E.g., organizational functions are represented in the KB as event types, adding 100 new instances of organization functions will result in the horizontal growth of the KB.

Definition of accumulation [9] as "collecting incompatible descriptions, for example, by forming the phrase "block or wedge" does not apply here. Horizontal knowledge increase is simply a "volume increase".

Definition 19: Vertical knowledge increase

Vertical increase in the amount of knowledge means adding knowledge that relates horizontal layers (new slots) or states facts, exceptions, balances between assertions within horizontal layers (rules). E.g., organizational functions are represented in the KB as event types that can have subevents of a certain type. Stating a fact that Payroll function never has Reserve event type as its subevent type results in the vertical growth of the KB.

Definition 20: The amount of knowledge (absolute, task-independent measure)

Given two knowledge bases KB1 and KB2 we assert that: "There is more knowledge in KB1 than in KB2" if there are more assertions (U-s-V) in the KB1 than in KB2. This is an absolute measure, independent of the problem solving situations and not taking into account the power (usefulness) of these assertions in achieving a solution to a problem P.

Definition 21: The amount of knowledge (task-specific measure)

We say that KB1 has more k knowledge useful in solving problem P if one or all of the following is true:

- a number of assertions related to P in KB1 is larger than in KB2
- a granularity level of assertions related to P in KB1 is finer that that in KB2 (we'll refer later to the knowledge from the lower granularity level as a more detailed knowledge)
- even if the number of P related assertions in KB1 and KB2 is equal, informational content of assertions in KB1 is more powerful for problem P than informational content of assertions from KB2.

16. Amount of Information and Its Quality and Usefulness

Definition 22: The amount of information is one assertion

There is no known method of quantifying the semantic information content of the assertion (message), so the measure of uncertainty of the message that is removed by the occurrence of the message is introduced. E.g., as assertion that is certain to occur (e.g., default value) does so with probability 1 no information is produced from the KB point of view. On the other hand, if a particular assertion is very improbable —Certainty Factor (CF) is low—the fact that it occurs (rather that some other assertion) conveys a great deal of information. If assertion A has probability of the occurrence P (A) then its information content I (A) is:

I (A) = –log(base2) P (A)

This means that one unit of information is associated with probability 0.5. So, if the facts in KB have CF = T (CF = 100) then is these facts are being used in the course of solving some problems, no information is produced from the information theory point of view.

Definition 23: Uso-quant (an idea for the unit of usefulness of a piece of knowledge)
Information theory does not deal with meaning, usefulness, and correctness of the message (assertion, observation) but only with uncertainty and randomness of it. Let's create a unit of usefulness of an assertion in the problem solving proccss by a specific KRA application. Let's call this unit uso-quant.

There are two most important aspects of KRA application's performance:

- **Adaptiveness** – how many significantly different novel problems an application can solve. This aspect is connected with the amount of horizontal knowledge
- **Accuracy** – how well the application performs the task. This is connected with the vertical knowledge and encoded regularities resulting in the problem solving method.

A concept of the uso-quant seems to be a useful approach to researching the power of knowledge (claimed by many but never measured precisely). We need an equivalent of Shanon's information theory based on usefulness of a message not its uncertainty.

Definition 24: A horizontal uso-quant
Unconstrained version:
One horizontal uso-quant is equal to the amount of additional knowledge (amount of assertions) that causes an increase in the KRA Application's scope of applicability by one novel problem (case).

Note that we only know that knowledge that effectively changed program's behavior is contained in the uso-quant but there is no way to identify a relevant part of this knowledge unless we constrain the definition to the relevant knowledge only. Another important thing is that the uso-quant varies in size from application to application and even within one application it depends on the developmental stage (e.g. do we measure knowledge needed to increase application's scope from one to two or from 100 to 101 novel cases). The constrained version of the horizontal uso-quant does not have the above shortcomings.

Constrained version:
One horizontal uso-quant is equal to the amount of additional knowledge (amount of assertions) that causes an increase in the system's scope of applicability by one, FIRST novel problem (case).

By referring to a specific application as a standard, we achieve constancy of the uso-quant size. Because of that, uso-quant can be used to compare different applications. For example, we can say that application X needed 5 horizontal uso-quants to increase its scope by 2, while application Y needed only 1 uso-quant to achieve the same result. This leads us straight to the concept of average usefulness of a piece of knowledge in application X in the situation S (solving problem P); it is 5 times smaller that that of a piece of knowledge of application Y. Constrained version of the horizontal uso-quant should be as useful in comparing power of knowledge as a kilogram is in comparing weight of objects. It is important to consider the first novel problem because of the amount of knowledge necessary to further increase adaptability may vary depending on the stage of development (e.g., it may be x for increasing the amount of novel cases covered from 0 o 1, but y from 1 to 2, and z from 2 to 3…).

Definition 24: A vertical uso-quant = Acu-quant
Unconstrained version: A vertical uso-quant is equal to the amount of additional knowledge (amount of assertions) that causes a unit increase in the accuracy of the solutions. E.g., causes an increase of the numeric solution's accuracy by 1%.

Constrained version: A vertical uso-quant is equal to the amount of additional knowledge (amount of assertions) that causes a unit increase in the accuracy of the solutions of the system. E.g., causes an increase of the estimate's accuracy by 1%.

Definition 25: Common-sense accuracy factor
A number of intuitively obviously correct KB suggestions presented to the user for verification divided by the number of all suggestions presented to the user.

17. Conclusions

Much more work is needed on measuring adaptive knowledge-rich systems performance and it is one of the most important research areas that can have a big pay-off in healthcare now and in the future. The non-repeating and personal nature of the healthcare makes it necessary to make systems that serve that sector continuously adaptive and meta-adaptive. AI should grow beyond research based on toy problems, which produce artifacts isolated from the complexities of real life. Methods that work for toy problems almost always have to be qualitatively changed when applied to similar problems of greater (real) magnitude. If we start form large subsets of real problems and coordinate groups of researchers to attack them, we will get better results. Comparing results obtained by various research groups working on similar problems will be more fruitful than learning about a success in x and a success in y, where x and y do not relate at all.

Bibliography

[1] Minsky, M., Logical vs. Analogical or Symbolic vs. Connectionist or Neat vs. Scruffy, In Winston, P., Expanding Frontiers: Artificial Intelligence at MIT, MIT Press, 1990.
[2] Minsky, M., Why People Think Computers Can't, Technology Review, November, 1983.
[3] Lenat, D., Prakash, M., and Shepard, M., CYC: Using Common-sense Knowledge to Overcome Knowledge Acquisition for Expert Systems, Kluwer, 1988.
[4] Greiner, R., Learning by Understanding Analogies, Artificial Intelligence 35, 81–125, 1988.
[5] Keane, M., Analogical Mechanisms, Artificial Intelligence Review 2, 229–250, 1988.
[6] Eliot, L.B., Investigating the Nature of Expertise: analogical thinking, expert systems, and ThinkBack, In Expert Systems, Vol. 4, No. 3. August 1987.
[7] Wellsch K. & Jones, M., Computational Analogy – an Algorithm for Detecting Analogies, Technical Report N2L 3G1, University of Waterloo, January, 1987.
[8] Davies T.R. & Russell S.J., A Logical Approach to Reasoning by Analogy, Technical Report 385, University of California, Berkeley, July 1987.
[9] Minsky, M., The Society of Mind, Simon and Schuster Inc., New York, NY, 1986.
[10] August, S. & Dyer, M.G., Understanding Analogies in Editorials, IN Proceedings of the Ninth International Joint Conference On Artificial Intelligence, August, 1985.
[11] Kedar-Cabelli, S.T., Purpose-Driedcted Analogy, In Proceeding of the Cognitive Science Society Conference, pages 150–159, Irvine, CA, August 1985.

[12] Winston, P., Learning New Principles from Precedents and Exercises: The Details, MIT AI Memo 632, 1981.
[13] Carbonell, J.G. & Minton, S., Metaphor and Common-Sense Reasoning, Technical Report, CMU-CS-83–11, 1983.
[14] Gentner, D., Structure Mapping: A Theoretical Framework for Analogy, Cognitive Science 7 (2): 155–170, April–June, 1983.
[15] McDermott, J., Learning to Use Analogies, IJCAL, pages 568–576, August, 1979.
[16] McDermott, J., A Preliminary Steps Toward a Taxonomy of Problem-Solving Methods, IN Automating Knowledge Acquisition for Expert Systems, Kluwer, 1988.
[17] McDermott, J., The World Would be a Better Place if Non-Programmers Could Program, Machine Learning, April, 1989.
[18] Bushko, R.G., KRA – Knowledge-Rich Analogy: Adaptive Estimation with Common Sense, MS Thesis, EECS Department, Massachusetts Institute of Technology, 1990.
[19] Clancey, W., The Knowledge Level Reinterpreted: Modeling How Systems Interact, Machine Learning, 4, 285–291, 1989.
[20] Newell, A., The Knowledge Level, Artificial Intelligence 18, 87–127, 1982.
[21] Lenat, D. and Guha, R.V., Building Large Knowledge-Based Systems: Representation and Inference in the CYC Project, Addison-Wesley Publishing Company, Inc., 1989.
[22] Eliot, L.B., Analogical Problem-Solving and Expert Systems, In IEEE Expert, pages 17–28, Summer 1986.
[23] Guha, r.V. and Lenat, D., CYC: A mid-Term Report; in preparation.
[24] Kedar-Cabelli, S.T., Analogy – from a unified perspective, Technical Report ML-TR-3, Rutgers University, December, 1985.
[25] Marques, D., Latto A., McDermott, J., A Comparison of Case Based Reasoning with Few Large vs. Many Small Features, In Proceedings of the Case-Based Reasoning Workshop, AAAI-88, August, 1988.
[26] Minsky, M., Finite and Infinite Machines, Prentice-Hall, 1967.
[27] Minsky, M., A Framework for Representing Knowledge, MIT AI Memo No. 306, 1974.
[28] Minton, S., Quantitative Results Concerning the Utility of Explanation-Based Learning, AI Journal, Vol. 42, 1990.
[29] Lazowska, E. and Zahorjan, J., and Sevcik, K., Quantitative System Performance: Computer System Analysis Using Queuing Networks Models, Prentice-Hall, 1984.
[30] Lenat, D., Guha, R.V., Pittman, K., Pratt, D., and Shepard, M., CYC: Toward Programs with Common Sense, Communications of the ACM, Vol. 33, No. 8, August, 1990.
[31] Lewis, B., The Evolution of Benchmarking as a Computer Performance Evaluation Technique, MIS Quarter/March 1985.
[32] Russell, S., Analogy by Similarity, In Analogical Reasoning, David Helman, ed., Reidel, Boston, 1988.
[33] Shen, W., Complementary Discrimination Learning: A duality between Generalization & Discrimination, In Proceedings of AAAI-90, pages 834–839, 1990.
[34] Sullivan, C.H. Jr. and Yates, C.E., Reasoning by Analogy – A Tool for Business Planning, In Sloan Management Review, No. 55, Spring, 1988.
[35] Winston, P., Learning by Understanding Analogies, MIT AI Lab Memo 520, 1979.

The Authors

Biographies of the Authors

Editor

Renata G. Bushko, M.S.

Renata G. Bushko, M.S., Director, Future of Health Technology Institute, www.fhti.org is an editor of the Future of Health Technology series, IOS Press. Ms. Bushko, after serving on boards of many national US healthcare organizations, international health standards organizations and 15 years as an executive in computer industry, founded Future of Health Technology Institute – health technology research and training organization that guides organizations in smart planning of investments in health technology. Since 1996 she has been leading an annual Future of Health Technology Summit(SM) – a unique interactive discussion forum defining future of health technology. She holds Master of Science in Electrical Engineering and Computer Science with specialization in intelligent systems from the Massachusetts Institute of Technology (MIT) and BA in Computer Science and Economics from Smith College and University of Warsaw. She applies her expertise in technology assessment and planning, intelligent agents, analogical reasoning, and computer intelligence to the health improvement area.

Chapter Authors

David Andre Ph.D.

Dr. David Andre is a scientist, an inventor, and an entrepreneur whose work emphasizes the role of learning in both artificial and natural intelligences. As the Director of Informatics at BodyMedia, he collects and analyzes clinical and user data and creates machine learning models to develop algorithms that provide detailed and specific statements about human physiology and activity, such as energy expenditure and sleep state. Dr. Andre earned B.S. and B.A. degrees in Symbolic Systems and Psychology from Stanford University and a Ph.D in Artificial Intelligence from Berkeley, where he was awarded a Hertz Fellowship. In addition to holding numerous patents, he is the author of more than 60 peer-reviewed publications in the areas of robotics, machine learning, reinforcement learning, evolutionary computation, and parallel processing, as well as a book on automatic circuit design. Dr. Andre also co-founded Just Passing Through, a company that creates and films multi-day puzzle adventures.

Timothy Bickmore Ph.D.

Timothy Bickmore is an Assistant Professor in the College of Computer and Information Science at Northeastern University. Dr. Bickmore's research focus is on the development of Relational Agents-computational artifacts designed to build long-term social-emotional relationships with their users. These agents have been deployed within the context of behavior change interventions in which they are designed to establish working alliance relationships with patients in order to maximize intervention outcomes. Prior to joining Northeastern, Dr. Bickmore was an Assistant Professor of Medicine at the Boston University School of Medicine. Dr. Bickmore received his PhD from the MIT Media Lab, studying under

Profs. Rosalind Picard (Affective Computing) and Justine Cassell (Gesture and Narrative Language).

Aubrey de Grey Ph.D.
Aubrey de Grey was born on 20th April 1963 in London, England. He obtained his B.A. in computer science and his Ph.D. in gerontology, both from the University of Cambridge, where he still works. He edits Rejuvenation Research, the world's only peer-reviewed journal focused specifically on reversal (repair) of the molecular and cellular changes that accumulate throughout life and eventually cause frailty, disease and death. He serves on the board of directors of the British Society for Research on Ageing, the American Aging Association and the International Association of Biomedical Gerontology. His contributions to the field have been recognised by Fellowship of the Gerontological Society of America and by the World Transhumanist Association's H.G. Wells award for outstanding contributions to transhumanism (the expansion of human potential through technology).

Alison S. Gottlieb, Ph.D.
Alison S. Gottlieb, Ph.D., is a Research Fellow at the Gerontology Institute, University of Massachusetts Boston. Her research interests include aging with chronic disability; the use of assistive technology, home modifications, and universal design among elders; and intergenerational residential decision-making. She received her Ph.D. from the Heller School of Social Policy at Brandeis University. Over the past ten years, she has published several scholarly articles and has taught aging policy and research methods on the college level.

Dave Gustafson Ph.D.
Dave Gustafson is a Research Professor at the University of Wisconsin-Madison, Director of the National Cancer Institute designated Center of Excellence in Cancer Communications and Director of the Network for the Improvement of Addiction Treatment funded by the Robert Wood Johnson Foundation and the federal government's Center for Substance Abuse Treatment. His research focuses on the use of systems engineering methods and models in individual and organizational change. Over the last ten years his individual change research centered on developing and evaluating eHealth systems using as the test vehicle CHESS (the Comprehensive Health Enhancement Support System), a computer system to help people facing serious health problems with a particular focus on cancer. His randomized control trials and field tests of CHESS help understand acceptance, use and impact of eHealth on quality of life, behavior change and health services utilization. His research also contributes to organizational improvement with a particular attention to models that predict and explain organizational change. The addiction treatment field is currently his primary test bed for these organizational change initiatives. Dave is a Fellow of the Association for Health Services Research and of the American Medical Informatics Association, a Fellow and past Vice-Chair of the Board of the Institute for Healthcare Improvement. He also chaired the Federal Science Panel on Interactive Communications in Health and is Chair of the eHealth Institute. He is a member of the Institute of Medicine Committee on Redesigning Health Insurance and the University of Wisconsin Athletic Board.

Teresita B. Hernández, Ph.D.
Teresita Hernández, PhD, is the President of Health Technomics, Inc., a small business firm in Northern Virginia engaged primarily in innovative research and development. She is also an Associate at the Frances Stern Nutrition Center in Boston. With advanced degrees in human nutrition from the University of Iowa, Dr. Hernández is one of the pioneers in the development of competency-based education in the health field, and in the application of computer technology in training. She has directed the development of computer-based

training programs for physicians and other health professionals. Dr. Hernández also pioneered the application of multimedia technology to dietary assessment, and has successfully led the development of 3 interactive picture prompted, bilingual dietary assessment programs for different cultural groups living in the US – American, Hispanics, and Chinese. Dr. Hernández has provided consulting services to the National Academy of Sciences' Food and Nutrition Board and has received grants from the US Department of Agriculture and the National Institutes of Health to conduct cognitive research on portion estimation using computer-based anchors. The Chapter contributed here is based on her recently completed research and development of digitized pictorial software for portioning anchors.

Bradford W. Hesse, Ph.D.

Chief of Health Communication and Informatics Research Branch, Behavioral Research Program, Division of Cancer Control and Population Sciences of the National Cancer Institute. Prior to that Dr. Hesse worked at Westat on *Health Information National Trends Survey*, or HINTS. Dr. Hesse joined the NCI to enlarge the HINTS survey to an ongoing program of data collection, analysis, and dissemination. Dr. Hesse also serves as the research director for the NCI's newly formed User-Centered Informatics Research laboratory. He co-founded the Center for Research on Technology at the American Institutes for Research in 1991. Before coming to NCI, he directed projects for the Departments of Education and Labor, the Centers for Disease Control and Prevention, and the National Institutes of Health.

Stephen Intille, Ph.D.

Stephen Intille, Ph.D., is Technology Director of the House_n Consortium in the MIT Department of Architecture. His research is focused on the development of context-recognition algorithms and interface design strategies for ubiquitous computing environments and devices. In current work he is developing systems for preventive health care that support healthy aging and well-being in the home by motivating longitudinal behavior change. He received his Ph.D. from MIT in 1999 working on computational vision at the MIT Media Laboratory, an S.M. from MIT in 1994, and a B.S.E. degree in Computer Science and Engineering from the University of Pennsylvania in 1992. He has published research on computational stereo depth recovery, real-time and multi-agent tracking, activity recognition, perceptually-based interactive environments, and technology for preventive healthcare. Dr. Intille has been principal investigator on two NSF ITR grants focused on automatic activity recognition from sensor data in the home, as well as the MIT principal investigator on sensor-enabled health technology grants from Intel, the National Institutes of Health, and the Robert Wood Johnson Foundation. He received an IBM Faculty award in 2003.

Thomas R. Kosten, M.D.

Thomas R. Kosten, M.D. is a Professor of Psychiatry and Medicine at Yale University Medical School and former Chief of Psychiatry at VA Connecticut. He was the founding Director of the Division of Substance Abuse in 1994 and has directed the Yale Medications Development Center for substance abuse since 1990. He is an international expert on medications development in substance abuse, been a Congressional Fellow, and a visiting Professor in Germany, Spain, Greece, China and Canada. He is the founding Vice Chair for Added Qualifications in Addiction Psychiatry of the American Board of Psychiatry and Neurology. He is Past President of the American Academy of Addiction Psychiatry, a Distinguished Fellow in the American Psychiatric Association, a fellow of the American College of Neuropsychopharmacology and the College on the Problems of Drug Dependence, and served on the National Academy of Sciences. He won several major clinical research awards, is Deputy Editor of two major Journals in substance abuse, been on the *American Journal of Psychiatry* editorial board, and published over 450 papers, books and reviews. His pharmacotherapy contributions include a cocaine vaccine, disulfiram for cocaine dependence, vasodilators for cocaine induced cerebral perfusion defects, and buprenorphine for opioid dependence. In addition to these pharmacotherapies, he has advanced our understanding of opiate and cocaine dependence mechanisms and treatment using SPECT and functional MRI neuroimaging.

Kent Larson

Kent Larson is a principal research scientist at MIT's School of Architecture and Planning. He is also director of the Changing Places Consortium and House_n research group introducing transformational ideas to the way we live and age. He is redefining the concept of home as a place for proactive health care, distributed energy, learning, communication, commerce, entertainment and work. Dr. Larson practiced architecture since 1981. His designs have won numerous awards, including American Institute of Architecture award for the design of the Graduate School of Business at Columbia University. His study of the unbuilt work of Louis Kahn was selected by Time magazine as a "best Design of the Year", and the related book was selected as one of the ten best books in architecture in the year 2000 by the New York Times Review of Books.

Alexander Libin, Ph.D.

Dr. Alexander Libin is an Affiliated Faculty member of the Department of Psychology at Georgetown University, as well as a founder of the Institute of Robotic Psychology and Robotherapy at the CyberAnthropology Research, Inc. (a non-profit company in Maryland). He specialized in both Information Sciences (MA) and Psychology (PhD). His research concentrates on the multi-dimensional evaluation of individual and group differences, the impact of a technological environment on human development through life span, and the psychological and psycho-physiological effects of people's engagement with the cyberworld. Among Libin's areas of specialization are behavioral health, human-computer interactions, personal robotics, and non-pharmacological interventions for children and adults with special needs. His professional experiences include both extensive academic training and diverse practical applications, incorporating education, computing entertainment, clinical, and cross-cultural studies. Drs. Alexander and Elena Libin's research on robotic psychology and robotherapy is presented at the www.robotherapy.org.

Elena Libin, Ph.D.

Dr. Elena Libin is an Affiliated Faculty member of the Department of Psychology at Georgetown University, as well as a Founder of the Institute of Robotic Psychology and Robotherapy at the CyberAnthropology Research, Inc. (a non-profit scientific company in Maryland, USA). While earning her MA in Information Sciences and PhD in Personality Psychology, Elena continued to work as a psychotherapist, educator and researcher. She developed an original concept of Coping Intelligence™, focused on the non–clinical management of psychological problems, the efficient resolution of every day difficulties, and situations with high level of uncertainty. Since 2001, together with Dr. Alexander Libin she has been developing an innovative concept of Robotic Psychology and Robotherapy, which emphasizes the human-centered aspects of person-robot communication. Practical application of this approach aims to design technology-mediated means for promoting psychological well-being in various populations. Her recent initiatives deal with the new field of cyber-anthropology, which applies humanistic principles to the merge of artificial and human worlds.

Cindy Mason

Cindy Mason is an Assistant Research Engineer at the University of California, Berkeley. Cindy's research interests include intelligent agents, distributed systems, and speech interfaces. She received her Ph. D in 1992 and was awarded Outstanding Student Contribution to the field of Distributed Artificial Intelligence for her work on collaborative belief revision. She was recipient of the National Research Council Research Associateship at NASA Ames Research Center from 1992 to 1995 and a Research Fellow in the Stanford School of Medicine in 1996. She joined the Berkeley Initiative on Soft Computing in 1995. She teaches courses on intelligent agents and is active in the area of multi-agent systems, and the development of human centered computing technologies, including speech interfaces and affective computing.

Benjamin L. Miller Ph.D.

Dr. Benjamin L. Miller is the leader of the Pathogen Detection Consortium of the Center for Future Health. Dr. Miller has focused on using his group's expertise in synthesis and molecular recognition chemistry to aid in the development of novel biosensors. He is currently Associate Professor of Dermatology, Biochemistry and Biophysics, and Biomedical Engineering at the University of Rochester. He carried out his undergraduate studies at Miami University, receiving degrees in Chemistry, Mathematics, and German in 1988. From there he moved to Stanford University, where he carried out his Ph.D. research under the direction of Paul Wender. This range of interests was further expanded during a stint as an NIH postdoctoral fellow in Stuart Schreiber's laboratories, where Ben synthesized nonpeptide combinatorial libraries. Ben joined the faculty of the University of Rochester in 1996; research in his group has included projects directed towards methods of non-biopolymeric molecular evolution, peptidomimesis, molecular recognition, computer-aided molecular design, and synthetic methodology.

George B. Moseley III, MBA, JD

George B. Moseley III, MBA, JD, is a Lecturer in Health Law and Management at the Harvard School of Public Healthy, where he teaches courses on legal and policy developments in the US health care system, managing people in health care organizations, and new venture creation in the health care and biotech industries. His recent research interests concern the adoption of new clinical medical evidence by health care providers. He is the author of books on Managed Care Strategies for Physicians, and Strategic Planning and Management in the Health Care and Biotech Industries. He also is a member of the Institute of Cybermedicine at the Harvard Medical School.

Aaron Oppenheimer

Aaron Oppenheimer leads product behavior design and development at Design Continuum, focusing on how functional, emotional, and conceptual elements of product use work together to create a cohesive experience for the consumer. Since joining Continuum in 2000, he has worked on a variety of projects for clients including Hewlett Packard, Sprint PCS, Polaroid, General Motors, and Sunbeam. His work synthesizes consumer research, strategic and tactical design, and product evaluation. He is an outspoken expert on product interaction, writing and presenting at business- and academically-focused conferences.

Salil Patel

Salil Patel's research experience and interests include molecular and cellular biology, clinical neurophysiology, particle physics, complex dynamical systems, biomedical engineering, and informatics. Mr. Patel is a graduate of Rice University and a recipient of the J. William

Fulbright Fellowship, under which he pursued work at the National University of Singapore. He is currently a Medical Doctor candidate at the Johns Hopkins School of Medicine.

Alex Pentland, Ph.D.

Alex (Sandy) Pentland is the Toshiba Professor of Media Arts and Sciences at MIT and heads the MIT Media Laboratory's Human Dynamics research group. His research interests include wearable computing, human-machine interfaces, computer graphics, artificial intelligence, and machine and human vision. Pentland is a cofounder of the IEEE Computer Society's Technical Committee on Wearable Information System and the IEEE NNS Autonomous Mental Development Technical Committee. He received a PhD from MIT.

Rosalind W. Picard, Sc.D.

Professor Rosalind W. Picard is founder and director of the Affective Computing Research Group at the Massachusetts Institute of Technology (MIT) Media Laboratory. She holds a Bachelors in Electrical Engineering from the Georgia Institute of Technology and Masters and Doctorate degrees, each in Electrical Engineering and Computer Science, from MIT. The author of over 100 peer-reviewed scientific articles in pattern recognition, multidimensional signal modeling, computer vision, and human-computer interaction, Picard is known internationally for pioneering research on content-based video retrieval and on giving computers the ability to recognize and respond to human emotional information. She is co-recipient with Tom Minka of a "best paper" prize (1998) from the Pattern Recognition Society for their work on interactive machine learning with a society of models. Her award-winning book, Affective Computing, (MIT Press, 1997) lays the groundwork for giving machines the skills of emotional intelligence. Her group's research on affective and wearable technologies has been featured in national and international public forums such as The New York Times, The London Independent, Scientific American Frontiers, Time, New Scientist, Vogue, as well as PBS and BBC specials. Picard is married and lives in Newton, Massachusetts with her husband, two sons, and seven non-affective computers.

Nina M. Silverstein, Ph.D.

Nina M. Silverstein, Ph.D., is Associate Professor of Gerontology at the University of Massachusetts Boston, College of Public and Community Service. Since 1984, she has worked closely with the Alzheimer's Association on projects relating to the Association's Helpline, its Safe Return Program, respite care, support groups for family caregivers, and home safety adaptations for people with dementia. She is a Fellow of the Gerontological Society of America. She has served as co-chair of the transportation track at the 2004 and 2005 joint meetings of the American Society on Aging and the National Council on the Aging. She has co-authored one book for Springer Publications entitled "Dementia and Wandering Behavior: Concern for the Lost Elder," and is working on her second, tentatively titled "Improving Hospital Care for Persons with Dementia." In 2004–05, she spent a sabbatical as a gerontology research fellow with the National Highway Traffic Safety Administration, Department of Transportation.

Richard Spivack Ph.D.

Richard Spivack is an economist in Advanced Technology Program's (ATP) Economic Assessment Office focusing on the long-term results of the ATP. ATP's mission of generating "broad-based economic impacts" occupies most of his time as it is his responsibility to oversee the development of the economic modeling necessary to evaluate the success(es) of the program. Richard's background includes over 18 years of college level teaching at both the undergraduate and graduate levels. Richard received his M.A. degree from the University of Rhode Island and his Ph.D. degree from the University of Connecticut. His areas of expertise include Healthcare economics as well as Urban/Regional economics in which he has published several scholarly articles.

Jeff Sutherland, Ph.D.

Dr. Sutherland is Chief Technology Officer of PatientKeeper Inc. He is currently providing mobile/wireless applications for patient care in physician practices and an interoperability architecture platform solution for healthcare enterprises. As CTO or VP of Engineering of 9 software companies (founder of two) Dr. Sutherland directed large software development projects in finance, aerospace, object databases, object design tools, compilers, and health-care web, wireless, and workflow platforms. He was a member of the faculty of the University of Colorado School of Medicine from 1975–1986. Beginning in 1986, he devoted himself exclusively to object-oriented software development and in 1993, invented the Scrum development process, now an industry standard Agile process. During 1996–2000, while CTO of IDX Systems he architected advanced Internet workflow systems, which led to his recent work as Co-Investigator of the University of Maryland Medical System Operating Room of the Future project.

Astro Teller, Ph.D.

A respected scientist, seasoned entrepreneur, and award-wining novelist, Dr. Astro Teller's endeavors all grow out of a passion for the transformative nature of intelligent technologies. Dr. Teller is currently the CEO of BodyMedia, Inc, the leading company in unobtrusive wearable body monitoring. Past work has taken Astro through a previous CEO position, teaching and researching at Stanford University, numerous patents, a Hertz fellowship, a range of technical and non-technical articles and books, and $23M in raised capital. Dr. Teller holds a BS in computer science and an MS in symbolic and heuristic computation, both from Stanford University. Dr. Teller completed his Ph.D. in artificial intelligence at Carnegie Mellon University.

Elizabeth Van Ranst, M.S.S.S

Elizabeth Van Ranst, M.S.S.S, a Research Fellow at the Gerontology Institute, University of Massachusetts Boston, is Co-Principal Investigator (with Nina M. Silverstein) and Project Coordinator of the research study "Promoting Safe Mobility among Elders by Increasing Awareness of Vehicle Modifications." Her background includes both gerontology and transportation. She has held direct service and administrative posts in agencies providing services to elders. She has also worked in mass transit, run a paratransit service for elders and people with disabilities, and worked on research projects related to human service transportation and both taxicab and boat accessibility issues.

Kevin Warwick, Ph.D.

Dr. Kevin Warwick is Professor of Cybernetics at the University of Reading, UK where he carries out research in artificial intelligence, control and robotics. His favourite topic is pushing back the frontiers of machine intelligence. Kevin began his career by joining British Telecom with whom he spent the next 6 years. At 22 he took his first degree at Aston University followed by a PhD and research post at Imperial College, London. He subsequently held positions at Oxford, Newcastle and Warwick Universities before being offered the Chair at Reading, at the age of 32.

Kevin has published over 350 research papers and his paperback "In the Mind of the Machine" gives a warning of a future in which machines are more intelligent than humans. He has been awarded higher doctorates both by Imperial College and the Czech Academy of Sciences, Prague and has been described (by Gillian Anderson of the X-Files) as Britain's leading prophet of the robot age. He appears in the 1999 Guinness Book of Records for an Internet robot learning experiment.

In 1998 he shocked the international scientific community by having a silicon chip transponder surgically implanted in his left arm. A series of further implant experiments is now planned in which Kevin's nervous system will be linked to a computer. This research led to him being featured in February 2000, as the cover story on the US magazine "Wired". He received the Future Health Technology 2000 Award from Future of Health Technology Institute, USA. Kevin had the honour of presenting the Year 2000 Royal Institution Christmas Lectures.

Stephan Wiet, Ph.D.

Dr. Stephan Wiet is a Consumer Psychologist within the Johnson & Johnson family of companies. He is currently Director of Consumer Sciences at McNeil Consumer and Specialty Pharmaceuticals, the over-the-counter pharmaceutical arm of J&J. He is responsible for leading R&D activities that enhance consumer understanding, translating consumer insights into new healthcare products, and optimizing the aesthetic features of these products. He also chairs McNeil's R&D Innovation Leadership Team, responsible for sustaining an innovative R&D culture, and measuring the Department's innovation contributions to topline growth. Dr. Wiet has held similar positions at J&J Consumer & Personal Products, and McNeil Nutritionals. He holds a Masters and Doctorate degree in Biopsychology from Rutgers University.

Jean A. Wooldridge, M.P.H.

Jean A. Wooldridge, M.P.H., is Strategic Advisor for Cancer Communication Technologies, Office of the Director, Division of Cancer Control and Population Sciences, National Cancer Institute, Bethesda, MD. She is on loan from the Cancer Prevention Research Program of the Fred Hutchinson Cancer Research Center, Seattle. She is Principal, St. Cloud Communications, whose mission is to link communities of shared imagination and practice for ensuring cross-sector dialogue supporting consumer e-health.

Future of Intelligent and Extelligent Health Environment
R.G. Bushko (Ed.)
IOS Press, 2005

Author Index

Andre, D.	89	Mason, C.	247
Bickmore, T.	132	Miller, B.L.	66
Burton, M.M.	278	Moseley III, G.B.	15
Bushko, R.G.	v, vi, viii, ix, 3, 273, 313	Oppenheimer, A.	111
Capoccia, V.A.	186	Palesh, T.E.	186
de Grey, A.	209	Patel, S.H.	43
Ganous, T.	278	Pentland, A.	55
Gottlieb, A.S.	231	Picard, R.W.	132, 186
Gustafson, D.H.	186	Plsek, P.E.	186
Hernández, T.B.	257	Silverstein, N.M.	231
Hesse, B.W.	159	Spivack, R.N.	32
Intille, S.S.	79	Sutherland, J.V.	278
Kosten, T.R.	177	Teller, A.	89
Kumar, A.	278	van den Heuvel, W.-J.	278
Larson, K.	79	van Ranst, E.	231
Libin, A.	146	Warwick, K.	125
Libin, E.	146	Wiet, S.G.	220
Maher, L.	186	Wooldridge, J.A.	263